Handbuch der experimentellen Pharmakologie

Vol. 47 Heffter-Heubner New Series

Handbook of Experimental Pharmacology

Kinetics of
Drug Action

Contributors

J. Blanck · F. G. van den Brink · C. A. M. van Ginneken
R. E. Gosselin · P. Th. Henderson · H. C. J. Ketelaars
E. Krüger-Thiemer · D. Mackay · J. M. van Rossum
W. Scheler · T. B. Vree

Editor

Jacques M. van Rossum

With 105 Figures

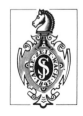

Springer-Verlag Berlin Heidelberg New York 1977

Prof. Dr. Jacques M. van Rossum, Katholieke Universiteit Nijmegen,
Farmacologisch Instituut, Faculteit der Geneeskunde, Geert Grooteplein Noord 21,
Nijmegen, The Netherlands

ISBN 3-540-08023-6 Springer-Verlag Berlin Heidelberg New York
ISBN 0-387-08023-6 Springer-Verlag New York Heidelberg Berlin

Library of Congress Cataloging in Publication Data. Main entry under title: Kinetics of drug action. (Handbuch der experimentellen Pharmakologie: New series; v. 47) Includes bibliographies and indexes. 1. Pharmacokinetics. 2. Pharmacology. I. Blanck, J. II. Van Rossum, J. M., 1930—III. Series. QP905.H3   Bd. 47   [RM301.5]   615'.1'08s [615'.7]   77—8315

Typesetting, printing, and binding: Brühlsche Universitätsdruckerei, Lahn-Giessen
2122/3130-543210

Dedicated to Dr. Ekkehard Krüger-Thiemer

Dr. EKKEHARD KRÜGER-THIEMER has been a world-leading authority in the field of pharmacokinetics. He was a brilliant intellectual, not only with a broad knowledge in medicine and the natural sciences, but also with a thorough background in cultural sciences. He was a world-leading scientist with a most sympathetic personality.

As a young physician he was forced to interrupt his career during World War II and for 5 years thereafter he was deprived of freedom by the Russian state. Finally, once again back in the free world he continued his studies in mathematics which he completed quite successfully in 1954.

Dr. KRÜGER-THIEMER was appointed to a research position at the Borstel Tuberculosis Research Institute in Northern Germany. Here he combined his broad knowledge in medicine, microbiology, and mathematics for the optimalization of chemotherapy in tuberculosis and other infectious diseases. He attacked practical problems in a fundamental way such that not only an elegant solution of the problem was offered but also general applications were presented. Within a few years he was known all over the world for his advanced studies in the new research area, called pharmacokinetics. With DOST and THEORELL he is the founder of modern pharmacokinetics in Europe.

His papers, not always easy to read, require a thorough study. Some of his work was so advanced that a full appreciation of their merits is just now beginning to come about. Dr. KRÜGER-THIEMER is certainly the first who made fundamental contributions to nonlinear pharmacokinetics that are just now being applied in therapy.

His original, fundamental, and practical approach to both pharmacokinetic and chemotherapeutic problems was highly appreciated among specialists all over the world. His accomplishments prompted invitations to lecture as a guest professor in Wisconsin and Boston and he was invited to many international symposia. He was also regarded as a consultant in difficult pharmacokinetic problems.

His sudden death is painfully felt by his wife and daughters and the scientific community. Those who have met Dr. KRÜGER-THIEMER will always remember this great scientist and warm personality. Those who read his papers will be impressed by his advanced knowledge in pharmacokinetics.

Preface

Most drugs, toxins, hormones, and the like bring about their biologic actions by reacting with specific receptors somewhere in the body.

Scientists working in all areas of biologic science have shown increasing interest in the analysis of drug-receptor interactions in the broadest sense. Studies of drugs (binding) to receptors in situ and to isolated and partly purified receptors are becoming common practice.

The action of a drug in the body is, however, a kinetic event not only with respect to transport of drug molecules to the environment of the receptors, but also with respect to the drug-receptor interaction itself.

Kinetics of Drug Action is an integrative approach to drug transport through the body, membrane transport toward the receptors, and the kinetics of drug-receptor interaction. This volume is aimed at providing a critical and penetrating study of the problems relevant to the kinetics or drug action from drug dosage to the final response.

It is felt that the critical surveys presented in this volume will contribute significantly to receptor study research in various biologic fields and to a better understanding of drug action.

I would like to express my gratitude to our secretary Miss MARGOT JANSSEN for the extensive typing of manuscripts and to our laboratory assistant Miss COBY HURKMANS for her dedicated assistance in the correcting some of the manuscripts and preparating the index.

Spring, 1977   J. M. VAN ROSSUM

Table of Contents

CHAPTER 2

Pharmacokinetics. Kinetic Aspects of Absorption, Distribution, and Elimination of Drugs. E. KRÜGER-THIEMER. With 21 Figures

CHAPTER 3

Pharmacokinetics of Biotransformation. J. M. VAN ROSSUM, C. A. M. VAN GINNEKEN, P. Th. HENDERSON, H. C. J. KETELAARS, and T. B. VREE. With 21 Figures

CHAPTER 4

General Theory of Drug-Receptor Interactions. Drug-Receptor Interaction Models. Calculation of Drug Parameters. F. G. VAN DEN BRINK. With 28 Figures

CHAPTER 5

A Critical Survey of Receptor Theories of Drug Action. D. MACKAY. With 7 Figures

List of Contributors

J. BLANCK, Dr. rer. nat., Akademie der Wissenschaften der DDR, Zentralinstitut für Molekularbiologie, Bereich Biokatalyse, DDR-1115 Berlin-Buch

F. G. VAN DEN BRINK, Dr., Katholieke Universiteit Nijmegen, Farmacologisch Instituut, Faculteit der Geneeskunde, Nijmegen, The Netherlands

C. A. M. VAN GINNEKEN, Dr., Katholieke Universiteit Nijmegen, Farmacologisch Instituut, Nijmegen, The Netherlands

R. E. GOSSELIN, M. D., Ph. D., Darmouth Medical School, Department of Pharmacology and Toxicology, Hanover, NH 03755/USA

P. TH. HENDERSON, Dr., Katholieke Universiteit Nijmegen, Farmacologisch Instituut, Nijmegen, The Netherlands

E. KAHRIG, Dr. sc. nat., Akademie der Wissenschaften der DDR, Zentralinstitut für Molekularbiologie, Bereich Biokatalyse, DDR-1115 Berlin-Buch

H. C. J. KETELAARS, Dr., Katholieke Universiteit Nijmegen, Farmacologisch Instituut, Nijmegen, The Netherlands

D. KIRSTEIN, Dr. rer. nat., Akademie der Wissenschaften der DDR, Zentralinstitut für Molekularbiologie, Bereich Biokatalyse, DDR-1115 Berlin-Buch

E. KRÜGER-THIEMER †, M. D., Ph. D.

D. MACKAY, Dr., Department of Pharmacology, University of Leeds, School of Medicine, Leeds 2, LS2 9NL, Great Britain

K.-U. MÖRITZ, Dr. rer. nat., Institut für Pharmakologie und Toxikologie der Universität, DDR-22 Greifswald

G. RAHMEL, Akademie der Wissenschaften der DDR, Zentralinstitut für Molekularbiologie, Bereich Biokatalyse, DDR-1115 Berlin-Buch

J. M. VAN ROSSUM, Prof. Dr., Katholieke Universiteit Nijmegen, Farmacologisch Instituut, Nijmegen, The Netherlands

W. SCHELER, Prof. Dr., Akademie der Wissenschaften der DDR, Zentralinstitut für Molekularbiologie, Bereich Biokatalyse, DDR-1115 Berlin-Buch

T. B. VREE, Dr., Katholieke Universiteit Nijmegen, Farmacologisch Instituut, Nijmegen, The Netherlands

General Introduction

J. M. VAN ROSSUM

Most drugs induce a spectrum of actions when given to man or animals. The intensity of each individual effect depends on the concentration of drug in the body and specifically the drug concentration in the target tissues. In general the intensity of effect increases with the concentration but the various effects may influence each other. This implies that drugs can best be studied in relative simple systems where the mutual interference is minimal.

The various effects induced by a drug may be based on the interactions of drug molecules with various types of receptors, although it is also possible that the same type of receptor in different tissues is involved in diverse effects. For instance, it is well-known that atropine causes mydriasis, intestinal relaxation, suppression of sweat production, thirst, and tachycardia by reacting with acetylcholine receptors in the various tissues.

Important aspects in drug action are:

1. the processes governing the drug concentration in the body and especially at the level of the receptors;

2. the interaction of drugs with the receptors;

3. the various events governing the generation of the ultimate effect once drug-receptor interaction has taken place;

4. the mutual interaction of the various effects caused by the drug.

The purpose of this volume is to present an integrated treatment of the kinetics of drug action, covering the principles of drug transport, the kinetics of drug absorption, distribution, and elimination via excretion and metabolism as well as the principles of drug-receptor interactions under steady-state conditions and the kinetics of the drug-receptor interaction.

The fundamental aspects of transport processes across membranes relevant to drug transport are treated by SCHELER et al.

Pharmacokinetics, including the kinetics of absorption, distribution, excretion, and metabolism under linear and nonlinear conditions, are treated by KRÜGER-THIEMER and by VAN ROSSUM. Dosage schedules are discussed in extenso.

The fundamentals of drug-receptor interactions are treated by VAN DEN BRINK, while MACKAY presents a critical survey of the existing drug-receptor theories.

The kinetics of drug-receptor interaction are presented by GOSSELIN, who offers a new model and by VAN GINNEKEN, who discusses, i.e., the relevance of the kinetics of drug transport and drug-receptor interaction for the effect as a time-dependent function.

The various aspects covering the fundamental processes in drug action are treated in a critical manner aimed at a fruitful use of the knowledge in drug research and drug therapy.

CHAPTER 1

Physicochemical Fundamentals and Thermodynamics of the Membrane Transport of Drugs

W. SCHELER and J. BLANCK
with the assistance of E. KAHRIG, D. KIRSTEIN, K.-U. MÖRITZ and G. RAHMEL

I. Introduction

Selectively acting drugs release their biological effects by reaction with specific receptor sites of nucleic acids, enzymes, and other active proteins or biomacro-molecules. As a rule these drug receptors are located some distance away from the body surfaces bordering on the milieu extérieur. Therefore, most drugs applied to the skin or the mucous membranes have to cross the cellular and intracellular membranes of several cells before interacting with the specific sites of reaction. These membranes are constructed for the purpose of transporting substrates, metabolites, ions, and other physiologic substances. Although most drugs are nonphysiologic molecules, their transport across the cell membrane and intracellular membranes involves the same systems and mechanisms as physiologic products, i.e. the same pathways, carriers, and energy sources [2, 62, 256]. In such cases the transport characteristics of drugs and of physiologic permeants are the same. In some cases drugs compete with substrates or metabolites for the carriers in the membranes. But the majority of drugs differ from the physiologic substances in their physicochemical properties, particularly in their solubility [35, 36, 247, 332]. This means they enter the cell interior via the lipid material of the cell membrane relatively readily, whilst the transport of the water-soluble substrates, metabolites, ions etc. is restricted to the aqueous pores and carrier systems of the membrane. Review articles on the transport of substances across biological membranes have been published by USSING [303], WILBRANDT and ROSENBERG [325], SCHANKER [256], CSÁKY [44], DIAMOND and WRIGHT [55], HAYDON and HLADKY [107], KOTYK [161], FISHMAN and VOLKENSTEIN [75], COLEMAN [42], and BRANTON and DEAMER [22].

II. Systems and Membrane Types

From the thermodynamic point of view there are several types of systems, which can be classified by their distribution of matter and their thermodynamic properties. For the description of the physicochemical fundamentals of membrane transport the following types of systems are of importance.

A. Homogeneous System

This type is characterized by a microscopically homogeneous distribution of all its components, of temperature, hydrostatic pressure, and other intensive properties. The homogeneity of solute concentration, of temperature, pressure etc. must be continuously maintained, though these parameters may change gradually, i.e. the rate of processes effecting changes in concentration, temperature, and pressure must always be slower than that of the local equilibration processes. An electrolyte-protein-water solution can be considered a prototype of such a homogeneous multicomponent system.

B. Heterogeneous Continuous System

This type of system is characterized by directed continuous changes of solute concentration or intensive properties like pressure, temperature etc. throughout the system. These gradients are described by the differential quotients dc/dx, (or $d\tilde{\mu}/dx$ for the case of activity coefficients < 1 of the solute), dp/dx, dT/dy, etc.

C. Heterogeneous Discontinuous System

A system of this type is composed of two or more homogeneous partial systems. The rate of the exchange of matter, of heat, or electric charge between the partial systems is lower than that within the subsystems. Prototypes of this system are non-miscible liquids like a heptane-water system or two liquid phases separated by a membrane. The latter constitutes the fundamental model for biological membranes. On first approximation cell membranes are diaphragms between two aqueous phases.

D. Membrane Types

Many physicochemical models of membranes are used for the investigation of transport processes. Several of them are suited to approximative description of single permeability properties of biological membranes. According to Solomon and his school, and also to other authors, they can be derived from two basic types, the liquid-phase membrane and the porous membrane [51, 274, 280]. The functional characteristics of biological membranes, however, especially those of the cell membranes, cannot be accounted for completely by a single one of the following types as they combine the main permeability characteristics of each model.

1. Liquid-Phase Membranes

The membrane consists of a liquid that is nonmiscible with both the adjacent aqueous phases, for example heptane, oil, lipids. Furthermore, there are no aqueous pores in it. Therefore the solvent, water, cannot penetrate the membrane. With respect to their permeability the solutes are differentiated according to their solubility in the membrane phase [55, 255]. Lipid membranes therefore exclude lipid-insoluble solutes from the exchange between the two aqueous phases, whereas lipophilic substances exchange readily.

2. Pore Membranes

The matrix of a porous membrane consists of an impermeable material traversed by solvent-filled capillaries or cavities connecting the two separated phases. All the components of the pore content are assumed to be distributed homogeneously across the pore diameter.

a) Narrow-Pore Membranes

In this type of porous membrane the pore diameter exceeds the diameter of the diffusing molecules, but both are within the same order of magnitude. If the pore size is about the same as the size of the permeant or is smaller, solute transport ceases whereas solvent transport continues. This is the case of the ideal semipermeable membrane. In a capillary membrane whose pore diameter is only slightly greater than the diameter of the permeants, the movement of each particle in the pore is coupled with that of the neighbouring ones, since neighbouring molecules cannot mutually change their places within the pore. Each particle proceeds only in the same ratio as the preceding one moves. This single file mechanism means that the transport of different permeants is tightly coupled, as observed in membranes of squid axon by HODGKIN and KEYNES [122].

b) Coarse-Pore Membranes

Porous membranes whose mean pore diameter is much greater than the diameter of the diffusing molecules do not discriminate between solutes of different sizes. The transport across such a membrane obeys the laws of free diffusion, the membrane matrix thus only restricting the diffusion area.

c) Charged Porous Membranes

Biological membranes contain regions with ion exchange character. At the walls of pores there are fixed charges in high concentrations (1–3 mol/l) [46, 233]. These charges modify the ion content and the diffusion of electrolytes in "ion exchange membranes" in comparison to uncharged membranes.

The fixed charges of such membranes are counterbalanced by mobile ions with opposite charge (counter-ions), according to the principle of electroneutrality. These counter-ions are readily exchangeable against ions of the same species (tracer fluxes) or against ions of the same charge (exchange-diffusion).

At low electrolyte concentrations in the surrounding solutions ($\leq$ two orders of magnitude of the fixed-charges concentration) the counter-ion concentration in the membrane is independent of the external concentrations and the coion concentration is negligibly small. The membrane is an ideal barrier for the diffusion of electrolytes in this case; only solvent and nonelectrolytes can diffuse through the matrix, charge transfer (excitation) occurs only by counter-ions. This behavior is changed by increasing the ratio of electrolyte concentration in the solutions to fixed-charges concentration.

There are two types of ion exchange membranes. Following a classification of EISENMAN et al. [65], we can define membranes of the dissociation type as having a more or less total dissociation of all fixed and counter-ions, and the association type where fixed charged groups and counter-ions are tightly associated. This strong ion-ion interaction can take place in a medium of low dielectric constant (lipophilic phases) or between ions which tend to form undissociated ion pairs. Weak ion exchangers with dissociation constants of $K_D \leqq 10^{-3}$ in the H^+-form (weak acids) or the OH^--form (weak bases) form association type membranes and are important for the modelling of regulatory phenomena. It is possible to regulate charge density, ion- and water-content, pore diameter, permeability, and selectivity of such membranes by changing the milieu conditions (pH, valency state of the counterions, ionic strength) in this way inducing a transition from the association- to the dissociation-type or vice versa.

Such mechanisms were observed both at glass electrodes [46] and biological membranes [330]. Milieu variations by chemical reactions could play a role in inducing special transport conformations of membrane proteins.

3. Composed Membranes

For characterizing the transport processes of biological membranes the simplified models both of the liquid phase membrane and the pore membranes are insufficient. Therefore several types of composed membranes are used for a closer approach to the behavior of biomembranes.

a) Composed Pore Membranes

Composed membranes which contain regions with cation and anion exchange properties exhibit a particular character. The arrangement of these regions may be mosaic-like or sandwich-like. Mosaic membranes are characterized by electrolyte permeabilities which exceed the diffusion velocity in solution. Such structures can be induced even in biological membranes by local different milieu conditions [15, 53, 214]. Sandwich membranes do not allow transports of electrolytes from one side of the membrane to the other (rectifying effect). They were used by BLUMENTHAL, et al. [16] for modeling the coupling between transport processes and chemical reactions, thus leading to the mechanism of active transport. A theoretical treatment with respect to composed charged membranes was presented by KEDEM and KATCHALSKY [148–150] and later by NAPARSTEK et al. [213].

Furthermore such arrangements can lead to instabilities and oscillations [263].

b) Composed Liquid Phase-Pore Membranes

According to what is known about the structure of biological membranes [63, 64], there exist some examples of model membranes consisting of lipid and protein regions [102, 103, 243, 244, 297].

It is impossible to explain the observed decrease of electrical resistance by the lipid layer being sandwiched between protein layers. Evidently, formation of a mosaic-like structure with water-filled pores inside "penetrating" proteins has to be assumed.

Transport processes in such membranes include two components: pore and matrix transport. As a borderline case, the uncoupling of solute and solvent transport or between two solute transports is possible. Polar solvents or solutes (ions or nonelectrolytes) are able to enter the pores (sieving effects excluded) whereas the liquid phase of the membrane matrix is only penetrable to matrix-soluble solutes [55, 171].

The permeability of hydrophilic pores can be regulated directly by ion exchange mechanisms (exchange of $Me^+ \rightleftarrows Me^{++}$, $H^+ \rightleftarrows Me^+$) or indirectly by addition of drugs, which dissolve in the lipid phase and change the interaction between lipids and hydrophilic protein side chains [71, 91, 97, 100, 225, 262, 283].

Structural alterations of the lipid matrix due to changes of composition or temperature cannot only influence the transport properties but also the structure of membrane bound enzymes and the active transport [11, 14, 67, 130, 159, 193, 224, 269].

Apart from the membrane types specified, passage through which can be treated theoretically by means of continuous statements, there are thin membranes composed of only a few layers of molecules, which require different treatment. In their case two sites of membrane resistance can be important; (a) the penetration of one of the two solution-membrane interfaces may be rate-limiting, whereas diffusion within the membrane is relatively rapid [70, 119, 168, 169]. Hence the supposition that H-bridging between solute and solvent is responsible for the resistance to the penetration of the permeant from the outside solution into the membrane [280]. This hypothesis is based on both the solid-state theory and the transition-state theory developed by GLASSTONE et al. [89], FRENKEL [81], and JOST [133]. (b) The interior of the membrane, which is thought to be built up of a series of barriers of potential that have to be overcome in a reaction in several stages, may be predominant (relaxation theory of DAVSON and DANIELLI [51]).

4. Biological Membranes

The membrane types with passive permeability described above can mimic only parts of the transport phenomena of biological membranes. The more complex behavior of biological membranes is a result of a combination of transport processes, chemical reactions, and structural variation due to specific action of binding states and milieu conditions. The mode of cooperation of these three effects is not fully understood:

1. The isolation of specific transport proteins is difficult because their amount in membrane preparations may be very small [21].

2. Biological transport processes are dynamic events in structure and function, while most of the modern physicochemical methods are static, or cannot be focussed at a sufficiently small area of the cell surfaces. Dynamic methods, such as experiments with fluorescence markers, can include influences of the marker on the structure of the object [21, 127, 132].

3. In contrast to unit-membrane-models, modern views of the structure of biological membranes emphasize the dominating role of highly specific proteins [22] traversing the lipid shell connected by hydrophobic interactions between side chains of proteins and the matrix [22, 94, 307].

The coupling between transport and chemical reaction is represented by two types of membranes; membranes with passive carrier transport and membranes with active transport.

a) Membranes with Passive Carrier Transport

The transport of a substance across the membrane may be facilitated by complex formation with specific membrane components, i.e. the carriers. This transport implies saturation characteristics because of the limited carrier concentration within the membranes; furthermore, no metabolic energy is needed for the process. The nature and the precise mechanism of function of the carriers are still unknown. Movable carriers such as macrocyclic compounds acting upon specific complex formation with cations [66, 107, 127, 162, 184, 207, 211, 234, 266], are not found in living cells. Recent reports about natural carriers postulate proteins and lipids with special binding sites for the transported solute [12, 38, 77, 249, 311]. Carrier transports are driven by concentration gradients of the permeants. The carrier transport ceases with the disappearance of these driving gradients.

b) Membranes with Active Transport

Membrane systems of biological organisms, especially cell membranes, are able to transport specific solutes by consumption of chemical energy. As in the case of coupling of vector phenomena, the coupling of transport with chemical reactions can lead to a transport even from lower to higher concentrations (uphill-transport). This active transport is coupled to the cell metabolism (ATPases or enzymes of the oxidative chain) and requires adequate energy sources like ATP. The energy from ATP or other compounds may serve:
    1. to induce conformational changes,
    2. to tie covalent bonds between membrane components
    3. to establish an electrochemical gradient [21].
The mechanism of active transport involves specific carriers [18, 77] or anisotropic membranes leading to vectorial transport [134, 248, 267]. A model was made of the latter mechanism by BROUN et al. [26], who used model membranes with sandwich-like arranged phosphorylating and dephosphorylating reticulated enzymes for an uphill glucose transport.

There are some references to the reversibility of active transport [41, 192, 298].

III. Classification of Membrane Transport

The exchange of matter between a biological system and its surroundings is an important life process. It is achieved via cell membranes and intercellular membranes. According to KEDEM [144] all the spontaneous transport processes are classified as *passive* ones. The driving force is the electrochemical potential gradient of a permeant and there is no coupling to energy supplying metabolic processes. In contrast to these, the *active* transport processes are coupled to exergonic chemical reactions within the cell and the net flux of the permeant may be in the opposite direction to its electrochemical gradient (uphill transport).

Both types of transport processes can be subdivided into carrier-free and carrier-mediated forms (Fig. 1). Several criteria make a distinction between the four main forms of membrane transport possible (Table 1).

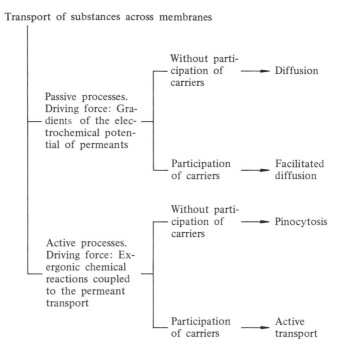

Fig. 1. Scheme of the basic types of transport processes

A. Diffusion Across Membranes

1. Driving Forces

Mass flow across a membrane is induced by differences of intensive properties between the two phases separated by the membrane, such as temperature (ΔT), pressure (Δp), chemical potential ($\Delta \mu$) or electrical potential ($\Delta \varphi$). $\Delta \mu$ and $\Delta \varphi$ are usually connected to the electrochemical potential ($\Delta \tilde{\mu}$). Furthermore, transport of particles can also be generated by external fields, e.g. magnetic, electrostatic, electrodynamic, and gravitation fields. Under physiologic conditions, however, this possibility is negligible.

If coupling with other vector phenomena is negligible, the diffusion of a solute across a membrane will cease if the driving concentration gradient becomes zero. If the permeant is continuously generated in one phase and in the other perpetually removed from the equilibrium, either by binding to components of the cytoplasm or by its metabolic conversion, the gradient will still persist. Apart from various substrates, which are metabolized within the cell, such chemical conversions are observed with some ions, like NO_3^-, NH_4^+, HCO_3^-, Fe^{2+} (reactions with porphyrines). In the mitochondria, Mg^{2+} is assumed to precipitate as magnesium phosphate, thereby maintaining a gradient between the surroundings and the inner mitochondrial compartment [23].

Fluxes can be generated not only by their own concentration gradient but also by coupling with other gradients. The observed phenomena are diffusion

Table 1. Characterization of the main forms of transport of a permeant A across membranes

Criterion	Diffusion	Facilitated diffusion	Pinocytosis	Active transport
Driving force	Gradient of the electrochemical potential of A	Gradient of the electrochemical potential of A and/or of permeant B (counter-transport)	Free energy from cell metabolism	Free energy from cell metabolism
Kinetics	Proportional to the concentration difference of A; nonsaturable	Changing with the concentration gradient of A; saturable; independent on the intensity of metabolism	Without precise mathematical equations; dependent on the intensity of metabolism	Like facilitated diffusion but dependent on the intensity of metabolism
Specificity	Dependent on solubility, charge and size of A; no structural specificity	Structural specificity	Unspecific	Structural specificity
Inhibition	Only limited; weak on temperature decrease	Competitive by permeantanalogs; noncompetitive by carrier poisons; on temperature decrease stronger; not by O_2 deficiency or by poisons of the cell metabolism	Under O_2 deficiency and in the presence of cell metabolism poisons; strong on temperature decrease	Like facilitated diffusion but strong with temperature decrease, O_2 deficiency and cell metabolism poisons

coupling or incongruent transport [136, 258], electrodialysis [170, 235], reverse osmosis [30, 170], and thermodiffusion [155, 170]. All these phenomena can lead to uphill transports.

2. Mechanism and Kinetics

The majority of nonelectrolyte drugs cross biological membranes by diffusion. Depending on the chemical nature and the physical properties of the drugs, the membranes act partly as lipid barriers and partly as porous molecular sieves. Ionic permeants may also cross the membrane by ion-exchange mechanisms. They are thought to move along the pore surface in exchange with other ions of identical charge jumping from one binding site to the next one (Fig. 2) [85, 183]. This mode of ion transport presupposes a continuity of ionic binding sites along the

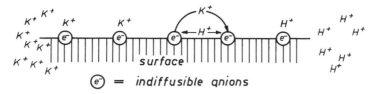

Fig. 2. Inverse movement of H^+ and K^+ in exchange diffusion along anion-engaged surface of membrane pore. According to [197]

pores and a continuous production of ions to be exchanged against the permeant ions in order to maintain the ion gradient as a driving force. The production of protons by the cell metabolism tends to support this hypothesis, which is particularly stressed by GONZALES and JENNY [93].

The mass flow across a membrane via diffusion obeys simple physical laws derived from the laws of diffusion in solutions. The application of Fick's laws to biological membranes is, however, restricted. Whereas in diffusion only solute-solvent and solute-solute interactions are of importance, in membrane diffusion solute-membrane and solvent-membrane interactions also have to be considered. Depending on the chemical composition and on the physical structure of the membrane, these interactions may cause a relative flow solute versus solvent within the membrane (exchange flow of solute and solvent). Solute flow and solvent flow across a membrane are therefore not independent of one another. Interrelationships of this kind have been recognized by FREY-WYSSLING [82], LAIDLER and SHULER [168, 169], USSING [301] and PAPPENHEIMER [226], and have been dealt with theoretically by STAVERMAN [277, 278] and KIRKWOOD [153], and more recently by KEDEM and KATCHALSKY [146, 147]. The kinetics of simple membrane diffusion is strictly proportional to the driving concentration gradient. Even at high gradients, there are no saturation phenomena of the mass flow.

3. Specificity

The size of lipophilic permeants is less important in membrane transport [8, 164, 256, 329] whereas lipid-insoluble drugs, especially ionic ones, are quite sharply differentiated according to their molar volume [8, 104, 164, 256, 257]. This molecular sieve property of the membrane is attributed to pores or capillaries of definite diameter in the membrane matrix, though it has never been possible to demonstrate permanent pores morphologically [87, 198]. Thus it may be assumed that pores are transient and dynamic structures of biological membranes [49, 51, 294]. Their mean radius is given as 3–5 Å [27, 72, 85, 198, 275], varying in different biological objects. The mean pore size is obviously dependent on the cell metabolism [238].

The effective diffusion coefficient in a porous membrane system is related to the bulk diffusivity in free solution D_0 by

$$D_{\text{eff}} = D_0 \, \Theta \, K_p K_r / \tau$$

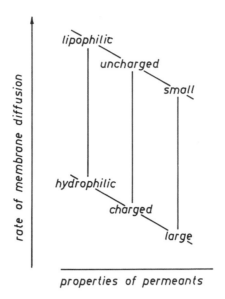

Fig. 3. Scheme of dependence of rate of membrane diffusion on physicochemical properties of permeants

where Θ is the pore volume fraction, τ is the tortuosity, and $K_p K_r$ is well approximated for λ up to 0.5 by

$$K_p K_r = (1 - \lambda)^2 \, (1 - 2.104\lambda + 2.09\lambda^3 - 0.95\lambda^5) \, .$$

λ is the ratio of the molecule diameter to the pore diameter.

This equation can be used to describe diffusion both through artificial membranes [9, 170] and biological ones [280]. Stereospecific differences between lipophilic permeants, for instance between stereoisomers, do not influence the penetration rate provided these stereochemical differences do not alter the lipid solubility [151]. In the case of hydrophilic drugs, stereochemical differences of a solute may slightly modify the transport rate because of the differences in the geometry of the permeant-pore interactions.

4. Inhibition Characteristics

There is no competitive inhibition between stereoisomers or chemical analogs. A fall in temperature reduces the permeant diffusion across the membrane to approximately the same small degree as in the case of free diffusion. The Q_{10} values amount to 1.1–1.4.

The mean pore size of cell membranes can be influenced by chemical agents [238]; bivalent cations diminish the membrane permeability. According to KAVANAU [142] these ions link lipid molecules, thereby decreasing the pore diameter; the influence of divalent cations on the structure of protein plugs is more direct due to the ion exchange character of these molecules [286]. Amphotericin and some other compounds increase the porous character of cell membranes [5]. This effect is thought to be due to an amphotericin membrane-cholesterol interaction.

B. Facilitated Diffusion

The structure of biological membranes permits only a limited transport of water-soluble, lipid-insoluble solutes of mean molecular weight into the cell interior. This class of substances does, however, include several essential energy-delivering substrates or components of biomacromolecules, e.g. sugars, amino acids, purine, or pyrimidine bases. Their entry is made possible by specific carrier molecules within the membrane [3, 4, 13, 161, 175, 177, 256, 311, 320–322, 325]. STEIN [280] calculates that glucose transport by this mechanism is accelerated by a factor of 10^4 and glycerol transport by 10^2. Therefore this type of membrane transport is called facilitated diffusion.

Most of the work on carrier transport has been concerned with sugars. The uptake and the release of glucose by erythrocytes obeys the passive carrier mechanism [4, 320, 321]. It also prevails in other mammalian cells [322], but in some cases it is replaced by active transport processes, e.g. in the kidneys [125].

There are transitions between facilitated diffusion and active transport to some extent. Escherichia coli, for example has a transport system for galactosides [79, 163, 326], which can be induced [77, 151, 158]. On induction a protein is augmented, which is essential for transport [151]. The inducible component is called "permease" [151, 156]. When it is absent the carrier cannot be loaded. Generally the permease is not identified with the carrier itself but is thought of as an enzyme catalyzing the permeant-carrier reaction [151, 322].

There is an experimentally well-established model of carrier transport that was first described by LE FEVRE and his school [177–181] and was systematically developed by WILBRANDT and co-workers [113, 251, 320, 321, 322, 325]. It allows a strict distinction between facilitated diffusion and other transport mechanisms. According to these authors and several others [19, 50, 178, 246, 252, 253, 279, 280, 282, 312, 322, 325], facilitated diffusion can be characterized as follows.

1. Mechanism

It is assumed that on the membrane surface the permeant molecule binds to specific membrane components, i.e. the carriers [212, 260]. The permeant-carrier complex crosses the membrane and, on the other side, the complex dissociates to release the free permeant into the next phase [19, 125, 222, 252, 312, 325]. There is no precise knowledge as to the nature of the carrier, but macromolecular components, especially proteins, are thought to be the stereospecific binding sites of the permeants [38, 79, 151, 158, 178, 227, 237, 281]. The free carrier and the permeant-carrier complex probably both move by simple diffusion within the membrane but rotation processes and other types of movement have been emphasized more recently [25, 70, 77, 108, 129, 156, 157, 306] and cannot be excluded. The diffusion velocity of the permeant-carrier complex exceeds that of the free carrier. Figure 4 gives a simple scheme of carrier transport.

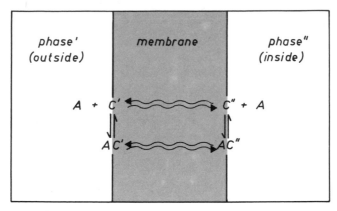

Fig. 4. Scheme of carrier transport. ⇌ equilibrium reactions; ⤳ diffusion processes (rate-limiting); A = permeant, C = carrier, AC = permeant-carrier complex

2. Driving Force

The driving force of facilitated diffusion of a permeant A is either its own gradient of chemical potential or that of a permeant B, which is competing with A for the carrier. In contrast to active transport, which also involves carrier mechanisms, facilitated diffusion is independent of the supply of free energy from exergonic chemical reactions [44, 62, 178, 230, 254]. The net flux of a single permeant stops when the concentration difference between the two phases separated by the membrane has been leveled out [44, 320].

3. Counter-Transport

The specific binding site of the carrier interacts with several permeants of similar structure. Therefore chemically related solutes mutually influence their transport across the membrane. The counter-transport is a special case of this interference. It is an uphill transport of permeant A arising from the downhill movement of permeant B. The driving force for the transport of A is the gradient of the chemical potential of permeant B.

The phenomenon of counter-transport presupposes movable carriers; it will not occur if the binding sites for the permeant are fixed in the membrane [253]. It has been studied with sugars and other permeants on various cell types [28, 40, 208, 230–232, 253, 322]. For example, when glucose- and xylose-equilibrated erythrocytes are transferred into a medium of identical glucose but lower xylose concentration, the resulting xylose outflux produces a corresponding glucose influx (counter-transport).

4. Kinetics

The kinetics of facilitated diffusion and of counter-transport was mainly derived by LE FEVRE [176, 180], WIDDAS [312], WILBRANDT and ROSENBERG [252, 319, 324, 325] and further developed by several authors [25, 128, 129, 178]. The kinetics of carrier transport reveals some peculiarities dependent on the permeant concentration on both sides of the membranes. (a) At low concentrations, i.e. at low saturation of the carrier system, both the unidirectional permeant fluxes, i.e. those into and out of the cell, are proportional to the respective external and internal concentrations. The resulting net flux is therefore proportional to the concentration difference, Δc, across the membrane. Under these conditions carrier transport cannot be distinguished from simple membrane diffusion; Fick's law is valid. (b) At medium concentrations the dependence of the transport rate of the unidirectional fluxes on concentration corresponds strictly to that of enzyme kinetics, conforming to the Michaelis-Menten equation. The net flux, however, commonly fails to follow simple Michaelis-Menten kinetics (cf. however IV.E.1.b). (c) At high concentrations (high saturation of the carrier system) the unidirectional fluxes become independent of the respective concentrations [280, 322, 325]. The net flux becomes proportional to the difference between the reciprocals of the two permeant concentrations.

5. Specificity

The permeant binding site of the carrier is highly stereospecific. Therefore the transport rates of structural analogs or stereoisomers may differ considerably. This characteristic of facilitated diffusion has been investigated in detail with different sugars [84, 178, 181, 182, 250, 316, 317, 320].

6. Competitive Inhibition

Permeant and binding site of the carrier interact reversibly and the reaction obeys the law of mass action. Provided one phase contains two (or more) permeants capable of reacting with the specific binding site of the carrier, they compete for this site according to their individual permeant-carrier equilibrium constants and their concentration gradients respectively. Phlorrhizin represents a specific competitive inhibitor of glucose transport [44, 62, 217, 317, 320], as it is bound to the glucose carrier but is not transported. The aglucone phloretin and the non-penetrating phloretin phosphate exert their action in the same way [176, 318, 323]. An excellent review on carrier inhibition is given by LE FEVRE [178].

Further types of inhibition: A fall in temperature lowers the rate of facilitated diffusion, the temperature coefficient Q_{10} having been shown to be >2 [230]. Carrier poisons like SH reagents such as organic Hg compounds and dinitrofluoro-benzene as well as guanethidine and anaesthetics can also inhibit facilitated diffusion [20, 29, 62, 175, 238, 254, 313, 314].

C. Active Transport

All the definitions of active transport [43, 154, 197, 215, 247 etc.] draw attention to the carrier mechanism of transport across the cell membrane and to its coupling with metabolic reactions. The driving force does not arise from differences of chemical potentials of permeants between phase' and phase'' but from exergonic chemical reactions. *Active transport is always based on the coupling of chemical*

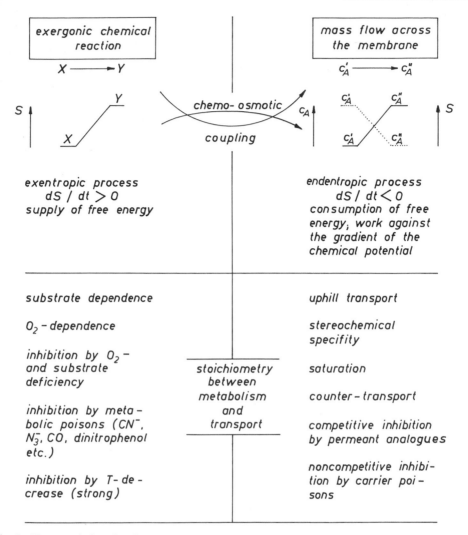

Fig. 5. Characteristics of active transport

reactions of the cell metabolism with the permeation process (= chemo-osmotic coupling). Metabolic energy is converted into work against the chemical potential gradient (Fig. 5).

Since the active transport follows the carrier mechanism it shares many characteristics with facilitated diffusion (cf. III.B.). Moreover, some further criteria of active transport [126, 268, 299–302, 304, 331] are concerned with its dependence on the intensity of cell metabolism [29, 112, 121, 125, 144, 228, 238, 259, 284], inhibition of it by a fall in temperature [261], and metabolic poisons [29, 209, 238], by O_2, and substrate deficiency. The accumulation of a permeant in the cell interior, as proposed by LING [187], TROSHIN [295], HARRIS and PRANKERD [106], SHAW et al. [264], and DAMADIAN et al. [47, 48] is possible in general terms because of its specific binding to cell components. The investigations of MITCHELL [202, 203], KEYNES [152], GLYNN [90], USSING and ZERAHN [304], MAIZELS [191], and KABACK and STADTMAN [135], however, prove that this mode of uphill movement can ultimately be excluded, because the actively transported particles are freely movable in the cytoplasm and osmotically effective. Furthermore, cells emptied of their cell content may nevertheless actively accumulate several permeants. On the subject of the active transport of amino acids, HEINZ [110] has summarized a series of results excluding the intracellular binding of amino acids as a reason for their accumulation. There are some models of the mechanism of the active transport [37, 95, 115–118, 143, 160, 229, 270, 308–310] but exact knowledge of the active transport, and in particular of chemo-osmotic coupling, is still lacking.

D. Pinocytosis

The membranes of many living cells form infoldings and invaginations associated with the uptake of fluid from the surrounding medium. This process is similar to the phagocytosis of particles and is called pinocytosis. Since the pioneering work of LEWIS [186], pinocytosis has been studied on different biological subjects. The bulk of our knowledge results from investigations on amoeba [328]. Pinocytosis can also be observed by means of the light microscope in the tubular cell of the kidney [125], in leukocytes [33] and tumourcell cultures [186] but not in the highly specific parenchyma cells of liver and pancreas [125]. For a review see FÜLLER [83]. Micropinocytosis, however, which can be observed in electron-microscope studies, is regarded as a ubiquitous faculty of living cells [58, 276]. There are close relations with phagocytosis, as was observed by DESSOLLE [54] in epididymia of rats.

1. Mechanism

Pinocytosis will only begin in vitro if the suspension fluid contains substances such as salts and proteins, which induce it [34, 327]. The process can be subdivided into two phases. Firstly, the inducer is absorbed onto the cell membrane. This reaction is independent of metabolism and temperature. The adsorption was clearly demonstrated by SCHUMAKER [261] and other authors by means of labeled proteins. The second phase is an energy-utilizing reaction linked to the cell metabolism. Membrane pseudopodia are formed and a fluid droplet is enclosed by wall fusion; it reaches the cell interior where it forms a vesicle within the cytoplasm [124]. When the content has been condensed by water withdrawal, the membrane of the vacuole disappears, probably by way of enzymatic degradation, and finally the components of the vescicle come into contact with the cytoplasm [68, 69].

BENNETT's theory [10] of membrane flow and membrane vesiculation is derived from electron-microscope investigations. Pinocytosis is a rhythmic process [124]. It is not known what factor is responsible for the periodicity. The breaks may be caused by the resynthesis of membrane material to replace the membrane segments that enclose the pinocytosis vacuoles [327].

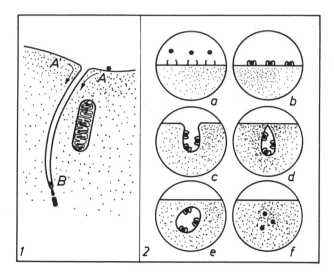

Fig. 6. Pinocytosis via membrane flow (1) and membrane vesiculation (2): (1) After adsorption in *A* the particle gets position *B* within the recessus by membrane flow. Here after vacuolization and wall lysis permeant is released into the cell interior. (2) Vesiculation occurs after invagination of cell membranes followed by permeant's release. According to [10]

2. Specificity

Pinocytosis is a nonselective transport process. It allows very different solutes of the medium to enter the cell. By this mechanism toxins, antitoxins, other proteins [73], and even glucose [34, 265] are taken up. Micropinocytosis may be of specific importance for the synthesis or resynthesis of transmitter substances [6, 7]. The general biological significance of pinocytosis, however, is still obscure.

3. Inhibition

As an active process, pinocytosis is inhibited both by metabolic poisons, such as dinitrophenol or KCN [261] and by a fall in temperature [261]. On the other hand microinjection of ATP into the cell leads to enhanced pinocytosis [92].

IV. Kinetics and Thermodynamics of Membrane Transport

A. Conventional Equations

The transport of substances across a membrane is generally governed by Fick's law [74], which states that the number of moles of a permeant crossing the membrane per unit time is proportional to its concentration gradient dc/dx across the membrane of thickness dx and surface area F:

$$\frac{dN}{dt} = D \cdot F \cdot \frac{dc}{dx}. \tag{1}$$

The factor D is the diffusion coefficient; it is specific with respect to the permeant and the membrane. Its dimension is $cm^2 \cdot sec^{-1}$.

If dx is unknown or cannot be exactly determined, the concentration difference dc or Δc can be inserted into the equation of transport:

$$\frac{dN}{dt} = P \cdot F \cdot dc. \tag{2}$$

The proportionality factor $P = D/dx$ is the permeability coefficient; its dimension is that of a velocity, $cm \cdot sec^{-1} \cdot P$ depends on the thickness of the membrane, its structure, and on the physicochemical properties of the permeant.

D_s or P_s of a compound S (solute) are determined by the estimation of its concentration in one phase or both phases separated by a membrane of known surface area at definite intervals. By analogy, the permeability coefficient of the membrane for the solvent (water), P_w, can be obtained by addition of small quantities of D_2O or ^3H_2O to one phase. P_w is commonly known as water permeability.

Description of the membrane permeability by two coefficients, P_s and P_w, proves to be inadequate, because solute and solvent molecules may interact with the membrane matrix with different affinities, thus generating a relative flow solute versus solvent. This exchange flow must be described by a third coefficient.

B. Introductory Remarks on the Thermodynamics of Irreversible Processes

Within a system in a state of nonequilibrium, the movement of particles continues until equilibrium is reached. As the system passes from the state of nonequilibrium to the state of equilibrium the entropy of the system increases:

$$\frac{dS}{dt} > 0. \tag{3}$$

This relation is valid for all irreversible processes. Therefore in recent years the theory of the thermodynamics of irreversible processes has been applied to the movement of substances within biological systems and especially to their membrane transport. Several authors and laboratories in particular have contributed to this work: DE DONDER [56, 57], ONSAGER [218, 219], ECKART [59, 60, 61], MEIXNER [195, 196], PRIGOGINE [239, 240], DE GROOT [98, 99], DENBIGH [52], STAVERMAN [278], and KIRKWOOD [153] (further monographs [76, 101]) should be mentioned, as should more recent publications, notably those by KEDEM, KATCHALSKY and co-workers [86, 137, 144–147]). Our treatment is based mainly on that described in [137, 144–147].

From a thermodynamic point of view, biological subjects must be regarded as partial systems, their surroundings being the complementary system. There is a continuous exchange of matter and energy between the two systems. The entropy change of a biological system is given by its spontaneous entropy production d_iS/dt

and the entropy exchange with the milieu $d_a S/dt$

$$\frac{dS}{dt} = \frac{d_i S}{dt} + \frac{d_a S}{dt}.$$ (4)

A living system that is continuously regenerating, growing and reproducing is characterized by the relation $dS/dt < 0$. Since $d_i S/dt > 0$ [Eq. (3)], it follows that $d_a S/dt < 0$ and $|d_a S/dt| > d_i S/dt$, i.e. the process only goes on when entropy is increasing in the environment. The extent of this entropy increase in the milieu must be greater than the extent of the entropy decrease of the biological system. Biological systems are characterized by their ability to overcompensate their spontaneous entropy production by a continuous uptake of substrates of low entropy content from the milieu and their chemical conversion into entropy-rich metabolites that they release into the milieu. Therefore the existence of cells or macro-organisms is linked to the constant exchange of matter and energy with the milieu through the cell membranes.

C. Passive Transport of Nonelectrolytes

1. Flux Equations

According to Figure 7, the treatment of the membrane transport can be restricted to the flow of the solvent (water, w) and of one solute (s) through a membrane of thickness Δx. The volumes of phase' and phase" are assumed to be large compared with the volume of the membrane.

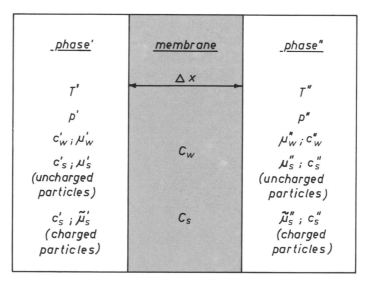

Fig. 7. Scheme of basic membrane transport system. Within heterogeneous discontinuous system two homogeneous subsystems, phase ' and phase ", are separated by membrane. (For notation of physicochemical parameters cf. text)

c_s and c_w denote the concentrations, μ_s and μ_w the chemical potentials, $\tilde{\mu}_s$ and $\tilde{\mu}_w$ the electrochemical potentials of solute and solvent in phase ' and phase "; C_s and C_w stand for the local concentrations of solute and water within the membrane, thus being functions of x, the spatial coordinate perpendicular to the membrane surface. T indicates the absolute temperature, p the hydrostatic pressure.

The thermodynamic treatment of a nonequilibrium system starts with the determination of the entropy production during the elapsing processes. The entropy increase per unit time of the phase-membrane-phase system as characterized in Figure 7 amounts to

$$\frac{d_i S}{dt} = \frac{1}{T} (\mu'_w - \mu''_w) \frac{dN''_w}{dt} + \frac{1}{T} (\mu'_s - \mu''_s) \frac{dN''_s}{dt} . \tag{5}$$

dN''_w/dt and dN''_s/dt stand for the number of moles of solvent (water, w) or solute (s) which penetrate per unit time into phase ". Related to the area F of the membrane the flux of solvent and solute are

$$J_w = \frac{1}{F} \frac{dN''_w}{dt} \quad \text{and} \quad J_s = \frac{1}{F} \frac{dN''_s}{dt} . \tag{6}$$

The rate of entropy production according to (5) can generally be expressed as the sum of products of fluxes J_i per unit area and generalized forces X_i, such as the gradients of chemical potential of the components i and the temperature gradient respectively. For isothermal systems it is convenient to use the dissipation function ψ, linking the fluxes J_i and the forces X_i in the same manner

$$\psi = \sum_i J_i X_i > 0 . \tag{7}$$

Application of this equation to the membrane transport of solvent and a solute gives

$$\psi = (\mu'_w - \mu''_w) J_w + (\mu'_s - \mu''_s) J_s . \tag{8}$$

If approximative chemical potentials of ideal solutions are referred to a highly dilute solution of the solute

$$\mu'_s - \mu''_s = \bar{v}_s \Delta p + RT \frac{\Delta c_s}{\bar{c}_s} ; \tag{9}$$

$$\mu'_w - \mu''_w = \bar{v}_w \Delta p - RT \frac{\Delta c_s}{c_w} . \tag{10}$$

$\bar{v}_s$ and $\bar{v}_w$ are the partial molar volume of solute and solvent, $\Delta p = p' - p''$, $\Delta c_s = c'_s - c''_s$, $\bar{c}_s$ being the mean concentration of solute in the phases according to $\Delta c_s/\bar{c}_s = \ln(c'_s/c''_s)$. If $\Delta c_s/c'' \ll 1$ then $\bar{c}_s = (c'_s + c''_s)/2$ is valid and from this it follows that $c_w = 1/\bar{v}_w$.

Introduction of (9) and (10) into (8) gives

$$\psi = (J_w \bar{v}_w + J_s \bar{v}_s)\,\Delta p + \frac{J_s}{\bar{c}_s} - \frac{J_w}{c_w}\,RT\Delta c_s. \tag{11}$$

Here the conjugated forces and fluxes are $X_v = \Delta p$, $X_D = RT\Delta c_s$ and J_v and J_D respectively. The fluxes are determined by

$$J_v = J_w \bar{v}_w + J_s \bar{v}_s \tag{12}$$

and

$$J_D = \frac{J_s}{\bar{c}_s} - \frac{J_w}{c_w}. \tag{13}$$

J_v is the volume flow, representing the total volume flow per unit area of the membrane; J_D is the exchange flow, this being a measure of the relative flow of solute versus solvent.

For slow transport processes a linear correlation between the driving forces X_i and the resulting fluxes J_i may be assumed:

$$(J_1, J_2, \ldots J_n) = f(X_1, X_2, \ldots X_n)$$
$$J_1 = L_{11}X_1 + L_{12}X_2 \ldots L_{1n}X_n$$
$$J_2 = L_{21}X_1 + L_{22}X_2 \ldots L_{2n}X_n \qquad J_i = \sum_j L_{ij}X_j \tag{14}$$
$$\vdots$$
$$J_n = L_{n1}X_1 + L_{n2}X_2 \ldots L_{nn}X_n$$

These homogeneous linear relations are called phenomenologic equations (ONSAGER), L_{ii} and L_{ij} being the phenomenologic coefficients. The straight coefficients L_{ii} are proportionality factors, characterizing the straight processes, such as diffusion, heat conduction, electricity conduction etc. The cross-coefficients L_{ij} describe the linked processes, such as the exchange flow solute versus solvent, thermodiffusion etc.

On the basis of the principle of microscopic reversibility ONSAGER demonstrated the equality of the cross-coefficients $L_{ij} = L_{ji}$. The matrix of coefficients is symmetrical, i.e. the number of independent coefficients L_{ij} reduces from n^2 to $n(n-1)/2$.

Application of Equations (14) to the fluxes (12) and (13) and their conjugated forces gives

$$\varphi J_v = L_p \Delta p + L_{pD} RT \Delta c_s, \tag{15}$$
$$J_D = L_{Dp} \Delta p + L_D RT \Delta c_s. \tag{16}$$

As mentioned before, $L_{Dp} = L_{pD}$. The second law of thermodynamics requires that the entropy production be positive. Therefore the straight coefficients must be positive, while $L_{pD} = L_{Dp}$ can be either positive or negative, though restricted by the condition $L_p L_D - L_{pD}^2 > 0$.

Table 2. Permeant fluxes and the corresponding phenomenologic coefficients

Conditions	Notation of the flux	Notation of the coefficient
$\Delta c_s \neq 0$, $\Delta p = 0$	J_D = Membrane diffusion (osmosis)	L_D = Diffusion coefficient (coefficient of exchange flow)
	J_v = Osmosis (osmotic volume flow)	L_{pD} = Osmotic coefficient
$\Delta p \neq 0$, $\Delta c_s = 0$	J_v = Permeation (hydrostatic volume flow)	L_p = Mechanical permeability coefficient (hydraulic permeability, pressure filtration coefficient)
	J_D = Ultrafiltration	L_{Dp} = Ultrafiltration coefficient

2. Significance of the Phenomenologic Coefficients

From (15) and (16) it can be concluded that in coarse unselective porous membranes the volume and the exchange flow are indepedent of each other and depend only on their conjugated forces; J_v is determined by Δp, and J_D by $\Delta \pi = RT \Delta c_s$, the hydrostatic pressure and the osmotic pressure differ respectively ($L_{pD} = L_{Dp} = 0$). For membranes with restricted permeability, however, J_v and J_D are coupled. Therefore, in addition to its conjugated volume flow, a pressure gradient Δp produces an exchange flow solute versus solvent, even in the case of concentration equilibrium between the two phases ($\Delta c_s = 0$). If the membrane is more permeable to the solute than to the solvent, ultrafiltration occurs. The ultrafiltration coefficient L_{Dp} characterizes the relative movement of solute versus solvent. Conversely, a concentration gradient Δc_s does not only cause an exchange flow but also a volume flow, even if $\Delta p = 0$. The coupling of the fluxes is represented by the osmotic coefficient L_{pD}. Under these conditions the following fluxes and their coefficients may be summarized:

a) Ideal Semipermeable Membrane

If these considerations are extended to a membrane permeable to the solvent but not to the solute $(J_s = 0)$, the application of a pressure difference $\Delta p \neq 0$ at $\Delta c_s = 0$ produces an exchange flow of $J_D = -J_w/c_w$ and a volume flow of $J_v = J_w \bar{v}_w$ [cf. (12), (13)]. For diluted solutions $c_w = 1/\bar{v}_w$, so that the ideal semipermeable membrane is characterized by

$$J_D = -J_v . \tag{17}$$

In this case volume flow and exchange flow are of equal magnitude but of opposite direction; both are due solely to the solvent.

Introduction of (15) and (16) into (17) at a solute flow $J_s = 0$ gives

$$(L_p + L_{pD}) \Delta p + (L_D + L_{pD}) RT \Delta c_s = 0 . \tag{18}$$

As Δp and Δc_s are finite quantities, Equation (18) holds only if $(L_p + L_{pD}) = 0$ and $(L_D + L_{Dp}) = 0$, in which case

$$L_p = -L_{pD} = L_D. \tag{19}$$

Substance transport across an ideal semipermeable membrane can therefore be completely described by a single coefficient, the filtration coefficient L_p.

b) Coarse Porous Membrane

When hydrostatic pressure is applied to a coarse nonselective membrane ($\Delta c_s = 0$), solute and solvent are moved to the same extent; no exchange flow is produced, and $J_D = 0$. From this it follows that

$$J_D = 0; \quad L_{pD}\Delta p = 0; \quad L_{pD} = 0. \tag{20}$$

Analogously, at $\Delta c_s \neq 0$ and $\Delta p = 0$ the volume flow J_v becomes zero and the transport takes place as an exchange flow.

c) Reflection Coefficient

From (19) and (20) it follows that in dependence on the permeability of the membrane, L_{pD} may vary between $-L_p$ and 0, i.e. $L_{pD} \leq 0$. If the solute, however, penetrates more easily than the solvent, L_{pD} will become positive.

STAVERMAN [278] introduced the reflection coefficient σ to characterize the semipermeability of a membrane, which can be calculated from the phenomenologic coefficients:

$$\sigma = -\frac{L_{pD}}{L_p}. \tag{21}$$

For an ideal semipermeable membrane $L_p = -L_{pD}$, and therefore $\sigma = 1$; for a non-selective membrane ($L_{pD} = 0$), $\sigma = 0$. In the special case of anomalous osmosis $\sigma < 0$. Experiments on anomalous osmosis have been performed by LOEB [188, 189], GRIM et al. [96, 271], and OSTERHOUT and MURRAY [223]; SÖLLNER [272, 273] presented the first extended theoretical treatment, whereas the full calculation has been developed by KEDEM and KATCHALSKY [147].

σ can be determined by measurement of Δp for a definite Δc_s, thereby suppressing the volume flow ($J_v = 0$):

$$\Delta p = -\frac{L_{pD}}{L_p} RT\Delta c_s \quad (J_v = 0);$$
$$\sigma = \frac{\Delta p}{RT\Delta c_s} \quad (J_v = 0). \tag{22}$$

d) Permeability Coefficient

In permeability studies, in addition to the volume flow, J_v, the solute flow, J_s, is measured instead of the exchange flow, J_D. In the case of diluted solutions J_s is given by

$$J_s = (J_v + J_D) \, \bar{c}_s . \tag{23}$$

J_s is determined at constant volume ($J_v = 0$), and Δp results from Equation (22), Introduction of (15), (16), and (22) into (23) gives

$$J_s = \frac{L_p L_D - L_{pD}^2}{L_p} \, \bar{c}_s R T \Delta c_s = (L_D - \sigma^2 L_p) \, \bar{c}_s R T \Delta c_s \quad (J_v = 0) . \tag{24}$$

Under these conditions J_s is directly proportional to the concentration difference between the phases, Δc_s. The proportionality factor is $\omega R T$, where

$$\omega = \frac{L_p L_D - L_{pD}^2}{L_p} \, \bar{c}_s = (L_D - \sigma^2 L_p) \, \bar{c}_s . ^{[1]}$$

Equation (24) therefore can be transformed to

$$J_s = \omega R T \Delta c_s \quad (J_v = 0) . \tag{25}$$

Comparison of (25) and (2) reveals a formal correspondence between $\omega R T$ and the conventional permeability coefficient P. For ideal semipermeable membranes, $\omega = 0$. Introduction of σ and ω into the equation of volume flow (15) and exchange flow (23) gives

$$J_v = L_p (\Delta p - \sigma R T \Delta c_s) ; \tag{26}$$

$$J_s = \bar{c}_s L_p (1 - \sigma) \, \Delta p + [\omega - \bar{c}_s L_p (1 - \sigma) \, \sigma] \, R T \Delta c_s . \tag{27}$$

Connecting (26) and (27) gives

$$J_s = \omega R T \Delta c_s + (1 - \sigma) \, \bar{c}_s J_v . \tag{28}$$

The membrane transport is described by a maximum of three independent coefficients. For practical use, the three coefficients L_p, σ and ω are preferred. In special cases, however, the number of coefficients necessary for the complete description of the membrane permeability can be reduced. For example, water transport, commonly measured by addition of $D_2 0$, is described by only two coefficients, L_p and ω, because $\sigma \approx 0$. Finally, the ideal semipermeable membrane is characterized by a single coefficient, L_p, since $\sigma = 1$ and $\omega = 0$.

Methods of determining the coefficients L_p, σ, ω experimentally are reviewed in [51, 280].

---

[1] ω is the permeability coefficient of the solute flow.

3. Coupling of Fluxes

If several irreversible processes coincide within a system, the total entropy increase per unit time is given by the sum of the entropy production of all individual processes according to Equation (7). The fluxes can be either independent of each other or structurally and energetically coupled. We can confine our attention to two processes

$$\frac{d_i S}{dt} = J_A X_A + J_B X_B > 0 . \tag{29}$$

If processes A and B are independent of each other, $J_A X_A > 0$, and $J_B X_B > 0$ will be valid. In the case of coupling, however, $J_A X_A$ can be negative provided $J_B X_B > |J_A X_A|$, and vice versa. If $J_A X_A < 0$ the direction of the flux J_A will be opposite to that of its conjugated force X_A.

According to (14) the fluxes can be taken as functions of forces X_A and X_B

$$
\begin{aligned}
J_A &= L_A X_A + L_{AB} X_B ; \\
J_B &= L_{BA} X_A + L_B X_B .
\end{aligned}
\tag{30}
$$

The ONSAGER relation sets $L_{AB} = L_{BA}$. For thermodynamic reasons the straight coefficients, L_A and L_B, are positive, whereas L_{AB} can be either positive or negative with the restriction $L_{AB}^2 < L_A \cdot L_B$.

The dependence of the flux ratio $J_A/J_B = j$ on the forces ratio $X_A/X_B = x$ is given by

$$\frac{j}{Z} = \frac{\dfrac{L_{AB}}{\sqrt{L_A \cdot L_B}} + Zx}{1 + \dfrac{L_{AB}}{\sqrt{L_A \cdot L_B}} Zx} = \frac{q + Zx}{1 + qZx} \tag{31}$$

where $Z = \sqrt{L_A/L_B}$ and $q = L_{AB}/\sqrt{L_A L_B}$. The coupling factor q represents a measure of the degree of linkage between the two processes and is confined to

$$-1 \leqq q \leqq 1 .$$

In the case $q = 0, j/Z = Zx$, i.e. j has become a function of x and the fluxes J_A and J_B are determined exclusively by their conjugated forces; no coupling occurs.

For $q = 1$ or $q = -1$, $j/Z = \pm 1$, i.e. the flux ratio is now independent of the forces ratio, X_A/X_B; there is a complete linkage between both the processes. When $q = 1$ both fluxes are in the same direction (positive coupling), while when $q = -1$ they are inversely directed (negative coupling). Taking as driving forces X_i the gradients of the chemical potentials $\Delta\mu_A$ and $\Delta\mu_B$ [172], the flux equations can also be written in the following form

$$
\begin{aligned}
J_A &= L_A [(1 - q^2) \Delta\mu_A + (q/\sqrt{L_A \cdot L_B}) J_B] ; \\
J_B &= L_B [(1 - q^2) \Delta\mu_B + (q/\sqrt{L_A \cdot L_B}) J_A] .
\end{aligned}
\tag{32}
$$

4. Interpretation of Membrane Transport by Means of Frictional Coefficients

a) General Equations

The permeant fluxes across a membrane (J_i) are conjugated with driving forces (X_i). On steady flow the driving forces X_i are counter-balanced by a sum of mechanical frictional forces F_{ij}; thus the acting forces on one mole of the penetrating solute (s) and solvent (w), respectively, are given by

$$X_s = -F_{sw} - F_{sm} \tag{33}$$

and

$$X_w = -F_{ws} - F_{wm} . \tag{34}$$

F_{sw} stands for the frictional force between 1 mole of solute and the membrane water, F_{sm} for that between solute and membrane matrix, F_{ws} and F_{wm} are the corresponding forces acting on the penetrating solvent. For intensively swollen membranes F_{sw} approaches F_{sw}^0, the frictional force between solute and solvent in free diffusion.

The frictional force F_{ij} is assumed to be linearly proportional to the relative velocity of both components i and $j(v_i - v_j)$

$$F_{ij} = -f_{ij}(v_i - v_j) . \tag{35}$$

The proportionality factor f_{ij} is the frictional coefficient per mole of the permeant i with respect to j. If the membrane matrix is taken as reference system v_m will become zero and the frictional forces will be $F_{sm} = -f_{sm}(v_s - v_m) = -f_{sm}v_s$ and $F_{wm} = -f_{wm}$ $\cdot (v_w - v_m) = -f_{wm}v_w$. The frictional coefficients obey the reciprocity relation

$$C_i f_{ij} = C_j f_{ji} . \tag{36}$$

By introducing (35) and (36) into (33) and (34) we obtain the driving forces at point x of the membrane as functions of the frictional coefficients

$$X_s = -\frac{d\mu_s}{dx} = v_s(f_{sw} + f_{sm}) - v_w f_{sw} \tag{37}$$

and

$$X_w = -\frac{d\mu_w}{dx} = -v_s \frac{C_s f_{sw}}{C_w} + v_w \left(f_{wm} + \frac{C_s}{C_w} f_{sw} \right) . \tag{38}$$

The driving forces X of Equations (37) and (38) can be related to their fluxes $J_s = C_s v_s$ and $J_w = C_w v_w$

$$X_s = \frac{f_{sw} + f_{sm}}{C_s} J_s - \frac{f_{sw}}{C_w} J_w ; \tag{39}$$

$$X_w = -\frac{f_{sw}}{C_w} J_s + \frac{C_w f_{wm} + C_s f_{sw}}{(C_w)^2} J_w . \tag{40}$$

Equations (39) and (40) represent inverse phenomenologic equations

$$X_s = R_s J_s + R_{sw} J_w;$$
$$X_w = R_w J_w + R_{ws} J_s.$$

(41)

Their inverse coefficients are

$$R_s = \frac{f_{sw} + f_{sm}}{C_s}; \quad R_{sw} = -\frac{f_{sw}}{C_w}; \quad R_w = \frac{C_w f_{wm} + C_s f_{sw}}{(C_w)^2}.$$

(42)

These equations refer to a point x of the membrane. They have to be integrated across the membrane ($x = 0$ to $x = \Delta x$) before they are suitable for practical use. After integration several simplifications and some further relations lead to

$$\Delta \pi = \Delta x \frac{f_{sw} + f_{sm}}{K} J_s - \Delta x \bar{c}_s \frac{f_{sw} \bar{v}_w}{\varphi_w^m} J_w;$$

(43)

$$\Delta p - \Delta \pi = \Delta x \frac{f_{sw}}{\varphi_w^m} J_s + \Delta x \left(\frac{f_{wm}}{\varphi_w^m} + K \frac{\bar{c}_s f_{sw}}{(\varphi_w^m)^2} \right) J_w.$$

(44)

$\Delta \pi = RT \Delta c_s$ is the osmotic pressure difference between phase $'$ and phase $''$, where $\varphi_s \Delta p \ll \Delta \pi$ is assumed to be valid. φ_s is the volume fraction of the solute, which is assumed to be low. K is the distribution coefficient of the solute between membrane and phases at equilibrium conditions; it is assumed to be independent of concentration and to be of the same quantity throughout the membrane, i.e. the membrane is assumed to be homogeneous. φ_w^m symbolizes the mean volume fraction of water within the membrane, whose value is also assumed to be independent of concentration.

b) Connections Between Frictional and Phenomenologic Coefficients

From (43) and (44) the correlations between frictional and the phenomenologie coefficients, ω and σ, can be derived as follows. (*a*) According to (28) the solute flow at a zero volume flow is $(J_s)_{J_v = 0} = \omega RT \Delta c_s = \omega \Delta \pi$. Since the solute flow for $J_w = 0$ and $J_v = 0$ has approximately the same value, Equation (43) can be transformed to

$$\Delta \pi = \Delta x \frac{f_{sw} + f_{sm}}{K} J_s \quad (J_w = 0).$$

(45)

From this the permeability coefficient ω is obtained at

$$\omega = \frac{K}{\Delta x (f_{sw} + f_{sm})}.$$

(46)

(b) For $J_v = 0$ Equation (26) leads to

$$\sigma = \Delta p / \Delta \pi \quad (J_v = 0).$$

(47)

The coefficient $\sigma'(J_w = 0)$ must not be equated with $\sigma\ (J_v = 0)$; both the coefficients are connected by the following relation

$$\sigma = \sigma' - \frac{\omega \bar{v} s}{L_p}. \tag{48}$$

From (43) and (44) σ' is obtained for $J_w = 0$:

$$\sigma' = 1 - \frac{K f_{sw}}{\varphi_w^m (f_{sw} + f_{sm})}. \tag{49}$$

From (49), (48), and (46) it follows that

$$\sigma = 1 - \frac{\omega \bar{v}_s}{L_p} - \frac{K f_{sw}}{\varphi_w^m (f_{sw} + f_{sm})} = 1 - \frac{\omega \bar{v}_s}{L_p} - \frac{\omega \Delta x f_{sw}}{\varphi_w^m}. \tag{50}$$

Equivalent relations between L_p, σ, ω and the frictional coefficients have been derived by VAIDHYANATHAN and PERKINS from their knowledge of statistical mechanics [305].

c) *Physical Significance of the Coefficients*

Equations (46) and (50) allow various conclusions:

The permeability coefficient ω becomes a constant characterizing the mobility of the solute within the membrane, provided K and the frictional coefficients are independent of the concentration.

a) In the case of lipid membrane and lipid-soluble solutes $f_{sm} \gg f_{sw}$; furthermore f_{sm} and K are relatively high. Increase of f_{sm} decreases ω, while increase of K raises ω. Generally the influence of K surmounts that of f_{sm}. Therefore the penetration rate of a solute increases with increasing lipid solubility in spite of the high f_{sm} values.

b) For a coarse nonselective membrane $f_{sw} > f_{sm}$, f_{sw} approximating the limiting value f_{sw}^0, the frictional coefficient between solute and solvent in free diffusion.

c) For porous membranes of medium permeability, f_{sm} increases, i.e. ω decreases. In regard to large solute molecules that are insoluble in the membrane material, f_{sm} approximates ∞ and therefore $\omega \to 0$ (ideal semipermeable membrane). If the solute is able to penetrate the membrane only via water-filled pores the solute concentration within the pores will equal that of the outer phases. The mean solute concentration within the pores is given by $\bar{C}_s = \bar{c}_s \cdot \varphi_w^m$. The distribution coefficient K amounts to $K = \bar{C}_s/\bar{c}_s = \varphi_w^m$, i.e. the distribution coefficient of the solute is identical with the distribution coefficient of the solvent or with the volume fraction of the solvent within the membrane. If the solute transport takes place exclusively via pores, Equation (46) can therefore be transformed to

$$\omega = \frac{\varphi_w^m}{\Delta x (f_{sw} + f_{sm})}. \tag{51}$$

In solute transport across a porous membrane, the membrane matrix may be assumed to be traversed by a tortuous and branched capillary system. The deviation from a straightchannel system normal to the membrane surface is accounted for by the tortuosity factor $\vartheta(\vartheta \leq 1)$. The mean length of the capillaries is given by $\Delta x/\vartheta$. According to MACKEY and MEARES [190] the effective frictional coefficient solute/water within the membrane is given by f_{sw}^0/ϑ. The solute flow across such a membrane is expressed by

$$J_s = \frac{\vartheta \varphi_w^m RT}{f_{sw}^0} \frac{\Delta c_s}{\Delta x} = \vartheta \varphi_w^m D^0 \frac{\Delta c_s}{\Delta x}. \tag{52}$$

$D^0 = RT/f_{sw}^0$ is the diffusion coefficient of free diffusion. In a few limiting cases the reflection coefficient σ shows the following values [cf. (50)]:

(a) In an ideal semipermeable membrane no solute penetrates, therefore $\omega = 0$ and $\sigma = 1$.

(b) For coarse nonselective porous membranes it holds that $\omega \bar{v}_s/L_p + \omega \Delta x f_{sw}/\varphi_w^m = 1$, and therefore $\sigma = 0$.

(c) In the case of lipid membranes and lipid-soluble solutes the values of ω are high and therefore those of σ are low. If the quotient $K/\varphi_w^m \gg 1$, σ will be negative. According to (22) there is $(\Delta p)_{J_v=0} = \sigma \Delta \pi$; i.e. for $\sigma < 0$, $\Delta p < 0$, too (anomalous osmosis, cf. p. 24, 25).

(d) If solute and solvent cross the membrane via separated routes $f_{sw} = 0$ and furthermore $\sigma = 1 - \omega \bar{v}_s/L_p$. This type of transport can therefore be described by only two coefficients. This is so, for example, if the solute is transported exclusively across the lipid phase of a combined lipid-porous membrane, whereas the solvent transport occurs only via the water-filled pores. In general the following is true: low values of f_{sw} indicate a separated solute and water transport, high values of f_{sw} are typical of a tight linkage of both the fluxes.

D. Passive Transport of Electrolytes Across Charged Membranes

1. General Relations

The ion transport across a membrane containing charged groups requires several extensions of the transport equations. There are several useful models to describe the peculiarities of electrolyte transport [105, 199, 200, 201, 287–290]. Let the net charge density of the fixed-charge groups within the membrane be X mole per unit volume, the concentration of counter-ions be C_1, that of the coions C_2. Electroneutrality at any point x of the membrane requires that

$$C_1 = X + C_2. \tag{53}$$

The total concentration of counter-ions is given by the sum of counter-ions provided by the membrane itself (concentration X) and those provided by the salt s in the membrane (concentration $C_2 = C_s$). Thus

$$C_1 = X + C_s. \tag{54}$$

For highly charged membranes $X \gg C_s$ and $C_1 \approx X$.

In the case of a salt dissociating into monovalent cations and monovalent anions, the mass flow is composed of the fluxes of the negative and the positive ions, J_1 and J_2 and also of the solvent flow, J_w. Their corresponding conjugated forces are represented by both the gradients of the electrochemical potentials, $-d\tilde{\mu}_1/dx$ and $-d\tilde{\mu}_2/dx$, and by the gradient of the chemical potential of water, $-d\mu_w/dx$. The dissipation function ψ can by written as

$$\psi = J_1\left(-\frac{d\tilde{\mu}_1}{dx}\right) + J_2\left(-\frac{d\tilde{\mu}_2}{dx}\right) + J_w\left(-\frac{d\mu_w}{dx}\right). \tag{55}$$

The phenomenologic equations require 6 independent coefficients to characterize the transport of electrolytes across a charged membrane.

A simplification is obtained if no electrical current flows across the membrane $(I = 0)$. Thus

$$J_1 = J_2 = J_s, \tag{56}$$

J_s being the flux of the neutral salt. Further simplification results from

$$\mu_s = \tilde{\mu}_1 + \tilde{\mu}_2 \quad \text{and} \quad -\frac{d\mu_s}{dx} = -\frac{d\tilde{\mu}_1}{dx} - \frac{d\tilde{\mu}_2}{dx}. \tag{57}$$

According to (56) and (57) the dissipation function (55) may be reduced to only two fluxes, the solute and the water flow

$$\psi = J_s\left(-\frac{d\mu_s}{dx}\right) + J_w\left(-\frac{d\mu_w}{dx}\right). \tag{58}$$

Therefore, the membrane transport of electrolyte solutions may be represented in the same way as that of nonelectrolytes, by the three coefficients L_p, ω and σ. It may be mentioned that in the case of electrolyte transport the mechanical permeability coefficient L_p is measured at zero electrical current, $I = 0$, whereas in the case of nonelectrolytes at zero electrical potential $\varphi = 0$.

2. Introduction of Frictional Coefficients

The transformation of the thermodynamic flux coefficients into frictional coefficients may be performed analogously to the procedure for nonelectrolytes. The driving forces X are again assumed to be counterbalanced by frictional forces

$$X_1 = -\frac{d\tilde{\mu}_1}{dx} = -F_{1w} - F_{1m} = f_{1w}(v_1 - v_w) + f_{1m}(v_1 - v_m). \tag{59}$$

Again $v_m = 0$ (the membrane being the reference system), and with respect to X_1 and X_2

$$X_1 = -\frac{d\tilde{\mu}_1}{dx} = \frac{f_{1w} + f_{1m}}{C_1} J_1 - \frac{f_{1w}}{C_w} J_w \, ;$$

$$X_2 = -\frac{d\tilde{\mu}_2}{dx} = \frac{f_{2w} + f_{2m}}{C_2} J_2 - \frac{f_{2w}}{C_w} J_w \, .$$

(60)

C_1, C_2, C_w are the respective concentrations of ion 1, ion 2, and water. In (60) the frictional force between ion 1 and ion 2 and therefore the coefficient f_{12} have been neglected since within a charged membrane the concentration of coions is small.

The thermodynamic driving force of the solute flow is given by

$$-\frac{d\tilde{\mu}_1}{dx} = \frac{d\tilde{\mu}_2}{dx} = -\frac{d\mu_s}{dx} = \left(\frac{f_{1w} + f_{1m}}{C_1} + \frac{f_{2w} + f_{2m}}{C_2} \right) J_s - \frac{f_{1w} + f_{2w}}{C_w} J_w \, .$$

(61)

Taking into consideration the Onsager reciprocity relation $f_{w1} = f_{1w} C_1 / C_w$ and $f_{w2} = f_{2w} C_2 / C_w$, the respective force of the water flow amounts to

$$-\frac{d\mu_w}{dx} = -\frac{f_{1w} + f_{2w}}{C_w} J_s + \left(\frac{C_1 f_{1w} + C_2 f_{2w}}{C_w} + f_{wm} \right) \frac{J_w}{C_w} \, .$$

(62)

In view of equation (54), Equations (61) and (62) can be reduced for $J_w = 0$ to

$$-C_s \frac{d\mu_s}{dx} = \left[(f_{2w} + f_{2m}) + \frac{C_s}{C_s + X} (f_{1w} + f_{1m}) \right] J_s \quad (J_w = 0) \, ;$$

(63)

$$-C_w \frac{d\mu_w}{dx} = -(f_{1w} + f_{2w}) J_s \quad (J_w = 0) \, .$$

(64)

In the case of $X = 0$ (uncharged membrane), Equations (63) and (64) correspond to (40) concerning the transport of nonelectrolytes if we set $(f_{1w} + f_{2w}) = f_{sw}$ and $(f_{1m} + f_{2m}) = f_{sm}$, i.e. the transport of electrolytes across uncharged membranes occurs analogously so that of nonelectrolytes.

The other limiting case is when $X \gg C_s$ and $C_1 \approx X$, i.e. in highly charged membranes. In this case the quotient $C_s / (C_s + X)$ of Equation (63) becomes very small, and, providing $(f_{2w} + f_{2m})$ and $(f_{1w} + f_{1m})$ are of the same magnitude, Equation (63) reduces to

$$-C_s \frac{d\mu_s}{dx} = (f_{2w} + f_{2m}) J_s \quad (J_w = 0) \, .$$

(65)

3. Permeability and Reflection Coefficients of 1 – 1-Valent Salts

In electrolyte transport the equations valid for a point x of the membrane have to be integrated in a similar way to those for nonelectrolyte transport. Assuming several simplifications the following expressions are obtained at $J_w = 0$:

$$\Delta \pi_s = \frac{J_s \Delta x}{K} (f_{2w} + f_{2m}) \qquad (J_w = 0). \tag{66}$$

$$\Delta p - \Delta \pi_s = -\frac{J_s \Delta x}{\varphi_w^m} (f_{1w} + f_{2w}) \qquad (J_w = 0). \tag{67}$$

$\Delta \pi_s$ denotes the gradient of osmotic pressure of the salt across the membrane, and K again represents the mean distribution coefficient of the salt between the membrane and the aqueous phases, while φ_w^m represents the volume fraction of water within the membrane. The permeability coefficient may be derived from Equation (66):

$$\omega \approx \omega' = \left(\frac{J_s}{\Delta \pi_s} \right)_{J_w = 0} = \frac{K}{\Delta x (f_{2w} + f_{2m})}. \tag{68}$$

According to (68) the electrolyte transport across a highly charged membrane is determined exclusively by the friction of the coions, whose concentration is low, while the counter-ions do not contribute to the friction although their concentration within the membrane is relatively high. The distribution coefficient K of non-electrolytes is approximately independent of the solute concentration. In the case of electrolytes, however, K is directly proportional to the average salt concentration in the external solutions. Therefore ω is also a function of the salt concentration, increasing as c_s increases.

The reflection coefficient σ is obtained according to Equations (47) and (48) at $J_w = 0$:

$$\sigma' = 1 - \frac{K}{\varphi_w^m} \frac{f_{1w} + f_{2w}}{f_{2w} + f_{2m}} \qquad (J_w = 0); \tag{69}$$

$$\sigma = \sigma' - \frac{\omega \bar{v}_s}{L_p} = 1 - \frac{\omega \bar{v}_s}{L_p} - \frac{K}{\varphi_w^m} \frac{f_{1w} + f_{2w}}{f_{2w} + f_{2m}} \qquad (J_w = 0). \tag{70}$$

Since σ is linearly correlated to ω, the reflection coefficient σ also changes with the salt concentration. With increasing c_s, σ decreases and may even shift to negative values (anomalous osmosis).

Considering the ion transport across membranes of high lipid content, the values of ω are relatively low and can be ignored, i.e. $\sigma \rightarrow 1$. This behaviour is common in biological membranes.

4. Permeability and Reflection Coefficients of 1 – 2- and 2 – 1-Valent Salts

For highly charged membranes characterized by $X \gg C_s$, analogous transport equations can be derived with respect to electrolytes composed of monovalent counter-ions and bivalent coions (1 – 2-valent salt) or such of bivalent counter-ions and monovalent coions (2 – 1-valent salt). The relations obtained for ω and σ and also the concentration dependence of K are summarized in Table 3. Electro-

Table 3. Permeability characteristics of highly charged membranes against different electrolytes

Parameter	Monovalent counter-ion monovalent coion	Monovalent counter-ion bivalent coion	Bivalent counter-ion monovalent coion
Chemical potential of the salt, $d\mu_s =$	$d\tilde{\mu}_1 + d\tilde{\mu}_2$	$2d\tilde{\mu}_1 + d\tilde{\mu}_2$	$d\tilde{\mu}_1 + 2d\tilde{\mu}_2$
Permeability coefficient, $\omega =$	$\dfrac{K}{\Delta x(f_{2w} + f_{2m})}$	$\dfrac{K}{\Delta x(f_{2w} + f_{2m})}$	$\dfrac{K}{2\Delta x(f_{2w} + f_{2m})}$
Reflection coefficient on $J_w = 0$, $\sigma' =$	$1 - \dfrac{K}{\varphi_w^m} \dfrac{f_{1w} + f_{2w}}{f_{2w} + f_{2m}}$	$1 - \dfrac{K}{\varphi_w^m} \dfrac{2f_{1w} + f_{2w}}{f_{2w} + f_{2m}}$	$1 - \dfrac{K}{\varphi_w^m} \dfrac{1/2 f_{1w} + f_{2w}}{f_{2w} + f_{2m}}$
Dependence of K on the outside salt-concentration[a]	$\dfrac{K}{\varphi_w^m} = \left(\dfrac{c_s}{X'}\right)$	$\dfrac{K}{\varphi_w^m} = \left(\dfrac{2c_s}{X'}\right)^2$	$\dfrac{K}{\varphi_w^m} = \left(\dfrac{2c_s}{X'}\right)^{1/2}$

[a] $X' = X/\varphi_w^m =$ charge density per unit volume of the aqueous solution within the membranes pores and capillaries respectively.

neutrality, zero electrical current, and ideal Donnan distribution are presupposed conditions.

The influence of the salt concentration on the distribution coefficient K and thereby on ω and σ is especially instructive. In the case of a salt containing monovalent counter-ions and bivalent coions, K increases with the square of salt concentration, i.e. the reflection coefficient of the membrane increases by bivalent coions. On the other hand, bivalent counter-ions diminish the reflection coefficient with the square root of the salt concentration. Thus a divalent coion increases and a divalent counter-ion diminishes the selectivity of the membrane in comparison to the respective monovalent ions of a $1 - 1$ salt.

E. Passive Carrier Transport

Kinetic Analysis and Flux Equations

a) Basic Equations

Kinetic derivations concerning carrier transport have repeatedly been discussed and extended [25, 128, 129, 176, 180, 245, 252, 312, 319, 324, 325]. In general they are based on the model of Figure 8.

If a complex is formed between the carrier C and the permeant A according to $A + C \rightleftharpoons AC$, the transport rate ($v$) is dependent on the concentration difference of AC across the membrane

$$v = \frac{dN}{dt} = P \cdot F(c'_{AC} - c''_{AC}). \tag{71}$$

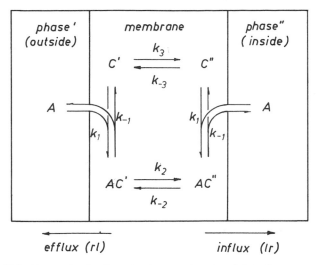

Fig. 8. Scheme of kinetic constants of carrier transport system (cf. text)

P is the conventional permeability coefficient, F the penetration area, c'_{AC} and c''_{AC} the concentrations of the carrier on the membrane surface facing phase' and phase" respectively. The movement of AC across the membrane can be viewed as a diffusion process. Since $J = v/F$ and $P \equiv k_{AC}$, the net flow is given by

$$J = k_{AC}(c'_{AC} - c''_{AC}).$$
(72)

k_{AC} represents the velocity constant of the AC transport.

Analysis of the kinetics of carrier transport involves both the complex formation and the corresponding complex dissociation reaction of AC on both sides of the membrane as well as the diffusion rates of the free carrier C and of the permeant carrier complex AC. The rate of the two diffusion processes is thought to limit the rate of the carrier transport. Furthermore, it is assumed that the membrane is symmetrical, that $k_2 = k_{-2}$ and that $k_3 = k_{-3}$. C and AC are not able to leave the membrane, and formation and dissociation of AC can only occur on the membrane surface facing phase' and phase" respectively. The diffusion rate of free solute within the membrane is assumed to be negligibly low. The ratio between the diffusion rate constants of AC and C may be

$$r = \frac{k_2}{k_3} = \frac{k_{-2}}{k_{-3}}.$$
(73)

The total carrier concentration within the membrane per unit area amounts to

$$C_{\text{tot}} = \frac{1}{2}(c'_C + c''_C + c'_{AC} + c''_{AC}).$$
(74)

The dissociation constant of AC is given by

$$K_{AC} = \frac{k_{-1}}{k_1} = \frac{c'_A \cdot c'_C}{c'_{AC}} = \frac{c''_A \cdot c''_C}{c''_{AC}}. \tag{75}$$

Assuming left-right (lr) and right-left (rl) transport of equal amounts of C_{tot} at steady-state conditions, it follows that

$$k_3 c'_C + k_2 c'_{AC} = k_{-3} c''_C + k_{-2} c''_{AC}; \tag{76}$$

$$c'_C + r \cdot c'_{AC} = c''_C + r \cdot c''_{AC}. \tag{77}$$

From (74), (75), and (76) the quantities c'_C, c''_C, c'_{AC}, and c''_{AC} are obtained:

$$c'_C = \frac{2 C_{tot} \cdot K_{AC}(K_{AC} + r c''_A)}{(K_{AC} + r c'_A)(K_{AC} + c''_A) + (K_{AC} + r c''_A)(K_{AC} + c'_A)}; \tag{78}$$

$$c'_{AC} = \frac{2 C_{tot} \cdot c'_A(K_{AC} + r c''_A)}{(K_{AC} + r c'_A)(K_{AC} + c''_A) + (K_{AC} + r c''_A)(K_{AC} + c'_A)}. \tag{79}$$

Analogous expressions for c''_C and c''_{AC} can be formulated by interchange of the labels $'$ and $''$.

For the influx (J_{lr}) and efflux (J_{rl}) of the permeant, the following equations are obtained

$$J_{lr} = k_2 c'_{AC} = \frac{2 \cdot k_2 \cdot C_{tot} \cdot c'_A(K_{AC} + r c''_A)}{(K_{AC} + r c'_A)(K_{AC} + c''_A) + (K_{AC} + r c''_A)(K_{AC} + c'_A)};$$

$$J_{rl} = k_{-2} c''_{AC} = \frac{2 \cdot k_{-2} \cdot C_{tot} \cdot c''_A(K_{AC} + r c'_A)}{(K_{AC} + r c''_A)(K_{AC} + c'_A) + (K_{AC} + r c'_A)(K_{AC} + c''_A)}. \tag{80}$$

If $r \neq 1$, J_{lr} is directly proportional to c'_A and also a function of c''_A. Conversely J_{rl} is directly proportional to c''_A and is a function of c'_A. The unidirectional fluxes are therefore not only determined by the concentration of the permeant in the phase of higher concentration (cis phase) but also by that in the trans phase.

Given $r = 1$, the flux equations reduce to

$$J_{lr} = \frac{k_2 \cdot C_{tot} \cdot c'_A}{(K_{AC} + c'_A)}; \quad J_{rl} = \frac{k_{-2} \cdot C_{tot} \cdot c''_A}{(K_{AC} + c''_A)} \quad (r = 1). \tag{81}$$

Thus the fluxes are determined only by the concentration in the cis phase. With respect to the net flux $J = J_{lr} - J_{rl}$, (assuming $k_2 = k_{-2} \equiv k_{AC}$),

$$\begin{aligned} J &= \frac{k_2 \cdot C_{tot} \cdot c'_A}{(K_{AC} + c'_A)} - \frac{k_{-2} \cdot C_{tot} \cdot c''_A}{(K_{AC} + c''_A)} \\ &= k_{AC} \cdot C_{tot} \left(\frac{c'_A}{K_{AC} + c'_A} - \frac{c''_A}{K_{AC} + c''_A} \right) \\ &= J_{max} \left(\frac{c'_A}{K_{AC} + c'_A} - \frac{c''_A}{K_{AC} + c''_A} \right) \end{aligned} \tag{82}$$

is obtained. J therefore depends on a capacity term $J_{max} = k_{AC} \cdot C_{tot}$ and on a saturation term $c'_A/(K_{AC}+c'_A) - c''_A/(K_{AC}+c''_A)$. $y' = c'_A/(K_{AC}+c'_A)$ represents the degree of saturation of the carrier at the phase '-membrane interphase, y'' that at the membrane-phase " interphase. If $c_A \gg K_{AC}$ and $c_A = 0$, $y' = 1$ and $y'' = 0$. In this case J reaches its maximum J_{max}; i.e. a further rise in c'_A does not increase the transport rate of A.

b) Limiting Cases

(a) For $r = 1$ and $y'' \approx 0$, transport kinetics corresponds to enzyme kinetics. This case is given during the initial period of the transport process, i.e. c'_A being relatively high and c''_A being small or even zero. It is also valid in the case of permeant consumption of A in phase ", e.g. of chemical conversion. Under these condition the total flux is almost identical with the unidirectional lr flux:

$$J = J_{max} \frac{c'_A}{K_{AC}+c'_A} \qquad (c''_A \to 0) . \tag{83}$$

Equation (83), containing the parameters J, J_{max}, K_{AC}, c'_A, corresponds to the well-known Michaelis-Menten equation of enzyme kinetics with the parameters v, v_{max}, K_m, and S. Therefore J_{max} and K_{AC} can be obtained by means of a Lineweaver-Burk plot.

(b) When $c'_A, c''_A \ll K_{AC}$ they can be derived from (82)

$$J = \frac{J_{max}}{K_{AC}} (c'_A - c''_A) \qquad (c'_A, c''_A \ll K_{AC}) . \tag{84}$$

At low concentrations of A, J becomes directly proportional to $c'_A - c''_A = \Delta c_A$ such as in the case of simple diffusion (when Fick's law is obeyed). Therefore transport by carrier mechanism and by diffusion are indistinguishable under these conditions (D kinetics according to WILBRANDT and ROSENBERG [325]). The differentiation between these two transport mechanisms is only possible at higher permeant concentrations. It should be noted at low concentrations of A the transport is inversely proportional to the dissociation constant K_{AC}.

(c) For $c'_A, c''_A \gg K_{AC}$, Equation (82) leads to

$$J = J_{max} \cdot \frac{K_{AC}(c'_A - c''_A)}{(K_{AC}+c'_A)(K_{AC}+c''_A)} = J_{max} \cdot K_{AC} \left(\frac{1}{c''_A} - \frac{1}{c'_A} \right) \qquad (c'_A, c''_A \gg K_{AC}) . \tag{85}$$

In this case the transport is directly proportional to K_{AC} and depends further on the difference of the reciprocals of the permeant concentrations. This type of transport kinetics is called E kinetics.

c) Counter-Transport and Competitive Exchange Diffusion

If a substance B competes with the solute A for the same carrier, each of the two permeants inhibit membrane transport of the other, with negative coupling of both fluxes. The distribution of A and B to the carrier C on the membrane interface is inversely proportional to the dissociation constants of AC and BC, and is directly proportional to the concentrations of A and B in the corresponding phases

$$\frac{c'_{AC}}{c'_{BC}} = \frac{c'_A \cdot K_{BC}}{c'_B \cdot K_{AC}} \quad \text{and} \quad \frac{c''_{AC}}{c''_{BC}} = \frac{c''_A \cdot K_{BC}}{c''_B \cdot K_{AC}}. \tag{86}$$

For definite values of c'_A and K_{AC} the concentration of the AC complex decreases if c'_B and the affinity of B for C increase. After equilibration of the system with respect to $A(c'_A = c''_A$ and $c'_{AC} = c''_{AC})$, addition of B into phase" produces an AC gradient across the membrane which drives an AC flux from interphase " to interphase ' and thereby a transport of A against the gradient of its chemical potential (counter-transport, incongruent transport).

In the case of $c''_A = c''_B = 0$, the transport of permeant A in the presence of B is described by

$$J_A = J_{max} \left(\frac{c'_A}{c'_A + K_{AC} + \dfrac{c'_B \cdot K_{AC}}{K_{BC}}} \right) \quad (c''_A = c''_B = 0). \tag{87}$$

This expression is valid for $(J_A)_{max} = (J_B)_{max} = J_{max}$. Assuming $c'_B = 0$, (83) is obtained, this equation describing the sole unidirectional flux of A. Comparison of (83) with (87) reveals the influence of c'_B and K_{BC} on A transport.

For $c'_A = c''_A = c_A$ and $c'_B \neq c''_B$ it follows that

$$J_A = J_{max} \frac{C_A(C''_B - C'_B)}{(C'_B + C_A + 1)(C''_B + C_A + 1)} \quad (c'_A = c''_A = c_A), \tag{88}$$

where $C_A = c_A/K_{AC}$ and $C'_B = c'_B/K_{BC}$ and $C''_B = c''_B/K_{BC}$. According to (88) counter-transport of A across the membrane occurs up to the point where $c'_B = c''_B$. The system is equilibrated if

$$\frac{c'_A}{c''_A} = \frac{(c'_B/K_{BC}) + 1}{(c''_B/K_{BC}) + 1}. \tag{89}$$

Equation (89) demonstrates that a greater accumulation of A against its concentration gradient is only possible if $c'_B/K_{BC} > 1$, i.e. the carrier operating close to the saturation limit. At complete saturation the coupling parameter q of both the fluxes J_A and J_B equals 1. The mechanism of the carrier transport with the principle of flux coupling is a guide to the understanding and the description of the phenomenon of competitive exchange diffusion (BRITTON [24, 109, 114, 167]). The efflux of glucose from erythrocytes e.g. can be accelerated by the addition of several sugars to the outer phase. They interact with the glucose carrier and therefore they competitively inhibit the reinflux of the glucose from the external solution (LACKO and BURGER [165]).

The concept of counter-transport and competitive exchange diffusion requires a physical separation of the influxes and the effluxes within the membrane, AC, BC, and C not being allowed to interact. This is only possible either (a) if the carrier is freely movable within the membrane or (b) if the membrane contains separated pores or channels for influx and efflux. Hypothesis (b) has been excluded by several authors [20, 166, 319]. If hypothesis (b) is correct, the addition of an inhibitor which is unable to penetrate the membrane to the outer phase would inhibit the influx more intensively than the efflux. In fact, however, both fluxes are inhibited to the same extent.

When $r > 1$, i.e. the free crrrier penetrates at a lower rate than the permeant-carrier complex, the unidirectional flux of a permeant can be increased by increasing the permeant concentration in the trans phase, the net flux, however, being relatively reduced. If glucose-equilibrated erythrocytes, in which some of the glucose is labeled, are added to a glucose-free salt medium, an efflux of the sugar takes place, which is easily measured by the occurrence of radioactivity in the medium. When unlabeled glucose is added to the external medium the efflux of radioactivity is increased. This effect is due to the accelerated membrane passage of the carrier loaded on the outside of the erythrocyte membrane with unlabeled glucose [114, 185, 194, 203]. In the limiting case $r = \infty$ only the loaded carrier penetrates the membrane and the unidirectional fluxes are given by ($k_2 = k_{-2}$, c'_A, $c''_A \neq 0$)

$$J_{lr} = J_{rl} = \frac{k_2 C_{tot} \cdot c'_A \cdot c''_A}{K_{AC}(c'_A + c''_A) + c'_A c''_A} \qquad (r = \infty). \tag{90}$$

The fluxes are of equal magnitude but of inverse direction. The net flux becomes zero, $J = J_{lr} - J_{rl} = 0$, i.e. equal amounts of the permeant are exchanged between phase ' and phase " (exchange diffusion according to USSING [299, 300]). It can easily be measured if a trace of labeled permeant is added to one phase of an equilibrated system ($c'_A = c''_A$). Exchange diffusion can furthermore be differentiated into the compulsory form ($r = \infty$) and the accelerative exchange diffusion ($\infty \gg r > 1$) [144, 185, 194, 204].

The phenomenologic treatment of the carrier transport follows that of simple diffusion. As is shown by the kinetics, the accelerated membrane passage of a solute A can be described as diffusion of the permeant-carrier complex AC. Therefore the solute flow J_A becomes an AC-specific flux, J_{AC}, the permeability coefficient of which, ω_{AC}, is greater than the A-specific quantity ω_A. If the driving force of $J_A = J_{AC}$ is expressed in terms of A concentrations, instead of $\Delta c_A = c'_A - c''_A$ in simple diffusion of A [cf. (25)], the more complex saturation term of (82) is valid. Apart from simple diffusion $J_A = J_{AC}$ is limited by C_{tot} within the capacity term of (82). Concerning the phenomenologic treatment of coupled fluxes J_A and J_B (as is specific with the carrier transport) cf. IV.C.3. and IV.E.1.c.

F. Active Transport

1. Kinetic Analysis and Conventional Flux Equations

Based on the kinetics and the equilibrium relations of passive carrier transport, modified equations have been developed for active transport. If the dissociation constant of the permeant-carrier complex is assumed to be different on the two sides of the membrane ($K'_{AC} \neq K''_{AC}$), Equation (82) becomes

$$J = J_{\max}\left(\frac{c'_A}{c'_A + K'_{AC}} - \frac{c''_A}{c''_A + K''_{AC}}\right). \tag{91}$$

If $K''_{AC} \gg K'_{AC}$, the permeant A is transported into phase $''$ and enriched there until a steady state is obtained, for which

$$c'_A/c''_A = K'_{AC}/K''_{AC} \quad (J = 0), \tag{92}$$

i.e. the distribution ratio of A is given by the ratio of the respective dissociation constants.

The dissociation constant of the permeant-carrier complex, however, is only altered by some additional reaction (or reactions) on one or the other side of the membrane, which changes (or change) the structure and conformation of the complex respectively. Contributions in this field come from ROSENBERG and WILBRANDT [252], CHRISTENSEN [39], SKOU [269, 270], and MITCHELL [206]. Accordingly we can assume that the carrier C reacts on the inside of the membrane enzymatically catalyzed with $X \sim P$, thereby being converted in an exergonic reaction (cleavage of the high energy bond $X \sim P$) into CX. Furthermore, the affinity of CX for A may be strongly decreased compared with the X affinity. As a result, A is released from the AC complex to enter phase $''$ inside the membrane. Now CX after diffusion from the inside to the outside of the membrane splits into C and X, which again takes place exergonically. Because of C having the higher affinity towards A (compared with CX), it reacts with the permeant to built up the complex AC, which again diffuses across the membrane to the inside border (Fig. 9).

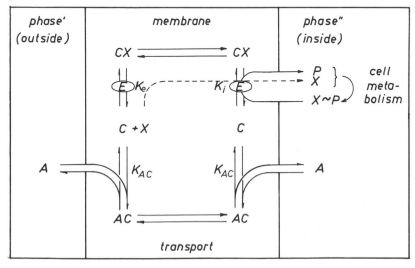

Fig. 9. Modified carrier scheme for active transport (cf. text)

Besides the equilibrium equations

$$K_{AC} = \frac{c'_A \cdot c'_C}{c'_{AC}} = \frac{c''_A \cdot c''_C}{c''_{AC}} \tag{93}$$

two further ones have to be taken into account

$$K_i = \frac{c''_{CX} \cdot c''_P}{c''_C \cdot c''_{X \sim P}} \quad \text{and} \quad K_e = \frac{c'_{CX}}{c'_C \cdot c'_X}. \tag{94}$$

These equations represent the competing reactions for the free carrier C on both sides of the membrane. The degrees of AC-complex formation at the border of the membrane with the respective phases, y' and y'', are given by

$$y' = \frac{c'_{AC}}{c'_{AC} + c'_C + c'_{CX}} = \frac{c'_A}{c'_A + K_{AC}(1 + K_e \cdot c'_X)} = \frac{c'_A}{c'_A + K_{AC}(1 + K_y)} \tag{95}$$

and

$$y'' = \frac{c''_{AC}}{c''_{AC} + c''_C + c''_{CX}} = \frac{c''_A}{c''_A + K_{AC}\left(1 + \dfrac{K_i \cdot c_{X \sim P}}{c_P}\right)} = \frac{c''_A}{c''_A + K_{AC}(1 + K_x)} \tag{96}$$

where $K_y = K_e \cdot c'_X$ and $K_x = K_i \cdot c''_{X \sim P}/c''_P$ can be assumed to be constants if by a permeant metabolic process both the formation rate of the $X \sim P$ compound and the dissociation rate of $X \sim P \rightarrow X + P$ are constant.

The net flux of permeant A then follows with

$$J = J_{max}(y' - y'') = J_{max}\left[\frac{c'_A}{c'_A + K_{AC}(1 + K_y)} - \frac{c''_A}{c''_A + K_{AC}(1 + K_x)}\right]. \tag{97}$$

This equation is the same as Equation (91) provided $K'_{AC} = K_{AC}(1 + K_y)$ and $K''_{AC} = K_A(1 + K_x)$.

2. Phenomenologic Treatment. Flux Equations

Being coupled to a chemical reaction, besides the solute and solvent fluxes, the flux equation of substance i transport also has to take account of the reaction

$$J_i = L_{ii}X_i + \sum_{\substack{j=0 \\ j \neq i}}^{n} L_{ij}X_j + L_{ir}X_r \tag{98}$$

where X_r represents the affinity of the chemical reaction, and $X_r = \sum_k v_k \mu_k$ according to DE DONDER [56]. The μ_k are the chemical potentials of the reactants k, v_k being their stoichiometric coefficients. With the reaction products, v_k is positive, whereas it is negative with the reacting species. The coefficient L_{ir} is a measure of coupling between the flux of component i and the driving force X_r of the chemical reaction.

Chemical reactions are generally unidirected with respect to the spatial coordinates. Therefore X_r is a scalar. On the other hand, the transmembranal flux J_i is a vectorial quantity. According to the Curie theorem [45], coupling between tensorial quantities of different degrees is not possible. However, because of the active transport underlying carrier mechanisms, and because the complex formation and dissociation reaction between permeant and carrier are locally separated, the restriction of the Curie theorem can be omitted with respect of the spatial directed overall reaction (JARDETZKY [131]). Similarly the concept of the acting enzymes in the carrier transport as anisotropic, as proposed by MITCHELL [203], may serve to interpret the invalidity of the Curie theorem in the chemo-osmotic coupling [1, 131, 139, 210]. Consequently the coefficient L_{ir} of Equation (98) then has the character of a vectorial operator.

The flux of the chemical reaction J_r can be obtained from the consumption of reactants, e.g. from that of metabolic substrates like glucose or O_2 in an aerobic reaction. J_r, the molar substrate conversion per cm^2 membrane area and unit time, and J_i, the flux of permeant i, are then determined by

$$J_r = \frac{-1}{R_{rr}}\left(\varDelta F + \sum_{i=0}^{n} R_{ri}J_i\right); \tag{99}$$

$$J_i = \frac{-1}{R_{ii}}\left(-\varDelta \mu_i + \sum_{\substack{j=0 \\ j \neq i}}^{n} R_{ij}J_j + R_{ir}J_r\right). \tag{100}$$

$\varDelta F$ is the change of Gibbs' free energy at constant temperature and pressure, $\varDelta \mu_i$ the difference of chemical potential of permeant i between the phases ($\varDelta \mu_i = \mu_i' - \mu_i''$), and the R's are generalized resistance coefficients. Again the Onsager reciprocity relation $R_{ij} = R_{ji}$ and $R_{ir} = R_{ri}$ is valid.

From Equation (99) it follows that the reaction flow J_r is not only a function of Gibbs' free energy change $\varDelta F$, but is also dependent on the flux J_i, coupled to the coefficient R_{ri}. That means the substrate conversion rate is controlled by the flux of component i. J_i and J_r being a vector and a scalar respectively demand again for R_{ri} to be a vector; i.e. the chemical reaction creates a directed flux.

Equation (100) shows clearly, that the flux of component i does not only depend on the chemical potential gradient of i across the membrane, but also on the fluxes of other components j, e.g. that of the solvent and those of other solutes respectively, as well as on the flux of the coupled chemical reaction.

The reciprocal of the coefficient R_{ii}, i.e. $1/R_{ii}$, characterizes the membrane's permeability to the solute i if all other fluxes are zero. R_{ij} is a measure of the coupling of J_i and the flux J_j of the components j (solvent, co-solutes). R_{ij} is negative on withdrawal of the components i and j, but positive with oppositely directed i and j fluxes (repulsion). The last term in Equation (100) again represents the coupling between the fluxes J_i and J_r, the latter being that of the chemical reaction. If $R_{ir} \neq 0$, coupling occurs. The condition $R_{ir} \neq 0$ therefore characterizes active transport. This formulation also involves the Ussing criterion, i.e. active transport is present if a stoichiometric relation between metabolism (substrate or O_2 consumption) and transport rate exists. Furthermore, even with $R_{ir}=0$, the transport of component i may depend on the reaction r. The conditions in which the i transport is correspondingly active are $R_{jr}\neq0$ and $R_{ij}\neq0$, i.e. the flux of component i is coupled to that of the component j (carrier) and the j transport is active, depending on the flux of a chemical reaction.

The effectivity of the chemo-osmotic coupling can be determined by an efficiency function η (KEDEM and CAPLAN [145]), where η represents the fraction of entropy production of the spontaneous chemical reaction $(J_r X_r)$ which is consumed by the metabolically driven permeant transport $(J_i X_i)$

$$\eta = -\frac{J_i X_i}{J_r X_r} = 1 - \frac{d_i S/dt}{J_r X_r}.$$
(101)

$0\leq\eta\leq1$ holds. Necessary and sufficient conditions are $-1\leq Zx/q\leq0$ and $0\leq j/Zq\leq1$, where according to IV.C.3. (flux coupling) $j=J_i/J_r$, $x=X_i/X_r$, $Z=\sqrt{L_{ii}/L_{rr}}=\sqrt{R_{rr}/R_{ii}}$ and $q=L_{ir}/\sqrt{L_{ii}\cdot L_{rr}}=-R_{ir}/\sqrt{R_{ii}\cdot R_{rr}}$. With isothermal systems instead of the entropy function $d_i S/dt$ the dissipation function $T(d_i S/dt)$ can be used to define η, the latter now representing the fraction of free energy of the chemical reaction consumed in the transport process of the permeant i.

With unstationary systems, η is a function of time where

$$\eta_{max} = q^2/(1+\sqrt{1-q^2})^2 .$$
(102)

The maximum output of free energy from the chemical reaction is therefore dependent only on the coupling parameter q. With isothermal systems and constant coefficients,

$$\eta_{max} = \eta'_{max} ,$$
(103)

where η'_{max} concerns the reverse process $(J_i X_i>0;\ J_r X_r<0)$, i.e. that by equilibrating the concentration gradients of a permeant i, a coupled chemical reaction may be driven endergonically with exactly the same efficiency (reversed chemo-osmotic coupling). Similar findings in biological systems have been reported [205]. This reversal has also been used by MITCHELL [204] to establish a new hypothesis of oxidative phosphorylation within the mitochondria.

G. Remarks on Nonlinear Thermodynamic Approach to Membrane Transport

1. Introduction

The linear thermodynamic approach to permeability of membranes is dominated by models of vast fixed equilibrium structures. Recently, biomembranes are increasingly regarded as dynamically organized systems in which transport, metabolism, and spatial arrangement are intimately correlated [140]. A membrane which undergoes structural changes, e.g. transition from the dissociation to the association type of an ion exchange membrane [65], caused by transport interaction or by chemico-diffusional coupling exhibits nonlinear behavior. This property may lead in the case of coupled vector phenomena to the well-known unstable stationary states of TEORELL's oscillator [291–293], and in the case of chemico-diffusional coupling to instabilities and spatial redistribution of matter as well as to time dependent oscillations [88, 140]. Since in such systems the phenomenologic coefficients depend on the parameters of state which are functions of the flows, they are no more independent of flows and forces and the linear equations are no longer valid.

As in the linear case the thermodynamic and kinetic treatment of nonlinear systems starts with the dissipation function. The balance equations for the different components have to be solved for far-from-equilibrium-conditions. The solution of these nonlinear partial differential equations is rather cumbersome. Recently, a helpful mathematical formalism was developed by noting the strict analogies between Kirchhoff's current and voltage laws in electrical network theory and the conservation laws of mass transport and chemical reactions: network thermodynamics [220, 221, 236]. The results are very close to the exact data obtained by solving the differential equations [236]. The stability of the steady state solutions must be studied by normal mode analysis [88]. The main purpose is to subject the conditions for time order or space order being set up in a system to the influence of dissipation. The excess entropy production $\sigma[\delta S] = \Sigma \delta J_\alpha \delta X_\alpha$ and the time dependence of each normal mode $\exp \varrho t$ (where ϱ is in general a complex quantity, $\varrho = \varrho_r + i\varrho_i$) are the basic quantities for characterizing the stability behavior (for more details see [88]).

2. Examples and Models

It is worth noting that a composite membrane with linear elements may already have nonlinear properties as discussed by KATCHALSKY [138]. Oscillatory behavior is expected in membranes which may undergo a "chemical melting" and a corresponding mechano-chemical contraction. KATCHALSKY and SPANGLER [141] showed that the accumulation of salt in ultrafine bilayers of polyelectrolytes may release a regenerative process based on the contraction of the macromolecular matrix. SHASHOUA [263] observed oscillatory behavior of a bilayer composed of a monolayer of polyacid mounted on a monolayer of polybase when a critical current is applied to the membrane.

Cooperativity in a membrane is related normally with metastable transitions. As shown by KATCHALSKY and OSTER [140], a conformational change of the membrane with a metastable transition leads to time-dependent concentration variations under the following conditions. Within a space surrounded by a membrane a metabolic reaction proceeds with the reaction flows $J_r = k_f C_M - k_r C_N$ (C_M = metabolite, C_N = end product concentration). If C_M = const. in the reaction space J_r decreases with C_N. Only N leaks out through the membrane at a rate proportional to the difference between the inner and outer concentration C_{N_0}, e.g. $J_d = P(C_N - C_{N_0})$. At a certain critical concentration, C_{N_c}, the membrane undergoes a conformational change and the permeability coefficient rises from P_1 to P_2. If the conformational change has the usual form with metastable states, the dependence of J_d on C_N is shown in Figure 10. J_r and J_d cross in the metastable

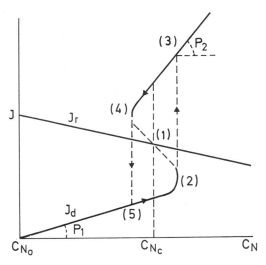

Fig. 10. Coupling between chemical reaction and diffusion leads under the conditions of a conformational change of the membrane with a metastable transition to concentration oscillations (see text)

range of concentrations. The change of C_N in the reaction space is given by $dC_N/dt = J_r - J_d$, and at the crossing point is $J_r = J_d$, so that $dC_N/dt = 0$. The crossing point (**1**) represents a stationary state, but the state is unstable. For if a slight fluctuation in C_N will occur to $C_{(N+dN)}$, the rate of reaction will be larger than the rate of diffusion or $dC_N/dt > 0$. Thus C_N will increase until the value of C_{N_2} is reached, and the state point will jump from (**2**) to (**3**). At (**3**) $J_d > J_r$ and $dC_N/dt < 0$. Hence from (**3**) C_N will decrease until point (**4**) is reached and the state point will jump over to (**5**) where again $dC_N/dt > 0$ and the concentration will increase to point (**2**), where the cycle proceeds anew. Thus a chemical oscillation (**2**)-(**3**)-(**4**)-(**5**) may continue as long as the supply of materials is unexhausted.

This example clearly demonstrates the unstable stationary state based on diffusion and reaction which can alter and influence rigorously the transport across a membrane. Otherwise such systems may play an important role in the cybernetic function of cells [140].

As was pointed out by NEUMANN [216] the metastable states of hysteretic enzymes can cause concentration oscillations by coupling with diffusion.

Furthermore, oscillations and hysteresis were observed experimentally in artificial membranes without structural changes of the membrane and without hysteretic effects in the enzyme activity. Periodic behavior and instability are induced only by changes in the activity caused by microenvironmental effects and correlated diffusion limitation [214, 333, 334]. Different kinetic models for passive transport, carrier transport, and active transport which take into account explicitly the interrelation between conformational states of the structural units of the membrane and the related transport properties have been derived by HILL and KEDEM [119, 120]. These models are not restricted to near-equilibrium steady states. The following model of BLUMENTHAL et al. [17] based on the Hill/Kedem-theory

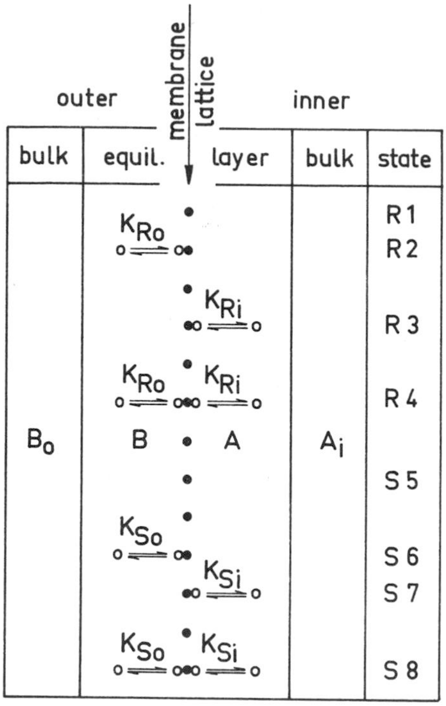

Fig. 11. The eight states of protomer. The permeant p is represented by a circle. In the R conformation state, p is both bound and transported. K_{Ro}, K_{Ri}, K_{So}, K_{Si} are equilibrium constants for adsorption-desorption of p in the R or S state

was developed for the membrane excitability. It includes, as an essential part, the treatment of nonelectrolyte transport across a membrane. The model (Figure 11) is characterized by the following parameters and conditions:

(i) The membrane consists of N equivalent lipoproteic units of protomers per unit of membrane area specialized in the selective translocation of the permeant p.

(ii) Each protomer carries two distinct specific sites for p, one on the outer face, the other inside the membrane. The permeant, therefore, binds and permeates across the membrane. Transport takes place by a jump of p from an internal to an external site, or vice versa.

(iii) The two conformations S and R of each protomer are reversibly accessible to each protomer, and both the affinity and permeability of p are altered when a transition occurs from one to the other conformation state. It is assumed that the R state favors the permeability and possesses a higher affinity for p than the S state.

Following CHANGEUX et al. [32], ε being the energy required to promote one protomer from S to R when all other protomers are in S state, the dependence of the free energy, ΔF, of the transition on the fraction $\langle r \rangle$ of protomers which are already in the R state is given by the linear relation $\Delta F = \varepsilon - \xi \langle r \rangle$ where ξ is a positive constant.

(iv) Cooperative interactions between protomers within the membrane are established by conformational coupling [31, 32].

(v) There exists on both sides of the membrane an "equilibration layer' [285], in which the concentration of the permeant p is a function both of the transport across the membrane and the rate of diffusion between the layer and bulk solution (Fig. 11).

The mathematical treatment, for simplicity, was restricted by additional assumptions: (a) p binds only to the R state and (b) the protomers are symmetrical, that means $K_{Ri} = K_{Ro}$ and $K_{Si} = K_{So}$.

Several procedures (details in [17]) lead to the basic equations:

$$\frac{d\alpha}{dt} = Z \cdot (\alpha - \beta) \langle r \rangle \cdot f(Z_i); \tag{104}$$

$$\frac{d}{dt} = Z \cdot (\beta - \alpha) \langle r \rangle \cdot f'(Z_i); \tag{105}$$

$$\frac{1}{\langle r \rangle} = 1 + l\Lambda^{\langle r \rangle} \cdot f''(Z_i). \tag{106}$$

$(Z, f(Z_i), f'(Z_i), f''(Z_i) =$ functions of the parameters of the model.

$\alpha = A/K$, $\beta = B/K$, A, B concentrations of p in the equilibration layer, $\langle r \rangle = \sum_1^4 n_i / \sum_1^5 n_i$, $l\Lambda^{\langle r \rangle} = \exp(\beta(\varepsilon - \xi \langle r \rangle)$ isomerisation constant of a protomer integrated in the membrane lattice. $Z =$ constant.

Equations (104)–(106) give the time-change of p concentration in the inner and outer equilibration layer, respectively, and the fraction of the membrane protomers which are in the R state for given values of these concentrations. The main outcomes of this model can be summarized as follows:

(i) $\langle r \rangle$ varies steeply with the difference $\Delta\alpha = \alpha - \beta$. The steepness depends on the cooperative interactions between protomers.

(ii) For certain values of the parameters a "negative" permeability occurs.

(iii) In the region where $\langle r \rangle$ varies steeply with the gradient, multi-steady state regimes are possible for a given value of the overall concentration difference $(\Delta\alpha)_t = \alpha_i - \beta_0$ between the two bulk solutions of the membrane $(B_0$ and $A_i)$. Three distinct values of $\langle r \rangle$ correspond to three states of the diffusion regime through the membrane, only two of them being stable.

This model is very instructive because (a) it shows that a flip-flop regime is related to the asymmetry in the boundary conditions (concentration difference between the bulk solutions inside and outside the membrane) and the existence of cooperative interactions between protomers, (b) it exemplifies that the constraints imposed by the outside world in biological systems bring them to states where their properties can no longer be understood solely on the basis of an extrapolation of the equilibrium situation [173, 174, 241, 242], and (c) the distinction between binding and permeation leads to the prediction of membrane effectors which might bind to the recognition site of the protomer without being transported thus preventing the transport of the physiologic permeant by steric hindrance.

Appendix

Glossary of Symbols

A, A (index)	permeant species A
AC, AC (index)	permeant-carrier complex AC
B, B (index)	permeant species B
BC, BC (index)	permeant-carrier complex BC
C, C (index)	membrane carrier
C_{tot}	total carrier concentration
C (with index)	permeant concentration within the membrane
$\bar{C}$ (with index)	mean permeant concentration within the membrane

$$\bar{C} = \frac{(C)_{x=0} + (C)_{x=\varDelta x}}{2}$$

C_A'; C_A'' [1]	c_A'/K_{AC}; c_A''/K_{AC} ⎱ in Equation (88)
C_B'; C_B''	c_B'/K_{BC}; c_B''/K_{BC} ⎰
c_A', c_B'; c_A'', c_B''	permeant A, B concentration within phase ' and phase "
c_C'; c_C''	carrier concentration within phase ' and phase "
c_{AC}', c_{BC}'; c_{AC}'', c_{BC}''	concentration of the permeant-carrier complex AC, BC within phase ' and phase "
$\bar{c}$ (with index)	mean permeant concentration outside the membrane

$$\bar{c} = \frac{c' + c''}{2}$$

D	conventional diffusion coefficient
D^0	conventional of free diffusion of the solute in aqueous solution
$\dfrac{dN}{dt}$ (with index)	number of moles of a permeant crossing the membrane per unit time
$\dfrac{dS}{dt}$	entropy change of a system
$\dfrac{d_i S}{dt}$	entropy production within a system
$\dfrac{d_a S}{dt}$	entropy exchange between a system and the surrounding milieu (complementary system)
F	membrane area
F (with index)	frictional force
f (with index)	frictional coefficient
f^0 (with index)	solute-water frictional coefficient of free diffusion
i (index)	permeant species i
J	mass flow, resp. generalized flow
J (with index)	mass flow
J_v	volume flow
J_D	exchange flow
J_{lr}, J_{rl}	fluxes from phase ' into phase " and vice versa

---

[1]   Notations referring to phase ' and phase " are generally termed with ' and ".

j	flux-ratio of two coupled fluxes ($j = J_A/J_B$)
j (index)	permeant species j
K	distribution coefficient of a solute s between membrane and solution $K = \bar{C}_s/\bar{c}_s$
K (with index)	dissociation constant
k (with index)	velocity constant
L (with index)	phenomenologic coefficients
L_D	diffusion coefficient
L_{Dp}	ultrafiltration coefficient
L_{pD}	osmotic coefficient
L_p	mechanical permeability coefficient (hydraulic permeability)
M	membrane
m (index)	membrane
P, P (with index)	conventional permeability coefficient
p	hydrostatic pressure
q	coupling coefficient
R	gas constant
R (with index)	phenomenologic resistance coefficient
r	ratio of the velocity constants of the loaded and the free carriers' membrane transfer
r (index)	chemical reaction r
S	entropy
s (index)	solute
T	absolute temperature (Kelvin)
t	time
v, v (with index)	velocity
$\bar{v}$ (with index)	partial molar volume
w (index)	solvent ($=$ water)
X	charge concentration per unit membrane volume (fixed charges)
X'	charge density per unit volume of the aqueous phase within the membrane
X (with index)	generalized force
x	spatial coordinate perpendicular to the membrane surface
x	ratio of the conjugated forces of two coupled fluxes ($x = X_A/X_B$)
y	degree of saturation of the carrier
$1, 2, 3 \ldots n$	permeant species $1, 2, 3 \ldots n$
Z	constant (see text)
Δ	difference of quantities between phase $'$ and phase $''$ (e.g. $\Delta c_s = c'_s - c''_s$)
η	efficiency function of coupled processes (η'-reverse processes)
ϑ	tortuosity factor of membrane capillaries
μ (with index)	chemical potential
$\tilde{\mu}$ (with index)	electrochemical potential
v (with index)	stoichiometric coefficient of reaction participants
π	osmotic pressure of a solute
ϱ	phase
σ	reflection coefficient (Staverman)

σ' reflection coefficient for $J_w = 0$
φ electrical potential
φ_w^m mean volume fraction of water within the membrane
ψ dissipation function
ω permeability coefficient for $J_v = 0$
ω' permeability coefficient for $J_w = 0$

References

1. Acland, J. D.: Active transfer and the Curie principle. J. theor. Biol. **13**, 318 (1966).
2. Albers, R. W.: Biochemical aspects of active transport. Ann. Rev. Biochem. **36**, 727 (1967).
3. Alvarado, F.: Transport of sugars and amino acids in the intestine: Evidence for a common carrier. Science **151**, 1010 (1966).
4. Alvarado, F.: Amino-acid transport in hamster small intestine: Site of inhibition by D-galactose. Nature (Lond.) **219**, 276 (1968).
5. Andreoli, T. E., Dennis, V. W., Weigl, A. M.: The effect of amphotericin B on the water and nonelectrolyte permeability of thin lipic membranes. J. gen. Physiol. **53**, 133 (1969).
6. Andres, K. H.: Mikropinozytose im Zentralnervensystem. Z. Zellforsch. **64**, 63 (1964).
7. Andres, K. H., Düring, M. von: Mikropinozytose in motorischen Endplatten. Naturwissenschaften **53**, 615 (1966).
8. Baker, J. B. E.: The effects of drugs on the foetus. Pharmacol. Rev. **12**, 37 (1960).
9. Beck, R. E., Schultz, J. S.: Hindrance of solute diffusion within membranes as measured with microporous membranes of known pore geometry. Biochim. biophys. Acta (Amst.) **255**, 273 (1972).
10. Bennett, H. St.: The concepts of membrane flow and membrane vesiculation as mechanisms for active transport and ion pumping. J. biophys. biochem. Cytol. **2**, Suppl. 99 (1956).
11. Benz, R., Stark, G., Janko, K., Läugner, P.: Valinomydin-mediated ion transport through neutral lipid membranes: Influence of hydrocarbon chain length and temperature. J. Membrane Biol. **14**, 339 (1973).
12. Berger, E. A., Weiner, J. H., Heppel, L. A.: Amino acid transport and binding proteins in E. coli. Fed. Proc. **30**, 1061 (abstract) (1971).
13. Bittner, J., Heinz, E.: Die Wirkung von g-Strophantin auf den Glyzintransport in Ehrlich-Ascites-Tumorzellen. Biochim. biophys. Acta (Amst.) **74**, 392 (1963).
14. Bloj, B., Morero, R. D., Farías, R. N.: Membrane fluidity cholesterol and allosteric transitions of membrane-bound Mg^{2+}-ATPase, $(Na^+ - K^+)$-ATPase and acetylcholinesterase from rat erythrocytes. FEBS Letters **38**, 101 (1973).
15. Blumenthal, R. P.: Dynamic patterns in active transport. Israel J. Chem. **11**, 341 (1973).
16. Blumenthal, R., Caplan, S. R., Kedem, O.: The coupling of an enzymic reaction to transmembrane flow of electric current in a synthetic "active transport" system. Biophys. J. **7**, 735 (1967).
17. Blumenthal, R., Changeux, J.-P., Lefever, R.: Membrane excitability and dissipative instabilities. J. Membrane Biol. **2**, 351 (1970).
18. Boos, W., Gordon, A., Hall, R. E.: Substrate induced conformational change of the galactose-binding protein of E. coli. Fed. Proc. **30**, 1062 (abstract) (1971).
19. Bowyer, F.: The kinetics of the penetration of nonelectrolytes into the mammalian erythrocyte. Int. Rev. Cytol. **6**, 469 (1957).
20. Bowyer, F., Widdas, W. F.: The action of inhibitors on the facilitated hexose transfer system in erythrocytes. J. Physiol. (Lond.) **141**, 219 (1958).
21. Boyer, P. D., Klein, W. L.: Energy-coupling mechanisms in transport. In: Fox, F., Keith, A. D. (Eds.): Membrane Molecular Biology, Stamford: Sinauer 1972, p. 323.
22. Branton, D., Deamer, D. W.: Membrane Structure (= Protoplasmatologia 2/E). Wien-New York: Springer 1972.
23. Brierley, G. P., Bachmann, E., Green, D. E.: Active transport of inorganic phosphate and magnesium ions by beef heart mitochondria. Proc. nat. Acad. Sci., (Wash.) **48**, 1928 (1962).

24. Britton, H. G.: Induced uphill and downhill transport: Relationship to the Ussing criterion. Nature (Lond.) **198**, 190 (1963).
25. Britton, H. G.: Fluxes in passive, monovalent and polyvalent carrier systems. J. theor. Biol. **10**, 28 (1966).
26. Broun, G., Thomas, D., Selegny, E.: Structured bienzymatical models formed by sequential enzymes bound into artificial supports: Active glucose transport effect. J. Membrane Biol. **8**, 313 (1972).
27. Bunch, W., Edwards, C.: The permeation of nonelectrolytes through the single barnacle muscle cell. J. Physiol. (Lond.) **202**, 683 (1969).
28. Burger, M., Hejmová, L., Kleinzeller, A.: Transport of some mono- and di-saccharides into yeast cells. Biochem. J. **71**, 233 (1959).
29. Caldwell, P. C., Hodgkin, A. L., Keynes, R. D., Shaw, T. I.: Effects of injecting energy-rich phosphate compounds on the active transport of ions in the giant axons of Loligo. J. Physiol. (Lond.) **152**, 561 (1960).
30. Carter, J. W.: Adsorption, solids drying and membrane permeation. Brit. chem. Eng. **11**, 718 (1966).
31. Changeux, J. P.: Remarks on the symmetry and cooperative properties of biological membranes. In: Engström, H., Strandberg, B. (Eds.): Symmetry and function of biological systems at the macromolecular level (= Nobel Symposium 11), p. 235, New York: Wiley Interscience 1969.
32. Changeux, J.-P., Thiéry, J., Tung, Y., Kittel, C.: On the cooperativity of biological membranes. Proc. nat. Acad. Sci. (Wash.) **57**, 335 (1967).
33. Chapman-Andresen, C.: Some observations on pinocytosis in leucocytes. Exp. Cell Res. **12**, 397 (1957).
34. Chapman-Andresen, C., Holter, H.: Differential uptake of protein and glucose by pinocytosis in Amoeba proteus. C. R. Lab. Carlsberg **34**, 211 (1964).
35. Chappell, J. B., Crofts, A. R.: Gramicidin and ion transport in isolated liver mitochondria. Biochem. J. **95**, 393 (1965).
36. Chappell, J. B., Crofts, A. R.: The effect of atraktylate and oligomycin on the behaviour of mitochondria towards adenine nucleotides. Biochem. J. **95**, 707 (1965).
37. Chizmadjev, Ju. A., Khodorov, B. I., Aityan, S. Kh.: The theory of ion transport through sodium channel of biological membranes. Dokl. Akad. Nauk SSSR **213**, 722 (1973).
38. Choke, Ho Coy: Genetical studies on active transport. Sci. Progr. **59**, 75 (1971).
39. Christensen, H. N.: Reactive sites and biological transport. Advanc. Protein Chem. **15**, 239 (1960).
40. Cirillo, V. P.: The transport of non-fermentable sugars across the yeast cell membrane. In: Kleinzeller, A., Kotyk, A. (Eds.): Membrane Transport and Metabolism, Prague: Czech. Acad. Sci. 1961, p. 343.
41. Cockrell, R. S., Harris, E. J., Pressman, B. C.: Synthesis of ATP driven by a potassium gradient in mitochondria. Nature (Lond.) **215**, 1487 (1967).
42. Coleman, R.: Membrane-bound enzymes and membrane ultrastructure. Biochim. biophys. Acta (Amst.) **300**, 1 (1973).
43. Conway, E. J.: Some aspects of ion transport through membranes. Symp. Soc. exp. Biol. **8**, 297 (1954).
44. Csáky, T. Z.: Transport through biological membranes. Ann. Rev. Physiol. **27**, 415 (1965).
45. Curie, P.: Oeuvres. Paris: Gauthier-Villars 1908, p. 118.
46. Damadian, R.: Biological ion exchanger resins. I. Quantitative electrostatic correspondence of fixed charge and mobile counter ion. Biophys. J. **11**, 739 (1971).
47. Damadian, R., Goldsmith, M., Zaner, K. S.: Biological ion exchanger resins. II. Querp water and ion exchange selectivity. Biophys. J. **11**, 761 (1971).
48. Damadian, R., Goldsmith, M., Zaner, K. S.: Biological ion exchanger resins. III. Molecular interpretation of cellular ion exchange. Biophys. J. **11**, 773 (1971).
49. Danielli, J. F.: Some properties of lipoid films in relation to structure of the plasma membrane. J. cell. comp. Physiol. **7**, 393 (1936).
50. Danielli, J. F.: The present position in the field of facilitated diffusion and selection active transport. In: Kitching, J. A. (Ed.): Recent Developments in Cell Physiology, Colston Papers Vol. 7, p. 1. London: Butterworth 1954.

51. Davson, H., Danielli, J. F.: The permeability of natural membranes, 2nd Ed. Cambridge: University Press 1952.
52. Denbigh, K. G.: The thermodynamics of the steady state. London: Methuen 1951.
53. Desimone, J. A., Beil, D. L., Scriven, L. E.: Ferroincollodion membranes: Dynamic concentration patterns in planar membranes. Science **180**, 946 (1973).
54. Dessolle, N.: Observation d'un comportement particulier de la cellule interstitielle testiculaire du rat. C. R. Soc. Acad. Sci. **258**, 2893 (1964).
55. Diamond, J. M., Wright, E. M.: Biological membranes: The physical basis of ion and nonelectrolyte selectivity. Ann. Rev. Physiol. **31**, 581 (1969).
56. Donder, T. de: L'Affinité. Paris: Gauthier-Villars 1927.
57. Donder, T. de: Bull. Acad. roy. Belg. Cl. Sci. **24**, 15 (1938), cited by Haase [101], p. 101 and 123.
58. Dorn, A.: Elektronenmikroskopische Untersuchungen über die licht- und submikroskopische Pinozytose an Fasern und Kapillaren des Skeletmuskels. Anat. Anz. **115**, 222 (1964).
59. Eckart, C.: The thermodynamic of irreversible processes. I. The simple fluid. Phys. Rev. **58**, 267 (1940).
60. Eckart, C.: The thermodynamics of irreversible processes. II. Fluid mixtures. Phys. Rev. **58**, 269 (1940).
61. Eckart, C.: The thermodynamics of irreversible processes. III. Relativistic theory of the simple fluid. Phys. Rev. **58**, 919 (1940).
62. Edelman, I. S.: Transport through biological membranes. Ann. Rev. Physiol. **23**, 37 (1961).
63. Eisenman, G.: Cation-selective glass electrodes and their mode of operation. Biophys. J. **2**, Part 2, 259 (1962).
64. Eisenman, G.: In: Kato, T. (Ed.): Physiology. Proc. 23rd Congress of the International Union of Physiological Sciences, Tokyo 1965, p. 489 (= International Congress Series No. 87). Amsterdam: Excerpta Medica Foundation 1965.
65. Eisenman, G., Sandblom, J. P., Walker, J. L., jr: Membrane structure and ion permeation. Science **155**, 965 (1967).
66. Eisenman, G., Szabo, G., McLaughlin, S. G. A.: Molecular basis for the action fo macrocyclic carriers on passive ionic translocation across lipid bilayer membranes structure. J. Bioenergetics **4**, 93 (1973).
67. Eletr, S., Williams, M. A., Watkins, T., Keith, A. D.: Perturbation of the dynamics of lipid alkyl chains in membrane systems: Effect on the activity of membrane-bound enzymes. Biochim. biophys. Acta (Amst.) **339**, 190 (1974).
68. Ericsson, J. L. E.: Transport and digestion of hemoglobin in proximal tubulus. I. Light microscopy and cytochemistry of acid phosphatases. Lab. Invest. **14**, 1 (1965).
69. Ericsson, J. L. E.: Transport and digestion of hemoglobin in proximal tubulus. II. Electron microscopy. Lab. Invest. **14**, 16 (1965).
70. Essig, A., Kedem, O., Hill, T. L.: Net flux and tracer flow in lattice and carrier models. J. theor. Biol. **13**, 72 (1966).
71. Famaey, J.-P., Whitehouse, M. W.: Interactions between non-steroidal anti-inflammatory drugs and biological membranes. 2. Swelling and membrane permeability changes induced in some immunocompetent cells by various non-steroidal anti-inflammatory drugs. Biochem. Pharmacol. **22**, 2707 (1973).
72. Farrant, J.: Permeability of guinea-pig smooth muscle to nonelectrolytes. J. gen. Physiol. **178**, 1 (1965).
73. Felton, M. H., Pomerat, C. M.: Antigen-antibody reaction in relation in pinocytosis. I. Cell injury and repair following Staphylococcus toxin and antiserum. Exp. Cell Res. **27**, 280 (1962).
74. Fick, A.: Über Diffusion. Ann. Phys. (Chem.) **94**, 59 (1855).
75. Fishman, S. N., Volkenstein, M. V.: The diffusion of ions across biological membranes. J. Membrane Biol. **12**, 189 (1973).
76. Fitts, D. D.: Nonequilibrium Thermodynamics. A Phenomenological Theory of Irreversible Processes in Fluid Systems. New York: McGraw-Hill 1962.

77. Fox, C. F., Carter, J. R., Kennedy, E. P.: Genetic control of the membrane protein component of the lactose transport system of Escherichia coli. Proc. nat. Acad. Sci. (Wash.) **57**, 698 (1967).
78. Fox, F., Keith, A. D., Ed.: Membrane Molecular Biology. Stamford: Sinuar 1972.
79. Fox, C. F., Kennedy, E. P.: Specific labelling and partial purification of the M protein, a component of the β-galactoside transport system of Escherichia coli. Proc. nat. Acad. Sci. (Wash.) **54**, 891 (1965).
80. Franck, U. F.: Über das elektronische Verhalten von porösen Ionenaustauschermembranen. Ber. Bunsenges. phys. Chem. **67**, 657 (1963).
81. Frenkel, J. I.: Kinetic Theory of Liquids. London-New York: Oxford University Press 1946.
82. Frey-Wyssling, A.: Zur Wasserpermeabilität des Protoplasmas. Experienta (Basel) **2**, 132 (1946).
83. Füller, H.: Die Pinocytose. Biol. Rdsch. **7**, 97 (1969).
84. Gachelin, G.: A new assay of the phosphotransferase system in Escherichia coli. Biochem. biophys. Res. Commun. **34**, 382 (1969).
85. Giebel, O., Passow, H.: Die Permeabilität der Erythrocytenmembran für anorganische Anionen. Pflügers Arch. ges. Physiol. **271**, 378 (1960).
86. Ginzburg, B. Z., Katchalsky, A.: Frictional coefficients of the flows of non-electrolytes through artificial membranes. J. gen. Physiol. **47**, 403 (1963).
87. Girbardt, M.: Probleme der Struktur, Dynamik und Genese zytoplasmatischer Membranen. Biol. Rdsch. **4**, 1 (1966).
88. Glansdorff, P., Prigogine, I.: Thermodynamic theory of structure, stability and fluctuations. London: Wiley 1971.
89. Glasstone, S., Laidler, K. J., Eyring, H.: The Theory of Rate Processes. New York: McGraw-Hill 1941.
90. Glynn, I. M.: Sodium and potassium movements in nerve, muscle, and red cells. Int. Rev. Cytol. **8**, 449 (1959).
91. Godin, D. V., Wan Ng, T.: Studies on the membrane-perturbational effects of drugs and divalent cations utilizing trinitrobenzenesulfonic acid. Molec. Pharmacol. **9**, 802 (1973).
92. Goldacre, R. J., Lorch, I. J.: Folding and unfolding of protein molecules in relation to cytoplasmic streaming, amoeboid movement and osmotic work. Nature (Lond.) **166**, 497 (1950).
93. Gonzales, J. de D. L., Jenny, H.: Modes of entry of strontium into plant roots. Science **128**, 90 (1958).
94. Green, D. E., Allmann, D. W., Bachmann, E., Baum, H., Kopaczyk, K., Korman, E. F., Lipton, S., Maclannan, D. H., McConnell, D. G., Perdue, J. F., Rieske, J. S., Tzagoloff, A.: Formation of membranes by repeating units. Arch. Biochem. Biophys. **119**, 312 (1967).
95. Green, D. E., Ji, S., Brucker, R. F.: Structure-function unitization model of biological membranes. J. Bioenergetics **4**, 253 (1973).
96. Grim, E., Sollner, K.: The contributions of normal and anomalous osmosis to the osmotic effects arising across charged membranes with solutions of electrolytes. J. gen. Physiol. **40**, 887 (1957).
97. Grisham, C. M., Barnett, R. E.: The effects of long-chain alcohols on membrane lipids and the $(Na^+ + K^+)$-ATPase. Biochim. biophys. Acta (Amst.) **311**, 417 (1973).
98. Groot, S. R. de: Thermodynamics of Irreversible Processes. Amsterdam: North-Holland 1951.
99. Groot, S. R. de, Mazur, P.: Non-equilibrium Thermodynamics. Amsterdam: North-Holland 1962.
100. Gross, E. L., Hess, S. C.: Correlation between calcium ion binding to chloroplast membranes and divalent cation-induced structural changes and changes in chlorophyll a fluorescence. Biochim. biophys. Acta (Amst.) **339**, 334 (1974).
101. Haase, R.: Thermodynamik der irreversiblen Prozesse. Darmstadt: Steinkopff 1963.
102. Hammes, G. G., Schullery, S. E.: Structure of macromolecular aggregates. II. Constriction of model membranes from phospholipids and polypeptides. Biochemistry **9**, 2555 (1970).

103. Hanai, T., Haydon, D. A., Taylor, J.: The influence of lipid composition and of some adsorbed proteins on the capacitance of black hydrocarbon membranes. J. theor. Biol. **9**, 422 (1965).

104. Hansson, E., Schmiterlöw, C. G.: A comparison of the distribution, excretion and metabolism of a tertiary (promethazine) and a quarternary (aprobit) phenothiazine compound labelled with S^{35}. Arch. int. Pharmacodyn. **131**, 309 (1961).

105. Harris, E. J.: Transport and Accumulation in Biological Systems. London: Butterworth 1956.

106. Harris, E. J., Prankerd, T. A. J.: Diffusion and permeation of cations in human and dog erythrocytes. J. gen. Physiol. **41**, 197 (1957).

107. Haydon, D. A., Hladky, S. B.: Ion transport across thin lipid membranes: A critical discussion of mechanisms in selected systems. Quart. Rev. Biophys. **5**, 187 (1972).

108. Heckmann, K.: Die Permeabilität biologischer Membranen. In: Karlson, P. (Ed.) Mechanisms of Hormone Action. Stuttgart: Thieme 1956, p. 41.

109. Heinz, E.: Kinetic studies on the "influx" of glycine-1-C^{14} into the Ehrlich mouse ascites carcinoma cell. J. biol. Chem. **211**, 781 (1954).

110. Heinz, E.: Aktiver Transport von Aminosäuren. In: Biochemie des aktiven Transports, Berlin-Heidelberg-New York: Springer 1961, p. 167.

111. Heinz, E.: Physiologie, Biochemie und Energetik des aktiven Transports. Naunyn-Schmiedebergs Arch. exp. Path. Pharmak. **245**, 10 (1963).

112. Heinz, E.: Transport through biological membranes. Ann. Rev. Physiol. **29**, 21 (1967).

113. Heinz, E., Geck, P., Wilbrandt, W.: Coupling in secondary active transport. Activation of transport by co-transport and/or counter-transport with the fluxes of other solutes. Biochim. biophys. Acta (Amst.) **255**, 442 (1972).

114. Heinz, E., Walsh, P. M.: Exchange diffusion, transport, and intracellular level of amino acids in Ehrlich carcinoma cells. J. biol. Chem. **233**, 1488 (1958).

115. Hill, T. L.: A proposed common allosteric mechanism for active transport, muscle contraction, and ribosomal translocation. Proc. nat. Acad. Sci. (Wash.) **64**, 267 (1969).

116. Hill, T. L.: Analysis of a model for active transport. Proc. nat. Acad. Sci. (Wash.) **65**, 409 (1970).

117. Hill, T. L., Chen, Yi-Der: Cooperative effects in models of steady-state transport across membranes. II. Oscillating phase transition. Proc. nat. Acad. Sci. (Wash.) **66**, 189 (1970).

118. Hill, T. L., Chen, Yi-Der: Cooperative effects in models of steady-state transport across membranes. I. Proc. nat. Acad. Sci. (Wash.) **65**, 1069 (1970).

119. Hill, T. L., Kedem, O.: Irreversible thermodynamics. III. Models for steady state and active transport across membranes. J. theor. Biol. **10**, 399 (1966).

120. Hill, T. L., Kedem, O.: Irreversible thermodynamics. IV. Diagrammatic representation of steady state fluxes for unimolar systems. J. theor. Biol. **10**, 422 (1966).

121. Hirschfeld, I., Fagarasan, M.: Action of sugars on methionine transfer in Ehrlich ascites carcinoma cells. Experientia (Basel) **25**, 363 (1969).

122. Hodgkin, A. L., Keynes, R. D.: The potassium permeability of a giant nerve fibre. J. Physiol. (Lond.) **128**, 61 (1955).

123. Hokin, L. E., Hokin, M. R.: Biological transport. Ann. Rev. Biochem. **32**, 553 (1963).

124. Holter, H.: Pinocytosis. Int. Rev. Cytol. **8**, 481 (1959).

125. Holter, H., Holtzer, H.: Pinocytotic uptake of fluorescein-labelled proteins by various tissue cells. Exp. Cell Res. **18**, 421 (1959).

126. Hoshiko, R., Lindley, B. D.: The relationship of Ussing's flux-ratio equation to the thermodynamic description of membrane permeability. Biochim. biophys. Acta (Amst.) **79**, 301 (1964).

127. Huang, H. W.: Kinetic theory of antibiotic ion carrier. I. and II. J. theor. Biol. **32**, 351 and 363 (1971).

128. Jacquez, J. A.: The kinetics of carrier-mediated active transport of amino acids. Proc. nat. Acad. Sci. (Wash.) **47**, 153 (1961).

129. Jacquez, J. A.: The kinetics of carrier-mediated transport: Stationary-state approximations. Biochim. biophys. Acta (Amst.) **79**, 318 (1964).

130. Janki, R. M., Aithal, H. N., McMurray, W. C., Tustanoff, E. R.: The effect of altered membrane-lipid composition on enzyme activities of outer and inner mitochondrial membranes of Saccharomyces cerevisiae. Biochem. biophys. Res. Commun. **56**, 1078 (1974).

131. Jardetzky, O.: The Curie principle and the problem of active transport. Biochim. biophys. Acta (Amst.) **79**, 631 (1964).
132. Jost, P. C., Griffith, O. H.: The molecular reorganization of lipid bilayers by osmium tetroxide. A spinlabel study of orientation and restricted y-axis anisotopic motion in model membrane systems. Arch. Biochem. Biophys. **159**, 70 (1973).
133. Jost, W.: Diffusion in Solids, Liquids, Gases. New York: Academic Press 1960.
134. Kaback, H. R.: The transport of sugars across isolated bacterial membranes. In: Bronner, F., Kleinzeller, A. (Eds.): Current Topics in Membranes and Transport, Vol. 1, p. 36. New York: Academic Press 1970.
135. Kaback, H. R., Stadtman, E. R.: Proline uptake by an isolated cytoplasmic membrane preparation of Escherichia coli. Proc. nat. Acad. Sci. (Wash.) **55**, 920 (1966).
136. Kahrig, E., Erpenbeck, J., Kirstein, D., Dreyer, G.: Zum Einfluß der Kationenhydratation, der Anionenhydratation und der Hydratation 2. Art auf die Diffusionskopplung. Teil I. Grundlagen. Stud. biophys. **55**, 163 (1976).
137. Katchalsky, A.: Membrane permeability and the thermodynamics of irreversible processes. In: Kleinzeller, A., Kotyk, A. (Eds.): Membrane Transport and Metabolism, p. 69. Prague: Czech. Acad. Sci. 1961.
138. Katchalsky, A.: Non-eqilibrium thermodynamics of biomembrane processes. In: Marois, M. (Ed.): Theoretical Physics and Biology. Proceedings of the First International Conference, Versailles 1967, p. 188. Amsterdam: North-Holland 1969.
139. Katchalsky, A., Kedem, O.: Thermodynamics of flow process in biological systems. Biophys. J. **2**, 53 (1962).
140. Katchalsky, A., Oster, G.: Chemico-diffusional coupling in biomembranes. In: Tosteson, D. C. (Ed.): The Molecular Basis of Membrane Function, Englewood Cliffs: Prentic Hall 1969, p. 1.
141. Katchalsky, A., Spangler, R.: Dynamics of membrane processes. Quart. Rev. Biophys. **1**, 127 (1968).
142. Kavanau, J. L.: Structure and Function in Biological Membranes. Part 1, p. 132. San Francisco: Holden-Day 1965.
143. Kavanau, J. L.: Membrane structure and function. Fed. Proc. **25**, 1096 (1966).
144. Kedem, O.: Criteria of active transport. In: Kleinzeller, A., Kotyk, A. (Eds.): Membrane Transport and Metabolism, p. 87. Prague: Czech. Acad. Sci. 1961.
145. Kedem, O., Caplan, R.: Degree of coupling and its relation to efficiency of energy conversion. Trans. Faraday Soc. **61**, 1897 (1965).
146. Kedem, O., Katchalsky, A.: Thermodynamic analysis of the permeability of biological membranes to non-electrolytes. Biochim. biophys. Acta (Amst.) **27**, 229 (1958).
147. Kedem, O., Katchalsky, A.: A physical interpretation of the phenomenological coefficients of membrane permeability. J. gen. Physiol. **45**, 143 (1962).
148. Kedem, O., Katchalsky, A.: Permeability of composite membranes. Part 1. Electric current, volume flow and flow of solute through membranes. Trans. Faraday Soc. **59**, 1918 (1963).
149. Kedem, O., Katchalsky, A.: Permeability of composite membranes. Part 2. Parallel elements. Trans. Faraday Soc. **59**, 1931 (1963).
150. Kedem, O., Katchalsky, A.: Permeability of composite membranes. Part 3. Series array of elements. Trans. Faraday Soc. **59**, 1941 (1963).
151. Kepes, A.: The place of permeases in cellular organization. In: Hoffman, J. F. (Ed.): The Cellular Function of Membrane Transport, p. 155. Englewood Cliffs, N.Y.: Prentice-Hall 1964.
152. Keynes, R. D.: Discussion. In: Kleinzeller, A., Kotyk, A. (Eds.): Membrane Transport and Metabolism, p. 104. Prague: Czech. Acad. Sci. 1961.
153. Kirkwood, J. G.: Transport of ions through biological membranes from the standpoint of irreversible thermodynamics. In: Clarke, H. T. (Ed.): Ion Transport across Membranes, p. 119. New York: Academic Press 1954.
154. Kirschener, L. B.: Phosphatidylserine as a possible participant in active sodium transport in erythrocytes. Arch. Biochem. Biophys. **68**, 499 (1957).
155. Kobatake, Y., Fujita, H.: Osmotic flows in charged membranes. II. Thermo-osmosis. J. chem. Phys. **41**, 2963 (1964).

156. Koch, A. L.: The role of permease in transport. Biochim. biophys. Acta (Amst.) **79**, 177 (1964).
157. Koch, A. L.: Kinetics of permease catalyzed transport. J. theor. Biol. **14**, 103 (1967).
158. Kolber, A. R., Stein, W. D.: Identification of a component of a transport "carrier" system: Isolation of the permease expression of the Lac operon of Escherichia coli. Nature (Lond.) **209**, 691 (1966).
159. Koltover, V. K., Blumenfeld, L. A.: Temperature induced conformational transition in electron-transporting biological membranes. Biofizika **18**, 827 (1973).
160. Korn, E. D.: Structure and function of the plasma membrane. A biochemical perspective. J. gen. Physiol. **52**, 257s (1968).
161. Kotyk, A.: Mechanisms of nonelectrolyte transport. Biochim. biophys. Acta (Amst.) **300**, 183 (1973).
162. Krasne, S., Eisenman, G., Szabo, G.: Freezing and melting of lipid bilayers and the mode of action of nonactin, valinomycin, and gramicidin. Science **174**, 412 (1971).
163. Kundig, W., Kundig, F. D., Anderson, B., Roseman, S.: Restoration of active transport of glycosides in Escherichia coli by a component of a phosphotransferase system. J. biol. Chem. **241**, 3243 (1966).
164. Kurz, H.: Lipid solubility as an important factor for the penetration of drugs into the liver. Biochem. Pharmac. **8**, 20 (1961).
165. Lacko, L., Burger, M.: Common carrier system for sugar transport in human red cells. Nature (Lond.) **191**, 881 (1961).
166. Lacko, L., Burger, M.: Interaction of some disaccharides with the carrier system for aldoses in erythrocytes. Biochem. J. **83**, 622 (1962).
167. Lacko, L., Burger, M., Hejmová, L., Rejnková, J.: Exchange transfer of sugars in human erythrocytes. In: Kleinzeller, A., Kotyk, A. (Eds.): Membrane Transport and Metabolism, p. 399, Prague: Czech. Acad. Sci. 1961.
168. Laidler, K. J., Shuler, K. E.: The kinetics of membrane processes. I. The mechanism and the kinetic laws for diffusion. J. chem. Phys. **17**, 851 (1949).
169. Laidler, K. J., Shuler, K. E.: The kinetics of membrane processes. II. Theoretical pressure-time relationship for permeable membranes. J. chem. Phys. **17**, 856 (1949).
170. Lakshminarayanaiah, N.: Transport Phenomena in Membranes, p. 329 New York: Academic Press 1969.
171. Lange, Y., Bobo, C. M. G., Solomon, A. K.: Nonelectrolyte diffusion through lecithin-water lamellar phases and red-cell membranes. Biochim. biophys. Acta (Amst.) **339**, 347 (1974).
172. Läuger, P.: Transportphänomene an Membranen. Angew. Chem. **81**, 56 (1969).
173. Lefever, R.: Disspative structures in chemical systems. J. chem. Phys. **49**, 4977 (1968).
174. Lefever, R., Nicolis, G., Prigogine, I.: On the occurrence of oscillations around the steady state in systems of chemical reactions far from equilibrium. J. chem. Phys. **47**, 1045 (1967).
175. Le Fevre, P. G.: Evidence of active transfer of certain non-electrolytes across the human red cell membrane. J. gen. Physiol. **31**, 505 (1948).
176. Le Fevre, P. G.: The evidence for active transport of monosaccharides across the red cell membrane. Symp. Soc. exp. Biol. **8**, 118 (1954).
177. Le Fevre, P. G.: Active transport across animal cell membranes. Protoplasmatologia **8**, 7 (1955).
178. Le Fevre, P. G.: Sugar transport in the red blood cell: Structure-activity relationship of substrates and antagonists. Pharmacol. Rev. **13**, 39 (1961).
179. Le Fevre, P. G., Habich, K. I., Hess, H. S., Hudson, M. R.: Phospholipid-sugar complexes in relation to cell membrane monosaccharide transport. Science **143**, 955 (1964).
180. Le Fevre, P. G., Le Fevre, M. E.: The mechanism of glucose transfer into and out of the human red cell. J. gen. Physiol. **35**, 891 (1952).
181. Le Fevre, P. G., Marshall, J. K.: Conformational specificity in a biological transport system. Amer. J. Physiol. **194**, 333 (1958).
182. Le Fevre, P. G., Marshall, J. K.: The attachment of phloretin and analogues to human erythrocytes in connection with inhibition of sugar transport. J. biol. Chem. **234**, 3022 (1959).

183. Lettvin, J. Y., Pickard, W. F., McCulloch, W. S., Pitts, W.: A theory of passive ion flux through axon membranes. Nature (Lond.) **202**, 1338 (1964).
184. Lev, A. A., Buzhinsky, E. P.: Cation specificity of the model bimolecular phospholipid membranes with incorporated valinomycin. Cytologiya **9**, 102 (1967).
185. Levine, M., Oxender, D. L., Stein, W. D.: The substrate-facilitated transport of the glucose carrier across the human erythrocyte membrane. Biochim. biophys. Acta (Amst.) **109**, 151 (1965).
186. Lewis, W. H.: Pinocytosis. Johns Hopk. Hosp. Bull. **49**, 17 (1931).
187. Ling, G. N.: A Physical Theory of the Living State. Waltham, Mass.: Blaisdell 1962.
188. Loeb, J.: Influence of the concentration of electrolytes on the electrification and the rate of diffusion of water through collodion membranes. J. gen. Physiol. **2**, 173 (1920).
189. Loeb, J.: Electrical charges of colloidal particles and anomalous osmosis. J. gen. Physiol. **4**, 463 (1922).
190. Mackay, D., Meares, P.: The electrical conductivity and electro-osmotic permeability of a cation-exchange resin. Trans. Faraday Soc. **55**, 1221 (1959).
191. Maizels, M.: Cation transfer in human red cells. In: Kleinzeller, A., Kotyk, A. (Eds.): Membrane Transport and Metabolism, p. 256. Prague: Czech. Acad. Sci. 1961.
192. Makinose, M., Hasselbach, W.: ATP synthesis by the reverse of the sarcoplasmic calcium pump. FEBS Letters **12**, 271 (1971).
193. Masotti, L., Lenaz, G., Spisni, A.: Effect of phospholipids on the protein conformation in the inner mitochondrial membranes. Biochem. biophys. Res. Commun. **56**, 892 (1974).
194. Mawe, R. C., Hempling, H. G.: The exchange of ^{14}C glucose across the membrane of the human erythrocyte. J. cell. comp. Physiol. **66**, 95 (1965).
195. Meixner, J.: Thermodynamik der irreversiblen Prozesse. Aachen: Author 1954.
196. Meixner, J., Reik, H. G.: Thermodynamik der irreversiblen Prozesse. In: Prinzipien der Thermodynamik und Statistik. Hdb. der Physik, Vol. III/2, p. 413. Berlin-Göttingen-Heidelberg: Springer 1959.
197. Mengel, K.: Stofftransport durch Zellgrenzflächen. In: Metzner, U. (Ed.): Die Zelle, Struktur und Funktion, p. 286. Stuttgart: Wiss. Verlagsgesellschaft 1966.
198. Metzner, U. (Ed.): Die Zelle, Struktur und Funktion. Stuttgart: Wiss. Verlagsgesellschaft 1966.
199. Meyer, K. H., Sievers, J.-F.: La perméabilité des membranes. I. Théorie de la perméabilité ionique. Helv. chim. Acta **19**, 649 (1936).
200. Meyer, K. H., Sievers, J.-F.: La perméabilité des membranes. II. Essais avec des membranes sélectives artificielles. Helv. chim. Acta **19**, 665 (1936).
201. Meyer, K. H., Sievers, J.-F.: La perméabilité des membranes. IV. Analyse de la structure de membranes végétales et animales. Helv. chim. Acta **19**, 987 (1936).
202. Mitchell, P.: Structure and function in microorganisms. In: Structure and Function of Subcellular Components. Proc. 16th Biochem. Soc. Symp., London 1957, p. 73. London-New York: Cambridge University Press 1959.
203. Mitchell, P.: Biological transport phenomena and the spatially anisotropic characteristics of enzyme systems causing a vector component of metabolism. In: Kleinzeller, A., Kotyk, A. (Eds.): Membrane Transport and Metabolism, p. 22. Prague: Czech. Acad. Sci. 1961.
204. Mitchell, P.: Coupling of phosphorylation to electron and hydrogen transfer by a chemo-osmotic type of mechanism. Nature (Lond.) **191**, 144 (1961).
205. Mitchell, P.: Molecule, group, and electron translocation through natural membranes. Biochem. Soc. Symp. **22**, 142 (1963).
206. Mitchell, P.: Chemiosmotic coupling in oxidative and photosynthetic phosphorylation. Biol. Rev. **41**, 445 (1966).
207. Moore, C., Pressman, B. C.: Mechanism of action of valinomycin on mitochondria. Biochem. biophys. Res. Commun. **15**, 562 (1964).
208. Morgan, H. E., Regen, D. M., Park, C. R.: Identification of a mobile carrier mediated sugar transport system in muscle. J. biol. Chem. **239**, 369 (1964).
209. Mossberg, S. M., Ross, G.: Ammonia movement in the small intestine: Preferential transport by the ileum. J. clin. Invest. **46**, 490 (1967).

210. Moszynski, J. R., Hoshiko, T., Lindley, B. D.: Note on the Curie principle. Biochim. biophys. Acta (Amst.) **75**, 447 (1963).
211. Mueller, P., Rudin, D. O.: Development of K^+-Na^+ discrimination in experimental bimolecular lipid membranes by macrocyclic antibiotics. Biochem. biophys. Res. Commun. **26**, 398 (1967).
212. Müller, E.: Aufbau und Funktion zellulärer Membranen. In: Bielka, H. (Ed.): Molekulare Biologie der Zelle. Jena: Fischer 1969.
213. Naparstek, A., Caplan, S. R., Katzir-Katchalsky, A.: Series arrays of ion-exchange membranes: Concentration profiles and rectification of electric current. Israel J. Chem. **11**, 255 (1973).
214. Naparstek, A., Thomas, D., Caplan, S. R.: An experimental enzyme-membrane oscillator. Biochim. biophys. Acta (Amst.) **323**, 643 (1973).
215. Nelles, A.: Kriterien des aktiven Transportes. Stud. biophys. **27**, 213 (1971).
216. Neumann, E.: Molekulare Hysterese und ihre kybernetische Bedeutung. Angew. Chem. **85**, 430 (1973).
217. Newey, H., Parsons, B. J., Smyth, D. H.: The site of phlorrhizin inhibition of intestinal glucose absorption. J. Physiol. (Lond.) **139**, 21P (1957).
218. Onsager, L.: Reciprocal relations in irreversible processes. I. Phys. Rev. **37**, 405 (1931).
219. Onsager, L.: Reciprocal relations in irreversible processes. II. Phys. Rev. **38**, 2265 (1931).
220. Oster, G., Perelson, A., Katchalsky, A.: Network thermodynamics. Nature (Lond.) **234**, 393 (1971).
221. Oster, G., Perelson, A., Katchalsky, A.: Network thermodynamics: Dynamic modelling of biophysical systems. Quart. Rev. Biophys. **6**, 1 (1973).
222. Osterhout, W. J. V.: How do electrolytes enter the cell? Proc. nat. Acad. Sci. (Wash.) **21**, 125 (1935).
223. Osterhout, W. J. V., Murray, J. W.: Behavior of water in certain heterogeneous systems. J. gen. Physiol. **23**, 365 (1940).
224. Pagano, R. E., Cherry, R. J., Chapman, D.: Phase transitions and heterogeneity in lipid bilayers. Science **181**, 557 (1973).
225. Papahadjopoulos, D., Cowden, M., Kimelberg, H.: Role of cholesterol in membranes. Effects on phospholipid-protein interactions, membrane permeability and enzymatic activity. Biochim. biophys. Acta (Amst.) **330**, 8 (1973).
226. Pappenheimer, J. R.: Passage of molecules through capillary walls. Physiol. Rev. **33**, 387 (1953).
227. Pardee, A. B.: Porification and properties of a sulfate-binding protein from Salmonella typhimurum. J. biol. Chem. **241**, 5886 (1966).
228. Pardee, A. B.: Biochemical studies on active transport. J. gen. Physiol. **52**, 2795 (1968).
229. Pardee, A. B.: Membrane transport proteins. Science **162**, 632 (1968).
230. Park, C. R., Crofford, O. B., Kono, T.: Mediated (nonactive) transport of glucose in mammalian cells and its regulation. J. gen. Physiol. **52**, 2965 (1968).
231. Park, C. R., Post, R. L., Kalman, C. F., Wright, J. H., Jr., Johnson, L. H., Morgan, H. E.: The transport of glucose and other sugars across cell membranes and the effect of insulin. In: Wolstenholme, G. E. W., O'Connor, C. M. (Eds.): Internal Secretions of the Pancreas (Ciba Foundation Colloquia on Endocrinology, Vol. 9). London: Churchill 1956, p. 240.
232. Park, C. R., Reinwein, D., Henderson, M. J., Cadenas, E., Morgan, H. E.: The action of insulin on the transport of glucose through the cell membrane. Amer. J. Med. **26**, 647 (1959).
233. Passow, H.: Passive ion permeability of the erythrocyte membrane. Progr. Biophys. molec. Biol. **19**, Part 2, 425 (1969).
234. Pedersen, C. J.: Ionic complexes of macrocyclic polyethers. Fed. Proc. **27**, 1305 (1968).
235. Peers, A. M.: Electrodialysis using ion-exchange membranes. II. Demineralization of solutions containing amino-acids. J. appl. Chem. **8**, 59 (1958).
236. Peusner, L.: The principles of network thermodynamics: Theory and biophysical applications. Ph. D. Thesis. Harvard University, Cambridge, Mass. 1970.
237. Piperno, J. R., Oxender, D. L.: Amino-acid-binding protein released from Escherichia coli by osmotic shock. J. biol. Chem. **241**, 5732 (1966).
238. Politoff, A. L., Socolar, S. J., Loewenstein, W. R.: Permeability of a cell membrane junction. Dependence on energy metabolism. J. gen. Physiol. **53**, 498 (1969).

239. Prigogine, I.: Étude Thermodynamique des Phénomènes irréversibles. Paris: Dunod; Liège: Desoer 1947.
240. Prigogine, I.: Introduction to Thermodynamics of Irreversible processes. Springfield, Ill.: Thomas 1955.
241. Prigogine, I., Lefever, R.: Symmetry breaking instabilities in dissipative systems. II. J. chem. Phys. **48**, 1695 (1968).
242. Prigogine, I., Nicolis, G.: On symmetry-breaking instabilities in dissipative systems. J. chem. Phys. **46**, 3542 (1967).
243. Redwood, W. R., Gibbes, D. C., Thompson, T. E.: Interaction of a solubilized membrane ATPase with lipid bilayer membranes. Biochim. biophys. Acta (Amst.) **318**, 10 (1973).
244. Redwood, W. R., Weis, P.: Interaction of a solubilized membrane ATPase with aqueous dispersions of bilayer lipid membranes. Biochim. biophys. Acta (Amst.) **332**, 11 (1974).
245. Regen, D. M., Morgan, H. E.: Studies of the glucose transport system in the rabbit erythrocyte. Biochim. biophys. Acta (Amst.) **79**, 151 (1964).
246. Regen, D. M., Tarpley, H. L.: Anomalous transport kinetics and the glucose carrier hypothesis. Biochim. biophys. Acta (Amst.) **339**, 218 (1974).
247. Rogers, A. I., Bachorik, P. S., Nunn, A. S.: Neomycin effects on glucose transport by rat small intestine. Digestion **1**, 159 (1968).
248. Roseman, S.: The transport of carbohydrates by a bacterial phosphotransferase system. J. gen. Physiol. **54**, 138s (1969).
249. Rosen, B. P.: Basic amino acid transport in Escherichia coli. J. biol. Chem. **246**, 3653 (1971).
250. Rosenberg, T.: Membrane transport of sugars. A survey of kinetical and chemical approaches. Path. et Biol. **9**, 795 (1961).
251. Rosenberg, T., Vestergaard-Bogind, B., Wilbrandt, W.: Modellversuch zur Trägerhypothese von Zuckertransporten. Helv. physiol. pharmacol. Acta **14**, 334 (1956).
252. Rosenberg, T., Wilbrandt, W.: The kinetics of membrane transports involving chemical reactions. Exp. Cell Res. **9**, 49 (1955).
253. Rosenberg, T., Wilbrandt, W.: Uphill transport induced by counter-flow. J. gen. Physiol. **41**, 289 (1957).
254. Rothstein, A.: Membrane phenomena. Ann. Rev. Physiol. **30**, 15 (1968).
255. Rubinstein, L. I.: On the sorption-diffusion model of the membrane transport of non-electrolytes. Citologija **15**, 519 (1973).
256. Schanker, L. S.: Passage of drugs across body membranes. Pharmacol. Rev. **14**, 501 (1962).
257. Schanker, L. S., Tocco, D. J., Brodie, B. B., Hogben, C. A. M.: Absorption of drugs from the rat small intestine. J. Pharmacol. exp. Ther. **123**, 81 (1958).
258. Schlögl, R.: Stofftransport durch Membranen (Fortschritte der physikalischen Chemie **9**). Darmstadt: Steinkopff 1964.
259. Scholefield, P. G.: The role of adenosine triphosphate in transport reactions. Canad. J. Biochem. **42**, 917 (1964).
260. Schön, R.: Äußere Zellabgrenzungen. In: Bielka, H. (Ed.): Molekulare Biologie der Zelle. Jena: Fischer 1969.
261. Schumaker, V. N.: Uptake of protein from solution by Amoeba proteus. Exp. Cell Res. **15**, 314 (1958).
262. Shami, Y., Messer, H. H., Copp, D. H.: Calcium binding to placental plasma membranes as measured by rate of diffusion in a flow dialysis system. Biochim. biophys. Acta (Amst.) **339**, 323 (1974).
263. Shashoua, V. E.: Electrically active polyelectrolyte membranes. Nature (Lond.) **215**, 846 (1967).
264. Shaw, F. H., Simon, S. E., Johnstone, B. M., Holman, M. E.: The effect of changes of environment on the electrical and ionic pattern of muscle. J. gen. Physiol. **40**, 263 (1956).
265. Siekevitz, P.: On the wearing of intracellular structure for metabolic regulation. In: Wolstenholme, G. E. W., O'Connor, C. M. (Eds.): Foundation Symposium on Regulation of Cell Metabolism. London: Churchill 1959, p. 17.
266. Simon, W., Morf, W. E.: Alkali cation specificity of carrier antibiotics and their behavior in bulk membranes. In: Eisenman, G. (Ed.): Membranes. Lipid Bilayer in Antibiotics, Vol. 2, Chapt. 4. p. 329. New York: Dekker 1973.

267. Simoni, R. D.: Macromolecular characterization of bacterial transport systems. In: Fox, F., Keith, A. D. (Eds.): Membrane Molecular Biology, p. 289. Stamford: Sinauer 1972.
268. Simons, R.: A thermodynamic analysis of particle flow through biological membranes. Biochim. biophys. Acta (Amst.) **173**, 34 (1969).
269. Skou, J. C.: The relationship of a $(Mg^{2+} + Na^+)$-activated, K^+-stimulated enzyme or enzyme system to the active, linked transport of Na^+ and K^+ across the cell membrane. In: Kleinzeller, A., Kotyk, A. (Eds.): Membrane Transport and Metabolism, p. 228. Prague: Czech. Acad. Sci. 1961.
270. Skou, J. C.: Enzymatic basis for active transport of Na^+ and K^+ across cell membranes. Physiol. Rev. **45**, 596 (1965).
271. Sollner, K., Dray, S., Grim, E., Nethof, R.: Electrochemical studies with model membranes: In: Clarke, H. T. (Ed.): Ion Transport across Membranes, p. 144. New York: Academic Press 1954.
272. Söllner, K.: Zur Klärung der abnormen Osmose an nicht quellbaren Membranen. (Part 1). Z. Elektrochem. angew. phys. Chem. **36**, 36 (1930).
273. Söllner, K.: Zur Klärung der abnormen Osmose an nicht quellbaren Membranen. (Part 2). Z. Elektrochem. angew. Chem. **36**, 234 (1930).
274. Solomon, A. K.: Pores in the living cell. Sci. Amer. **203**, 146 (1960).
275. Solomon, A. K.: Characterisation of biological membranes by equivalent pores. J. gen. Physiol. **51**, 335^S (1968).
276. Staubesand, J.: Experimentelle elektronenmikroskopische Untersuchungen zum Phänomen der Membranvesikulation (Pinocytose). Klin. Wschr. **38**, 1248 (1960).
277. Staverman, A. J.: The theory of measurement of osmotic pressure. Rec. Trav. chim. Pays-Bas **70**, 344 (1951).
278. Staverman, A. J.: Non-equilibrium thermodynamics of membrane processes. Trans. Faraday Soc. **48**, 176 (1952).
279. Stein, W. D.: Facilitated diffusion. Recent Progr. Surface Sci. **1**, 300 (1964).
280. Stein, W. D.: The Movement of Molecules across Cell Membranes. New York-London: Academic Press 1967.
281. Stein, W. D.: Some properties of carrier substances isolated from bacterial and erythrocyte membranes. Biochem. J. **105**, 3P (1967).
282. Stein, W. D., Lieb, W. R.: A necessary simplification of the kinetics of carrier transport. Israel J. Chem. **11**, 325 (1973).
283. Stillwell, W., Winter, H. C.: The stimulation of diffusion of adenine nucleotides across bimolecular lipid membranes by divalent metal ions. Biochem. biophys. Res. Commun. **56**, 617 (1974).
284. Straub, F. B.: Kaliumakkumulation und Adenosintriphosphat. Folia Haemat. (Lpz.) **74**, 237 (1956).
285. Tasaki, I.: Nerve Excitation: A Macromolecular Approach. Springfield: Thomas 1968, p. 201.
286. Tasaki, I., Takenaka, T., Yamagishi, S.: Abrupt depolarization and bi-ionic action potentials in internally perfused squid giant axons. Amer. J. Physiol. **215**, 152 (1968).
287. Teorell, T.: An attempt to formulate a quantitative theory of membrane permeability. Proc. Soc. exp. Biol. (N.Y.) **33**, 282 (1935).
288. Teorell, T.: Discussion. The Properties and Functions of Membranes, Natural and Artificial, p. 911. Trans. Faraday Soc. **33**, 1053 and 1086 (1937).
289. Teorell, T.: Transport process and electrical phenomona in ionic membranes. Progr. Biophys. **3**, 305 (1953).
290. Teorell, T.: Transport phenomena in membranes. Discuss. Faraday Soc. **21**, 9 (1956).
291. Teorell, T.: A contribution to the knowledge of rhythmical transport processes of water and salts. Exp. Cell Res. Suppl. **3**, 339 (1955).
292. Teorell, T.: Elektrokinetic membrane processes in relation to properties of excitable tissues. I. Experiments on oscillatory transport phenomena in artificial membranes, and II. Some theoretical considerations. J. gen. Physiol. **42**, 831, 847 (1959).
293. Teorell, T.: Oscillatory electrophoresis in ion exchange membranes. Ark. Kemi **18**, 401 (1961).

294. Troschin, A. S.: Das Problem der Zellpermeabilität. Jena: Fischer 1958.
295. Troschin, A. S.: Sorption properties of protoplasm and their role in cell permeability. In: Kleinzeller, A., Kotyk, A. (Eds.): Membrane Transport and Metabolism, p. 45. Prague: Czech. Acad. Sci. 1961.
296. Träuble, H., Eibl, H.: Electrostatic effects in lipid phase transitions: Membrane structure and ionic environment. Proc. nat. Acad. Sci. (Wash.) 71, 214 (1974).
297. Tsofina, L. M., Liberman, E. A., Babakov, A. V.: Production of bimolecular protein-lipid membranes in aqueous solution. Nature (Lond.) 212, 681 (1966).
298. Uribe, E. G.: ATP synthesis driven by a K^+-valinomycin-induced charge imbalence across chloroplast grana membranes. FEBS Letters 36, 143 (1973).
299. Ussing, H. H.: The active transport through the isolated frog skin in the light of tracer studies. Acta physiol. scand. 17, 1 (1949).
300. Ussing, H. H.: Distinction by means of tracers between active transport and diffusion. The transfer of iodide across the isolated frog skin. Acta physiol. scand. 19, 43 (1949).
301. Ussing, H. H.: Some aspects of the application of tracers in permeability studies. Advanc. Enzymol. 13, 21 (1952).
302. Ussing, H. H.: Ionic movements in cell membranes in relation to the activity of the nervous system. Proc. 4th Int. Congr. Biochem., Vienna 1958, Vol. 3, p. 1. Oxford: Pergamon 1959,
303. Ussing, H. H.: The alkali metal ions in biology. I. The alkali metal ions in isolated systems and tissues. (= Hdb. exp. Pharmakol. Vol. 13, p. 1). Berlin-Göttingen-Heidelberg: Springer 1960.
304. Ussing, H. H., Zerahn, K.: Active transport of sodium as the source of the electric current in the short-circuited isolated frog skin. Acta physiol. scand. 23, Suppl. 80, 110 (1951).
305. Vaidhyanathan, V. S., Perkins, W. H.: On the permeability of nonelectrolytes through biological membranes. J. theor. Biol. 7, 329 (1964).
306. Vidaver, G. A.: The inhibition of parallel flux and augmentation of counter flux shown by transport models not involving a mobile carrier. J. theor. Biol. 10, 301 (1966).
307. Wallach, D. F. H., Gordon, A. S.: Lipid-protein interactions in cellular membranes. In: Järnefelt, J. (Ed.): Regulatory Functions of Biological Membranes (= BBA Library, Vol. 11, p. 87). Amsterdam: Elsevier 1968.
308. Weiss, D. E.: Energy-transducing reactions in biological Membranes. I. Energy transducing in ion- and electron-exchange polymers. Aust. J. biol. Sci. 22, 1337 (1969).
309. Weiss, D. E.: Energy-transducing reactions in biological Membranes. II. A molecular mechanism for the permeability changes in nerve during the passage of an action potential. Aust. J. biol. Sci. 22, 1355 (1969).
310. Weiss, D. E.: Energy-transducing reactions in biological membranes. V. A model of oxidative phosphorylation and ion accumulation in mitochondria based on a thioacylation mechanism. Aust. J. biol. Sci. 22, 1389 (1969).
311. Whittam, R., Wheeler, K. P.: Transport across cell membranes. Ann. Rev. Physiol. 32, 21 (1970).
312. Widdas, W. F.: Inability of diffusion to account for placental glucose transfer in the sheep and consideration of the kinetics of a possible carrier transfer. J. Physiol. (Lond.) 118, 23 (1952).
313. Widdas, W. F.: Kinetics of glucose transfer across the human erythrocyte membrane. J. Physiol. (Lond.) 120, 23p (1953).
314. Widdas, W. F.: Facilitated transfer of hexose across the human erythrocyte membrane. J. Physiol. (Lond.) 125, 163 (1954).
315. Wilbrandt, W.: The significance of the structure of a membrane for its selective permeability. J. gen. Physiol. 18, 933 (1935).
316. Wilbrandt, W.: Die Permeabilität der roten Blutkörperchen für einfache Zucker. Pflügers Arch. ges. Physiol. 241, 302 (1938).
317. Wilbrandt, W.: Die Wirkung des Phlorizins auf die Permeabilität der menschlichen Erythrocyten für Glukose und Pentosen. Helv. physiol. pharmacol. Acta 5, C64 (1947).

318. Wilbrandt, W.: Permeabilitätsprobleme. Naunyn-Schmiedebergs Arch. exp. Path. Pharmak. **212**, 9 (1950).
319. Wilbrandt, W.: Secretion and transport of non-electrolytes. Symp. Soc. exp. Biol. **8**, 136 (1954).
320. Wilbrandt, W.: Permeabilität, aktiver Transport und Trägermechanismus. Dtsch. med. Wschr. **82**, 1153 (1957).
321. Wilbrandt, W.: Permeability and transport systems in living cells. J. Pharm. Pharmacol. **11**, 65 (1959).
322. Wilbrandt, W.: Zuckertransporte. In: Biochemie des aktiven Transports, p. 112. Berlin: Springer 1961.
323. Wilbrandt, W., Rosenberg, T.: Weitere Untersuchungen über die Glukosepenetration durch die Erythrocytenmembran. Helv. physiol. pharmacol. Acta **8**, C82 (1950).
324. Wilbrandt, W., Rosenberg, T.: Die Kinetik des enzymatischen Transports. Helv. physiol. pharmacol. Acta **9**, C86 (1951).
325. Wilbrandt, W., Rosenberg, T.: The concept of carrier transport and its corollaries in pharmacology. Pharmacol. Rev. **13**, 109 (1961).
326. Winkler, H. H., Wilson, T. H.: The role of energy coupling in the transport of β-galactosides by Escherichia coli. J. biol. Chem. **241**, 2200 (1966).
327. Wittekind, D.: Pinozytose. Naturwissenschaften **50**, 270 (1963).
328. Wohlfarth-Bottermann, K. E., Stockem, W.: Pinocytose und Bewegung von Amöben. II. Permanente und induzierte Pinocytose bei Amoeba proteus. Z. Zellforsch. **73**, 444 (1966).
329. Wolfe, L. S.: Cell membrane constituents concerned with transport mechanisms. Canad. J. Biochem. **42**, 971 (1964).
330. Wright, E. M., Diamond, J. M.: Effects of pH and polyvalent cations on the selective permeability of gall-bladder epithelium to monovalent ions. Biochim. biophys. Acta (Amst.) **163**, 57 (1968).
331. Zerahn, K.: Oxygen consumption and active sodium transport in the isolated and short-circuited frog skin. Acta physiol. scand. **36**, 300 (1956).
332. Zörbel, P.: Untersuchungen über den Einfluß der Stoffwechselinhibitoren auf das Adenylsäuresystem und die Pyruvatverwertung bei intakten Ehrlich-Ascites-Tumorzellen. Diss. Med. Akad. Magdeburg, 1968.
333. Caplan, S. R., Naparstek, A., Zabusky, N. J.: Chemical oscillations in a membrane. Nature (Lond.) **245**, 364 (1973).
334. Naparstek, A., Romette, J. L., Kernevez, J. P., Thomas, D.: Memory in enzyme membranes. Nature (Lond.) **249**, 490 (1974).

CHAPTER 2

Pharmacokinetics
Kinetic Aspects of Absorption, Distribution, and Elimination of Drugs

E. KRÜGER-THIEMER[1]

I. Introduction

Pharmacokinetics has been initiated by the classical paper of TEORELL in 1937 and received attention in pharmacotherapy through the monograph *Der Blutspiegel* by DOST in 1953. General interest in pharmacokinetics started early in the 1960s (KRÜGER-THIEMER, 1960a, b, RESCIGNO and SEGRE, 1961).

The present chapter on pharmacokinetics is preceded by a list of definitions of relevant basic terms, and a brief historical outline.

A. Basic Definitions

Pharmacokinetics constitutes the study of all processes involved in time-dependent concentration changes of drugs, poisons, other foreign substances, and their metabolites in human and animal bodies and in isolated tissues and their description by mathematical equations. Most of the experimental procedures used in this field are common to other areas of fundamental medicine, as biochemistry, clinical chemistry, physiology, experimental and clinical pharmacology, and pharmaceutical chemistry. Therefore, experimental details will be mentioned in this review as far as it seems to be necessary only for understanding of certain arguments or situations. There is a recent tendency among authors not actively engaged in pharmacokinetics to use this term for anything being modern or progressive in pharmacology. This is an inappropriate misuse of the term pharmacokinetics which should be restricted to the mathematical treatment of concentration changes and their physicochemical and biochemical causes. Therefore, this term should be clearly discriminated from other terms, as *pharmacodynamics*, which is used for the study of drug action on the body or its parts.

Pharmacodynamics deal with the action of drugs on the body and pharmacokinetics with the rate processes of the action of the body on the drugs. In the following fields pharmacokinetics may be of use:

a) *clinical pharmacology*, which deals with quantitative aspects of drugs in the clinical situation and in which pharmacokinetics may be used as one of the tools, b) *biochemical* and *molecular pharmacology*, which deals with action of drugs on biochemical and enzymatic processes in the body, the interaction of drug molecules with receptors and other molecular processes, c) *biopharmaceutics* (WAGNER, 1961,

---

[1]   Dr. E. Krüger-Thiemer died suddenly in 1969. The manuscript left by him has been organized into the present form by the editor.

1971; LEVY, 1963) which is the study of the influence of dosage forms on the therapeutic and toxic activity of a drug, and d) *biostatistics* (GOLDSTEIN, 1964).

Definitions of basic terms, used in pharmacokinetics, are following in alphabetical order.

Absorption — the transport from the site of administration into the general circulation, e.g., intestinal absorption.

Accumulation — Increase in the plasma or tissue concentration, i.e., the total amount of drug in the body following repetitive drug administration when intake exceeds elimination.

Activity — measure for the intensity of a certain action of a drug. See also *intrinsic activity*.

Affinity constant (K, 1/mol) — reciprocal of the *dissociation constant* of a chemical or enzymatic reaction described by the law of Mass action or the Michaelis and Menten equation.

After-effect — a biological drug effect which lasts longer than the drug concentration at the site of action, usually the result of any type of irreversible or slowly reversible reaction.

Biotransformation — chemical alteration of a drug that occurs by virtue of the sojourn of the drug in a biological system. Biotransformation, involving the chemical effects of the body on a drug, should be distinguished from *metabolism*, *detoxication*, and *pharmacodynamics*. Biotransformation constitutes one of the "driving forces" responsible for the concentration changes described in pharmacokinetics.

Biotranslocation — this uncommon term might be used for the experimental substrate of pharmacokinetics.

Catenary system — a pharmacokinetic model consisting of a chain of compartments, each of which is connected to one or two other compartment(s), namely the preceding and (or) the succesive one(s) by reversible (symmetric system) or irreversible (asymmetric system) reactions.

Ceiling — the maximum biological effect that can be induced in a tissue or body by a given drug, regardless of how large a dose is administered; it is analogous to the maximum reaction velocity of an enzymatic reaction when the enzyme is saturated with substrate.

Clearance — the ratio of the drug amount eliminated from a compartment per unit of time to the drug concentration in the compartment ($\dot{V}$, volume/time). It may be formally identified as that volume from which the drug is totally cleared in one unit of time. The term clearance has a more general meaning in that it also applies to distribution between compartments. It comprises the flow of body fluids containing the drug.

Compartment — distribution volume of anatomic or physiologic homogeneity with respect to the pharmacokinetics of a drug or one of its biotransformation products. A compartment may be identical to, for instance, the blood plasma but in general has no morphologic basis.

Concentration — ratio of drug amount to the volume of fluid in which the drug exists in true solution. *See content.*

Confidence limits — range of values of a repeatedly measured quantity or a parameter, calculated from various measured quantities, comprising a given percentage of probability that the true value lies within these limits according to the *t*-test of STUDENT.

Content — ratio of drug amount in relation to the volume of an anatomic entity or a compartment which contains the drug in different physicochemical states (e.g., unbound and bound to certain molecules).

$C \times t$ *Index* — the product of the concentration, *C*, of a drug administered to a biological system and the duration, *t*, of application required to produce a specified effect, implying an irreversible or slowly reversible reaction of the drug at the site of action.

Detoxication — a biotransformation process for a drug or poison resulting in a product of lower toxicity than that of the original substance.

Dissociation constant — (amount in molar units per volume) — ratio of the rate constants of the backward reaction and the foreward reaction as defined by the law of mass action. The MICHAELIS *constant* in the Michaelis and Menten equation may be assumed to be a dissociation constant only if the original equilibrium assumption of MICHAELIS and MENTEN (1913) is valid. See *steady state*.

Distribution — the amount of drug in various parts of the body.

Distribution coefficient — (volume per body mass) — ratio of the relative drug amount in the body (amount divided by body weight) to the drug concentration in the central compartment.

Distribution function — (volume per body mass) — a variable *distribution coefficient*, usually dependent on the drug concentration in the central or other body compartments.

Dosage flow — (amount per time) — infusion rate of a drug for continuous intravenous infusion ($\dot{D}$ or D/T).

Dosage form — the pharmaceutic preparation of a drug for therapeutic use (tablets, capsules, sterile solution, etc.).

Dosage interval (time) — time between two successive drug doses during a multiple-dose therapy (Δt).

Dosage regimen (or schedule) — the schedule of drug doses and dosage intervals for specific therapeutic use.

Dose (amount) — drug amount administered to a subject at a given time (*D*). See *dosage flow*.

Dose-effect curve — the graph which relates dose to the intensity of effect for any drug-object system.

Driving force — the physical or chemical cause for changing the drug concentration in a compartment.

Elimination — sum of metabolic and excretory processes (WIDMARK and TANDBERG, 1924) causing the disappearance of pharmacologically active drug from the body fluids.

Entrance — term used by DOST (1953, 1968) for that fraction of the plasma volume formally achieving the final drug concentration per minute (neglecting drug elimination).

Equilibrium constant — ratio of the rate constants of a process and its reversal, defining the state of zero net transfer between the two compartments or forms of the drug.

Excretion — a process causing the drug to finally leave the body.

First-order reaction — reaction in which the rate of a change in drug amount is proportional to the first power of the concentration of a drug.

Freedom, degrees of — difference between the number of measured values and the number of parameters to be calculated from the measured values.

Half-life — binary time constant, it is the period in which a time-dependent process is half way. See also *time constant of half elimination*.

Initial dose — first dose of a multiple-dose regimen of treatment, alternatively called priming or loading dose.

Intrinsic activity — the property of a drug determining the amount of biological effect produced per unit of drug-receptor complex formed (ARIËNS, 1954).

Maintenance dose — one of the doses following the initial dose in a multiple-dose regimen of treatment, designed to maintain a certain minimal or average drug concentration in blood plasma throughout the duration of therapy.

Mammillary system — multicompartment model consisting of a central compartment connected by reversible transfer reactions to a number of outer compartments, each adjacent to the central one only. The central compartment may have an irreversible exit (RESCIGNO and SEGRE, 1966).

Median effective dose — the dose of a drug predicted (by statistical techniques) to produce a characteristic effect in 50% of the subjects to whom the dose is given.

Metabolism — biotransformation of materials essential to an adequate nutritional state of the body. According to this definition the term metabolism would be inappropriate for the biotransformation of most drugs.

Parameter — variable terms of an equation that determine the overall configuration and position within the axes of the line or figure described by the equation. Parameters should be distinguished from the independent and dependent variables and from constants. In pharmacokinetic equations, parameters are the volume of distribution, rate-constants, clearance constants, and time constants.

Pharmacodynamics — the study of the action (activity) of drug in the mammalian body or other organisms.

Pharmacogenetics — the study of genetic differences of the kinetics and dynamics of drugs and related substances.

Plasma concentration — the concentration of the drug in the blood plasma, i.e., the sum of plasma protein bound and free drug concentration.

Plasma water concentration — the concentration of a drug or metabolite in the plasma ultrafiltrate also called the free drug concentration.

Plateau concentration — the concentration of a drug in the plasma or tissues finally obtained following chronic medication when, as a result of accumulation, a steady-state is reached between intake and elimination of drug (see Ceiling).

Potency — Quantitative measure for the activity of a drug, i.e., how potent is the drug.

Protein binding — binding of drug to plasma proteins or other proteins in the body.

Rate constant — a parameter governing the rate of drug translocation (per unit of time), e.g., rate constant for drug elimination, distribution, etc.

Receptor — entity of approximately the size of a drug molecule with which the drug molecule interacts in order to induce its particular effect, e.g., cholinergic receptors.

Second-order reaction — a reaction in which rate of change in drug amount is proportional to the second power of concentration, e.g., dependent on drug concentration and concentration of plasma proteins.

Steady-state — dynamic equilibrium, e.g., when intake of drug is equal to elimination and the amount in the body remains constant.

Therapeutic index — index of therapeutic efficacy often in relation to absence of toxicity.

Threshold dose, subliminal dose: The smallest dose that causes a measurable effect.

Time-concentration curve — the relation between the drug concentration in the blood plasma, or the tissues as function of time, e.g., the plasma concentration decay curve.

Time constant — the parameter governing the rate of drug translocation (in time units, e.g., hours), e.g., the time constants for elimination, distribution, etc. The time constant is the reciprocal of the rate constant.

Time of half- elimination — binary time constant of drug elimination or the period in which half the amount of drug is eliminated.

Transport function — function by which a transport process can be described, e.g., a linear differential equation.

Volume of distribution — volume of a tissue or compartment in which a drug is distributed. Also seen in relation to the concentration of drug in the central compartment, i.e., the apparent volume of distribution.

Zero-order reaction — reaction that proceeds at a constant rate independent of the drug concentration.

B. Historical Outline

Since the very beginning of drug therapy the causal relationship between the dose of a drug and its therapeutic and toxic activity has been well understood. Accordingly, PARACELSUS wrote: "...*allein die Dosis macht, daß ein Ding kein Gift ist* (...the dosis alone makes that a substance is not a poison)." Similar remarks may be found in the previous century. But only late in the second decade of this century the trend to quantitate scientific observation was introduced in the dose-concentration-activity relationships by the Swedish research worker WIDMARK (1919), to whom the credit for the first scientific approach in this field belongs, because he introduced the mathematical language to these problems. The basic ideas may be traced farther back, as shown by the first "analog computer", namely a hydrokinetic apparatus designed by BRUNTON (1899) for simulating absorption and excretion kinetics of drugs.

The use of the mathematical language is one of the causes of the rapid development of pharmacokinetics (TEORELL, 1937; DRUCKREY and KÜPFMÜLLER, 1949; DOST, 1953). But mathematical equations make the field incomprehensible for the majority of physicians. The results of developments in pharmacokinetics are applied in pharmacotherapy by the physician. It is therefore necessary that the results of pharmacokinetic calculations are conveyed to the medical profession as rules of thumb. The mathematical symbolism is a kind of convenient and effective shorthand connecting the field under study with other scientific fields, in which similar problems may have been formulated and solved by analogous equations. This refers also to mathematics itself, comprising a wealth of solved problems, waiting for their use in other fields of science.

II. Pharmacokinetic Models

Drug concentration changes in time may readily be described with data tables, graphs, or words for those body fluids and tissues in which the drug concentration may be estimated. Such descriptions of experimental data are valid under the specific experimental conditions, but do allow only qualitative conclusions or generalizations with respect to the influence of certain conditions. It is the challenge of a kinetic analysis of dose-concentration relationships of drugs to provide a description of the experimental data by meaningful parameters, which may characterize the behavior of the drugs in patients, test subjects under certain experimental conditions, and which may be used for scientific predictions, e.g., dosage regimen calculations, forecast of multiple-dose concentration curves from single-dose experiments, evaluation of the toxic risk of certain dosage regimens, etc.

The performance of a complete kinetic analysis of experimental data consists of three steps, namely:
1. Choice of a pertinent pharmacokinetic model.
2. Curve fitting of the model curve(s) to experimental data.
3. Usage of the achieved model parameters for predictions.

This review is mainly devoted to details of the first and third step of the kinetic analysis, while for the second step only brief notes and references are given. The three steps are strongly interdependent and limited by the reliability of the experimental data, the availability of computer programs, and the scope of desired predictions. It is the same philosophy which prevails in pharmacokinetics as in other fields of science. ROSSOTTI and ROSSOTTI (1961) have expressed it in their monograph on the determination of stability constants as follows: "As much care should be taken in computing the stability constants as in making the actual measurements. It is stupid to waste good experimental work by using inadequate methods of computing. The best methods are those which make the fullest use of the experimental measurements and give realistic limits of error in the stability constants obtained. On the other hand, the data should be interpreted in terms of the minimum number of parameters consistent with the precision of the measurements."

A. Choice of Models

The first step of a kinetic analysis, namely the choice of a pertinent model, is treated in a vast selection of literature (see references). A model may consist of:
1. *words* describing the process,
2. *symbols* with defined meaning,
3. *mathematical equations*,
4. *physical analogs*, e.g., hydro- and gaskinetic apparatus, electrical networks, electronic analog computers.

To describe verbally an experimental situation will often be the beginning of model building, but it will not have essential inferences unless one proceeds to a scheme of defined symbols, to the corresponding mathematical equations, and/or to physical analogs. The most important principle in the choice of a pertinent model is that physically meaningful models should be preferred and that merely phenomenologic models such as polynomials, the FREUNDLICH isotherme (1907), should be avoided. As far as possible the model building has to start with the description of the driving forces which are, or may be, responsible for the observed concentration changes in time. Most of the elementary processes, from which pharmacokinetic models may be constructed, are described by differential equations. It is hazardous to avoid the description of the driving forces, proceeding from a graphic data analysis by intuition to a mathematical relationship for the measured quantities. The result may not be much more meaningful than data fitting by a polynomial. This refers, e.g., to the common practice of fitting a sum of exponential functions to data of a decay process without assigning a physical meaning to the model parameters.

A dose-concentration relationship may be defined simply by the formal equation

$$C = F(D, t, \pi_i) = D \cdot f(t, \pi_i...) \tag{1}$$

where C is the therapeutically essential concentration of drug in the blood plasma, D is the amount of the administered dose, and $F(t, \pi_i...)$ is a function of time, t, and of one or more parameters, $\pi_i...$, which describe the pharmacokinetic properties of the drug with respect to absorption, distribution, biotransformation, and excretion. A dose-concentration relationship is linear only if the time function $F(t)$ is independent of the dose, D, and of the drug concentration in the plasma, implying that all pharmacokinetic parameters, $\pi_i...$, involved in $f(t, ...)$, are also independent of D and C or that any dependency of the parameters, $\pi_i...$, on D, and/or C cancels out because of the special form of the function $F(t, ...)$. A linear dose-concentration relationship means that the entire curve of the concentration of the drug in plasma water with respect to time would be directly proportional to the administered dose, D. Therefore, in a semilogarithmic plot, the time concentration curves for different doses would have the same shape, merely shifting up or down parallel to the logarithmic concentration axis for higher or lower doses according to Equation (2)

$$\log C = \log D + \log F(t, \pi_i, ...) . \tag{2}$$

An example is given in Figure 1 for different doses of ampicilline from data by DAEHNE et al. (1970). In general there is little proof that the function F is dose independent. For multiple-dose therapy, Equation (1) may be understood in terms of the dosage regimen theory (KRÜGER-THIEMER, 1960a, b; KRÜGER-THIEMER and BÜNGER, 1965/66a, b) assuring the maintenance of the therapeutically effective minimum concentration of the drug C_f^{min}, in plasma water. In this case, D is the maintenance dose, while the dose ratio, R^*, determining the proper initial dose, D^*, is contained in the time function $F(t, \Delta t, \pi_i, ...)$, which depends also on the chosen

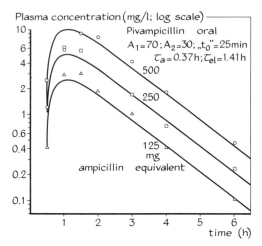

Fig. 1. Curves representing logarithm of plasma concentration of ampicilline as function of time after administration of three different doses to same subject. These curves obey equation 2 and are typical examples of linear elimination kinetics. (Data adopted from DAEHNE et al., 1970)

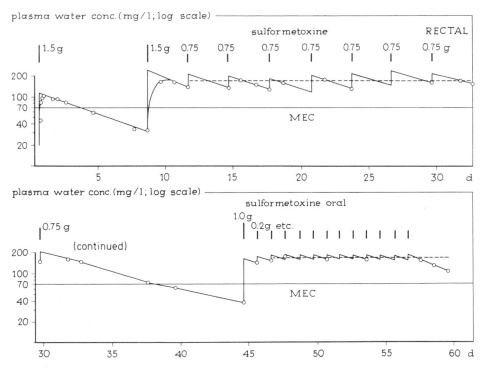

Fig. 2. Plasma concentration curves of sulfonamide following repetitive intake via two different routes. Level is directly proportional to dosage flow $(D/\Delta t)$ according to Equation (3). (Data from DILLER and BÜNGER, 1965)

dosage interval Δt, as shown in Equation (3)

$$C = D \cdot F(t, \Delta t, \pi_i, \ldots) \,. \qquad (3)$$

An example is given for different routes of administration of a sulfonamide from data by DILLER and BÜNGER, 1965 (Fig. 2) and for ampicilline from data by DAEHNE et al., 1970 (Fig. 1).

B. Critique of Models

The assumptions, on which the calculations for linear dose-concentration relationships are based, are summarized in the following:

1. Drug distribution is achieved rapidly as compared with the rate of elimination.

2. Drug elimination, comprising biotransformation and excretion, may be sufficiently described as a first-order process.

3. Drug absorption may be described as a first-order process or may be neglected because of its rapidity.

If the dose-concentration relationship is nonlinear, then the dependency of the pharmacokinetic parameters on dose and/or concentration has to be checked in experiments using different doses or dosage regimens, resulting different steady-state levels.

Thus, the experimental work for dosage regimen estimation would be much more difficult and tedious for drugs showing nonlinear rather than linear dose-concentration relationships.

If the pharmacokinetic behavior of a drug is not consistent with assumptions 1., 2., and 3., deviations from linearity of the dose-concentration relationships may be expected. From a phenomenologic viewpoint one may distinguish four cases of nonlinearity of dose-concentration relationships, namely:

1. The peak concentration will be higher with increasing dose than would be expected in the linear case. This occurs when the capacity of elimination is reached.

2. The peak concentration will be lower with increasing dose than would be expected in the linear case. This occurs when absorption is dose dependent, e.g., for ascorbic acid.

3. The nonlinearity occurs mainly in the descending branch of the curve, e.g., in case of protein binding.

4. The nonlinearity occurs mainly in the ascending branch of the curve, e.g., in case of capacity limited absorption.

For quantification of the various influences they should be (as much as possible) studied separately. Certain aspects will be discussed in the following for drug elimination, distribution, and absorption.

III. Models for Single-Dose Administration

The study of single-dose administration is used mainly as the basis for the study of multiple-dose administration. Most drugs are given repetitively as antiepileptics, sulfa-amides, etc. In certain forms of therapy single doses are given as acetosal in

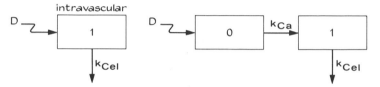

Fig. 3. Block diagram demonstrating single compartment kinetics both for intravascular and extravascular administration. Important kinetic parameters are elimination clearance constant k_{Cel} and apparent volume of distribution V_f

case of headache. But in some of these cases the concentration activity relationship is not as well understood as in the cases where multiple-dose therapy is necessary for achieving the desired therapeutic result. A possible objection to the use of single-dose studies as the basis for multiple-dose therapy is that the pharmacokinetic parameters may change during a multiple-dose therapy, so that the drug behavior in multiple-dose experiments may not be predicted from single-dose experiments. For example, the rate of metabolism of a drug may be increased by the prior administration of that drug or other structurally related and unrelated drugs (GILLETTE, 1971). Still other ways in which compounds may affect their own kinetics have been discussed by DOST (1953). However, this problem does not exist for most drugs and, therefore, the following discussions may be applied to many compounds which are nonautoreactive with respect to their pharmacokinetics.

The most simple model in which the body is comprised as a single compartment is given in Figure 3 for intravascular (i.v.) and extravascular (oral, rectal etc.) administration.

A. Intra- and Extravascular Administration

A complete pharmacokinetic model, taking into account all known processes in the most correct way, would be of no practical use because of mathematical difficulties. For special studies it is, therefore, necessary to make a choice of the experimental conditions so that the experimental data may be interpreted by meaningful models.

Considering the body as a single compartment in which the drug in a dose D is introduced momentarily (i.v. injection) leads to the following differential equation:

$$\frac{dQ_1}{dt} = -k_{Cel} \cdot C \quad \text{or} \quad \frac{dC}{dt} = \frac{k_{Cel}}{V_f} \cdot C = -k \cdot C. \tag{4}$$

Where k_{Cel} is the clearance constant governing elimination of the drug from the body, V_f is the apparent volume of distribution, and k the rate constant for elimination. Integration of equation gives:

$$C = A e^{-k \cdot t} = A e^{-t/\tau_{el}} = A 2^{-t/t_{\frac{1}{2}}}. \tag{5}$$

Where A is a dose-dependent constant representing the concentration at the moment just after injection ($t = 0$), k is the rate constant for elimination, τ_{el} the

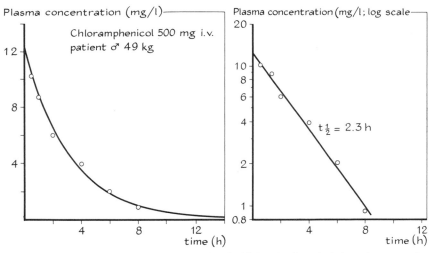

Fig. 4. Plasma concentration curves of chloramphenicol following i.v. administration. Experimental data agree well with equations 4 and 5. Elimination clearance constant is 160 ml/min and volume of distribution is about 25 l. (Data adopted from AZZOLINI et al., 1972)

time constant of elimination, and $t_{\frac{1}{2}}$ the half value time of elimination (Fig. 4). The kinetic behavior of a drug in the human body is likely to be more complex as different distribution processes are involved. In case of extravascular administration at least the absorption process has to be taken into account.

For the discussion of dose-concentration relationships, several processes are unimportant. Practical experience with dosage regimen calculations (BÜNGER, 1962; BÜNGER et al., 1961, 1964; KRÜGER-THIEMER and BÜNGER, 1965a, b) as well as theoretical reasons (KRÜGER-THIEMER, 1961) have revealed that the well-known equation of TEORELL [1937, pg. 220, Eq. (25)], widely used by DOST (1953, 1968) and others is very useful for practical purposes if one carefully interprets the included parameters and the results. This equation reads in the symbolism used in this article as follows:

$$C = A\{e^{-k \cdot t^*} - e^{k_a \cdot t^*}\} = A\{e^{-t^*/\tau_{el}} - e^{t^*/\tau_a}\} . \tag{6}$$

Where A is a dose-related coefficient being dependent on plasma protein binding, volume of distribution, etc., while $t^* = (t - t_0)$, that is, the time after administration minus the zero time shift t_0 (Fig. 5). If C is the concentration in the plasma water this coefficient may be described as follows:

$$A = \frac{D \cdot F \cdot k_a}{G \cdot d \cdot (k_a - k)} = \frac{D \cdot F}{G \cdot d} \cdot \frac{\tau_{el}}{(\tau_{el} - \tau_a)} . \tag{7}$$

Where D is the dose, F the fraction of the dose that ultimately becomes absorbed, k_a and τ_a the rate constant and time constant for absorption, k and τ_{el} the rate constant and time constant for elimination, G the weight of the subject, and d a coefficient of distribution which may be a complicated function when protein binding is involved. t^* is the time from the moment of onset of absorption. So $t^* = (t - t_0)$ if t is the time after administration and t_0 the time needed for disintegration of a tablet and the passage from stomach to intestine (Fig. 5). For details of the interpretation see the cited literature and NELSON (1961) and KRÜGER-THIEMER (1964a).

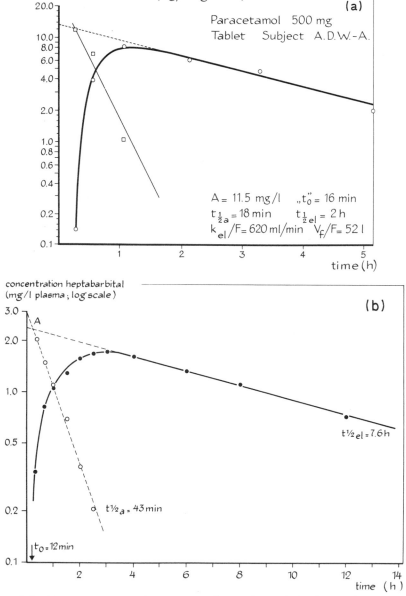

Fig. 5a and b. Plasma concentration curves of two drugs following oral administration. (a) Paracetamol (VAN GINNEKEN, 1976). (b) heptabarbital (data by BREIMER, 1974). It may be noted that absorption starts some time after administration. This is so-called zero-time-shift

B. Elimination

The disappearance of the active drug from body fluids may occur mainly in two ways, namely by biotransformation (metabolism) and by excretion through kidneys, lungs, etc. From the viewpoint of most pharmacokinetic models the drug amount within the gastrointestinal tract is considered to be "outside" of the body. Therefore that drug amount which leaves the body with the feces without having been absorbed is not considered as being eliminated. The same does not apply to drug which is lost during the enterohepatic cycle, which may or may not include biotransformation of the drug. From the following discussion all minor processes are excluded that do not substantially contribute to the change of concentration of active drug in the body fluids.

The concept of biological half-life is widely used in pharmacokinetics. However, the term "biological half-life" may be used pharmacodynamically to refer to the decay of pharmacologic or toxicologic activity. Therefore, for pharmacokinetics, a more specific term to use would be "plasma half-life" or the more general term for dose-concentration relationships, "elimination half-life." This half-life concept describes the observation that a drug concentration at zero time (exactly only after drug equilibration throughout the body fluids), falls down to half of the initial value within the time $t_{\frac{1}{2}}$. It will diminish to one-quarter of the initial value after the next time interval $t_{\frac{1}{2}}$, to one-eight of the initial value after the third interval $t_{\frac{1}{2}}$, etc. A plot of time vs. log concentration data will show a straight line. (Fig. 4). The negative slope of this straight line is directly related to the rate constant for elimination, k, and inversely related to the time constant for elimination τ_{el} which are connected with the plasma half-life, $t_{\frac{1}{2}}$ also called the time of half elimination, by the following equation:

$$\tau_{el} = 1/k \quad \text{and} \quad t_{\frac{1}{2}} = \tau_{el} \cdot \ln 2. \tag{8}$$

The rate constant for elimination, k, is the quotient of the elimination clearance or total body clearance and the volume of the central compartment, V_f from which the clearance occurs. In formula:

$$k = k_{Cel}/V_f \quad \text{and} \quad \tau_{el} = V_f/k_{Cel}. \tag{9}$$

The total body clearance comprises the renal clearance constant k_{Cr}, the metabolic clearance constant, k_{Cm}, and possible other clearance constants.

$$k_{Cel} = k_{Cm} + k_{Cr} + \cdots. \tag{10}$$

These ideas have been put forward already by WIDMARK and TANDBERG (1924).

Innumerable experiments have revealed that the concept of the elimination half-life describes with sufficient accuracy the behavior of many drugs in the blood plasma or serum. DOST (1953), v. WILBRANDT (1964), and RITSCHEL (1970) have collected half-life values of many drugs. It will be shown later that the elimination half-life is the most important pharmacokinetic parameter for dosage evaluation.

From the theoretical viewpoint the concept of the elimination half-life may be derived from FICK's law of diffusion (1855), which may be written for a system of two compartments, in which concentration gradients are negligible because of perfect mixing, separated by a thin membrane, which is permeable for the drug:

$$-\frac{dQ_1}{dt} = \frac{dQ_2}{dt} = +k_{C12}(C_1 - C_2).$$ (11)

The index denoted the body fluids and the environment of the body, connected with the body fluids by the liver and the kidney. As the drug is introduced into the body (compartment) and eliminated from it into the environment, the concentration in the second compartment may always be neglectably small, so that diffusion may occur only in one direction. In fact, clearance occurs only in one direction and the model may be simplified to a single open compartment (Figure 3). The final equation then reduces to Equation (4).

In other words, the infinitively small amount of drug, dQ_1, eliminated in the short time interval, dt, is proportional to the drug concentration C in the body fluids. Integration of this differential equation results in the well-known exponential function: Equation (12), which is the logarithm of Equation (5).

$$\ln C = \ln A - t/\tau_{el} \quad \text{or} \quad \log C = \log A - 0.301 t/t_{\frac{1}{2}}.$$ (12)

The logarithm of the concentration decreases linearly with time. Consequently the rate constant for elimination, the time constant for elimination and the half-life for elimination may be calculated from plasma decay curve (Fig. 4).

The pharmacokinetic model described by Equations (4) and (5) is symbolized in Figure 3. That is, the drug is given i.v. while the body may be regarded as a single, open compartment. This model contains another important concept, namely that of the so-called volume of distribution, denoted in Equations (4) and (9) by V_f. Under the assumptions of intravascular administration or rapid oral absorption and immediate drug equilibration between blood plasma and body fluids, the initial drug concentration will be given by

$$A = C^0 = D/V_f \quad \text{and} \quad V_f = D/A.$$ (13)

A is the apparent initial plasma concentration. If a drug preferentially accumulates in the extravascular space as muscle, body fat, etc., the concentration in the blood plasma may be very small and the volume of distribution very large. If, on the other hand, a drug preferentially binds to plasma proteins, the volume of distribution is very small provided that the blood plasma is taken as a reference point. Obviously if the plasma water is taken as a reference different volumes of distribution may be encountered. The volume of distribution could be separated into the body weight, G, and the coefficient of distribution, d, for reasons discussed in Section IV.

In general $V_f = G \cdot d$ (KRÜGER-THIEMER, 1964b, 1968e). Since the body may be considered as a single compartment when absorption and distribution occur very rapidly with regard to elimination, the volume of that compartment is equal to the apparent volume of distribution.

The coefficient of distribution has the dimension of l/kg. Under certain circumstances the coefficient of distribution, d, is fairly independent from the administered dose, D, so that d may be regarded as a pharmacokinetic parameter.

The final form of Equation (4) and (12) then becomes:

$$C = \frac{D}{G \cdot d} \cdot 2^{-t/t_{\frac{1}{2}}} \cdot \quad \text{or} \quad \log C = \log D - \log G \cdot d - 0.301\, t/t_{\frac{1}{2}} \qquad (14)$$

where 0.301 stands for $\log 2$.

This equation represents the relationship between the administered dose, D, and the drug concentration, C, in the body fluids, changing with time under the two previously mentioned assumptions. If one knows the values of half-time for elimination, the distribution coefficient, d, and the body weight, G, one may predict the drug concentration, C in the body fluids at any time, t, after the administration of the dose, D. The coefficient of distribution of a drug bound to plasma proteins may be substantially smaller than one. On the other hand, in the case of extensive tissue binding, d may be larger than one. That the actual situation is often more complicated than assumed will be shown in the following paragraphs. It may be anticipated that it is therefore advisable to call $t_{\frac{1}{2}}$ the apparent elimination half-life and d the apparent coefficient of distribution.

1. Biotransformation

The majority of drugs in common usage are biotransformed in the mammalian body but the extent of this metabolism varies widely even for drugs which are closely related structurally. From the viewpoint of dose-concentration relationships it is more important that the metabolism of a drug may vary between different individuals and during the lifetime of one individual. Some of these observations have been claimed to be caused by genetical differences (BÖNICKE and LISBOA, 1957; KALOW, 1962; MEIER, 1963), while others may be explained by enzyme maturation or by enzyme induction (REMMER, 1959). Differences of this type are one important cause of interindividual differences of the apparent elimination half-life (BÜNGER et al., 1961; SWINTOSKY, 1961).

Many metabolic processes may be described with sufficient accuracy by the simple first-order model according to Equations (5), (9), and (14), provided that the rate of metabolism is proportional to the drug concentration. The corresponding pharmacokinetic models are shown in Figure 6. The clearance constant for metabolism,

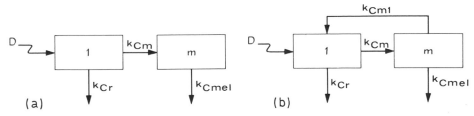

Fig. 6a and b. Block diagram representing drug elimination by renal excretion and biotransformation. (a) first order metabolism, (b) second order metabolism. The metabolite is again eliminated from body, having its own drug parameters: elimination clearance, volume of distribution and half-life

k_{Cm}, may be calculated from drug and metabolite concentrations in blood plasma (PORTWICH and BÜTTNER, 1956; KRÜGER-THIEMER, 1961) or from drug and metabolite amounts in urine (NELSON and O'REILLY, 1960, 1961). The values of clearance constants for metabolism, k_{Cm}, are more useful for research work than for practical dosage regimen evaluations, since for the latter purpose it is often unnecessary to separate k_{Cm} from k_{Cel} [Eq. (10)]. This is especially true for drugs having several metabolites whose analytical separation is difficult. In some cases the previously mentioned metabolism model is only a first approximation; for example, the acetylation of sulfa drugs is indeed a reversible process (KREBS et al., 1947), while tolbutamide (NELSON et al., 1962), ethanol (LINDQUIST and WOLTHERS, 1958; WAGNER and PATEL, 1972), and salicylic acid (LEVY, 1965a) are oxidized by the human body with an apparent zero-order reaction. For some purposes it suffices to know the fraction, f, of the given (or absorbed) dose, that is excreted into urine unchanged (NELSON and O'REILLY, 1960):

$$amount\ excreted\ \text{dose} = f = k_{Cr}/k_{Cel} = k_{Cr}/(k_{Cr} + k_{Cm}).\qquad(15)$$

This implies that if the renal clearance is known the total body clearance and the metabolic clearance can be determined. In these cases the apparent plasma half-life of the drugs does not depend on the dose of the drug. The above type of description has been successfully used by many authors (e.g., for sulfa drug acetylation by PORTWICH and BÜTTNER, 1956; NELSON and O'REILLY, 1960, 1961) but it should be understood as an approximation, because enzymatic reactions, which in most cases mediate the biotransformation, are neither irreversible nor truly monomolecular processes.

The acetylation of sulfa drugs is known to be a reversible process (KREBS et al., 1947; SMITH and WILLIAMS, 1948; ROEPKE et al., 1957). The second model of Figure 6 is designed for the description of such processes. The differential equations of this model and of their solutions have been given by KRÜGER-THIEMER (1961, pp. 353–356) and RESCIGNO and SEGRE (1961, 1966, pp. 27–29). The equation for the drug concentration in plasma water c_f, in this model corresponds formally to Equation (5). Therefore the dose-concentration relationship of a drug, the kinetic behavior of which may be described with sufficient accuracy by this reversible model, is supposed to be linear. But this model does not account for the saturability of enzymatic reactions.

The equation of MICHAELIS and MENTEN (1913) has been used for the description of metabolic reactions (TEPHLY et al., 1964; LEVY, 1965b; LEVY and MATSUZAWA, 1967; LEVY et al., 1969a, b) because it accounts for the saturability of metabolic reactions. But one should bear in mind, that this equation assumes irreversibility of the reaction. This assumption may be a valid approximation of the real situation if the reverse reaction is much slower than removal of drug from the body fluid. In this respect it may be noted that many biotransformations, carried out by enzymes of the intermediary metabolism of body constituents or nutrients, tend to make the substances more polar and more soluble in water than in lipids, thereby enhancing renal excretion of the metabolites.

Since the rate of biotransformation may be reasonably well described by the Michaelis-Menten equation, the rate of elimination of drug may be described in the following equation:

$$\frac{dQ}{dt} = -\frac{\dot{Q}_m + C}{C + K_M} - k_{Cr}C.$$ (16)

Where the first term is the Michaelis Menten term which introduces a nonlinear aspect. (See also Chap. 3 by VAN ROSSUM in this volume.) Its solution, which has been given by LUNDQUIST and WOLTHERS (1958) is implicit with respect to the drug concentration, C. This equation is also transcendental for the initial drug concentration, $A = D/V_f$. Therefore, it obviously does not correspond to Equation (12), i.e., the dose-concentration relationship of this is nonlinear.

The model has some interesting properties. For drug concentrations, C, much lower than Michaelis constant, K_M, it approaches the linear model [Eq. (4)] and shows the expected first-order decay function with the rate constant for elimination of Equations (5), (12). The other extreme is the situation where the concentration greatly exceeds the dissociation constant K_M. In this case elimination is zero order provided that renal clearance is neglectable in formula:

$$\frac{dQ}{dt} = -\dot{Q}_m - k_{Cr}C.$$ (17)

When renal elimination may be neglected, $(k_{Cr} \rightarrow 0)$ integration of Equation (17) yields the following equation:

$$C = A - \frac{\dot{Q}_m}{V_f} \cdot t.$$ (18)

This result has an important consequence. If one finds a nearly linear drug elimination (zero-order decay of the concentration curve in plasma) for an appreciable duration of time, then this means that an irreversible and saturable metabolism process, is the main route of elimination and that other routes, e.g., renal excretion, are negligible. This seems to apply to the data of LARSEN (1963a, b) on the elimination of ethanol and glycerol, even though ethanol is excreted by the kidneys, too. (The renal clearance is very small.)

According to the MICHAELIS and MENTEN (1913), equation a kinetic process displays competitive inhibition by other drugs or intermediate metabolites which may undergo the same biotransformation, as shown for tolbutamide by NELSON et al. (1962), ethanol by LUNDQUIST and WOLTERS (1958) and for salicylic and benzoic acids competing for glycerine (LEVY and AMSEL, 1966). LEVY (1965a) has drawn attention to the possibility of simultaneous apparent zero-and first-order kinetics occurring in the in vivo formation of a single drug metabolite. This may be due to the formation of that metabolite by two different tissues. In such a case it is likely that, at sufficiently high drug concentration in body fluids, biotransformation in one tissue proceeds at maximum rate while the same process in another tissue follows apparent first-order kinetics. Such a dissociation of the order of reaction rate may occur, if the Michaelis constants of the process in the two tissues differ appreciably from each other.

2. Renal Excretion

The second component of drug elimination is excretion, and the major role in excretion is carried out by the kidneys. Renal excretion of drugs is generally described with sufficient accuracy as an irreversible first-order process (WIDMARK and TANDBERG, 1924; TEORELL, 1937; DOST, 1953; and many others) according to the model of Figure 6. This is in some respects surprising, since the clearance constant for renal excretion, k_{Cr}, stands up for three different processes, namely glomerular filtration, tubular secretion, and/or tubular reabsorption.

So the renal clearance, k_{Cr}, consists of the glomerular filtration rate, $\dot{V}_{gl}$, the tubular secretion rate, $\dot{V}_{ts}$, and the negative tubular reabsorption rate, $\dot{V}_{ra}$:

$$k_{Cr} = \dot{V}_{gl} + \dot{V}_{ts} - \dot{V}_{ra} . \tag{19}$$

The three constituents of renal clearance are subject to changes by several physiologic conditions which may influence the rate of renal excretion of the drug. Up to now a full quantitative understanding of all renal functions has not been achieved. However, interesting models for several partial functions are known (e.g., WALSER, 1966a, b; WOOLF et al., 1966; KOIZUMI et al., 1964). Some of the more important influences on renal excretion of drugs may be explained using a model of KRÜGER-THIEMER and BÜNGER (1965), which is a generalization of the model of KOIZUMI et al. (1964) (see also KRÜGER-THIEMER, 1968b). The tubular secretion may be described by the Michaelis-Menten equation:

$$\dot{V}_{ts} = T_m/(K_{ts} + C) \tag{20}$$

where T_m is the maximal tubular secretion rate (e.g., mg/min) and K_{ts} the dissociation constant (e.g., mg/ml). The generalized model corresponds to the following equation:

$$\dot{V}_{ra} = \bar{V}_{ra} \cdot P_a \left[\frac{\dot{V}_{gl} + \dot{V}_{ts}}{\dot{V}_u(1 + Q_u)} - \frac{1}{(1 + Q_{pl})} \right] \tag{21}$$

where $\bar{V}_{ra}$ is a drug independent renal reabsorption flow (dependent on bloodflow), P_a the partition-coefficient of the neutral form, $\dot{V}_u$ the urinary production rate, and $1/(1 + Q_u)$ and $1/(1 + Q_{pl})$ the fraction of neutral drug in relation to total drug concentration in the primary urine and the blood plasma, respectively (KRÜGER-THIEMER, 1968b).

$$Q_u = 10^{pH_u - pK_a} \quad \text{and} \quad Q_{pl} = 10^{7.4 - pK_a} \tag{22}$$

where pH_u is urine pH and K_a the dissociation of the acidic drug. This model is derived from the following assumptions:

1. The glomerular filtration rate of the drug is identical with the glomerular filtration rate, $\dot{V}_{gl}$, of the plasma water, usually measured as the inulin clearance. This includes the assumption that the rate of glomerular filtration of the drug is proportional to the concentration, C_f, of the freely dissolved drug in plasma water (not bound to proteins).

2. The tubular secretion of the drug is assumed to be an active process which may be described by a Michaelis-Menten term, characterized by the dissociation constant of the drug-enzyme complex, K_{ts}, and by the maximum secretion rate, T_m.

3. According to KOIZUMI et al. (1964) (cf. PITTS, 1963, p. 113), it is assumed that nearly all water reabsorption ($\dot{V}_{gl} - \dot{V}_u$) occurs before the site of the passive reabsorption in the collecting tube. Thereby the initial drug concentration, C_f, in the glomerular filtrate is enlarged by the tubular secretion and multiplied by the water reabsorption (factor $(\dot{V}_{gl} + \dot{V}_{ts})/\dot{V}_u$).

4. The drug reabsorption is assumed to be a passive process which may be described by FICK's law of diffusion (1855) according to KOIZUMI et al. (1964). This process is characterized by the permeability constant for reabsorption, $\bar{V}_{ra} \cdot P_a$, having the dimension of a clearance.

5. In addition to the foregoing it is assumed that only the nonionized molecules of the drug are able to permeate through the tubule cells. That is supported by observations of PORTNOFF et al., 1961; KOSTENBAUDER et al., 1962; DETTLI and SPRING, 1964; BECKETT et al., 1965; and others on the dependency of the renal excretion rate of weak acids and bases from urinary pH, which changes diurnally between pH 5 and pH 7 (BECKETT et al., 1965).

For example, although assumption 2 is correct for most drugs, some organic bases may be secreted by nonionic diffusion. Naturally, this model is merely a first approximation to the much more complicated renal processes. The large pH difference which may exist between plasma and acid urine theoretically allows for secretion of organic bases to occur by nonionic diffusion alone. Ammonia formed in the tubular cells also is secreted by diffusion into the tubular urine. Drug reabsorption, assumed to be a passive process in assumption 4, has been shown to be active for at least some compounds, i.e., uric acid. Despite the exceptions, this model is useful since it points out the direction of the glomerular filtration rate, the renal clearance by influences, the water reabsorption, the specifity and the maximum rate of tubular secretion, and the pH changes. These processes may be altered artificially or by pathologic situations. Therefore all of these processes are important for the dose-concentration relationship under drug therapy. KOIZUMI et al. (1964) have used a similar relation as pointed out in Equations 19–22. They did not take into account protein binding, tubular secretion, and pH influences. Under such conditions the following equation is obtained:

$$k_{Cr} = \dot{V}_{gl} - \dot{V}_{ra} \cdot P_a \left(\frac{\dot{V}_{gl}}{\dot{V}_u} - 1 \right) \tag{23}$$

According to this equation, KOIZUMI et al. (1964) have tried to describe the relationship between the clearance constant, k_{Cr}, the glomerular filtration rate, and the rate of drug reabsorption in the distal tubules, as influenced by the glomerular filtration rate and the water reabsorption rate ($k_{gl} - \dot{V}_u$).

In this model the drug reabsorption is described by the diffusion law of FICK (1855). They found a good correlation between corrected renal clearance and the partition coefficient in chloroform: buffer pH 5 for a series of sulfa drugs.

For the current discussion it is only necessary to note that the renal clearance, k_{Cr}, will be constant, if the glomerular filtration rate, $\dot{V}_{gl}$, the urinary flow, $\dot{V}_u$, and the urinary pH are kept constant and if no tubular secretion occurs, or if tubular secretion occurs at concentrations when C_f is small with respect to k_{ts}. Changes of the first three conditions will cause a dependency on drug concentration in plasma water, C_f. Wagner (1967) has extended the equations derived by Krüger-Thiemer and Bünger (1965) so that it might describe also the tubular reabsorption of ionized molecules. The only example given is phenol red.

3. Extrarenal Excretion

Enterohepatic cycle. The excretion of drugs, vitamins, and other substances by the liver is a well-known phenomenon (see Jusko and Levy, 1967). Because bile production and gallbladder emptying depend on ingestion of certain foods and on psychic influences, it is difficult to describe these processes by mathematical equations (Fig. 7). This difficulty becomes somewhat less, however, for experiments carried out with the rat since this animal has no gallbladder and, therefore, the emptying of this organ does not have to be taken into consideration. If the compound may be absorbed from the small intestine, this may occur also after hepatic excretion resulting in enterohepatic cycling of the drug. Jusko and Levy (1967) have shown that this may cause a second maximum of urinary excretion of riboflavin. Even when the drug is conjugated in the liver to form a less lipoid soluble material, enterohepatic cycling may occur because the conjugate may be acted upon by intestinal bacteria to yield the active drug which is then reabsorbed.

Recently, the pharmacokinetic behavior of a new rifamycin derivative has been studied (Keberle et al., 1967). This group of antibiotics is known to be excreted mainly by the liver. It turned out that in a study with single doses from 100 to 900 mg of rifamycin per person, the apparent half-lives of elimination, $t\frac{1}{2}$, increased from 1.53 to 5.28 h and the plasma distribution coefficient, d, decreased from 0.784 to 0.447 ml/g with increasing doses. Up to now no explanation for this behavior is available. It may, however, be that with increasing dose the

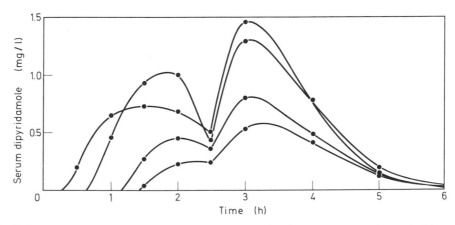

Fig. 7. Serum curves of dipyridamole. A second peak in plasma concentration coincides with emptying of gallbladder because of fatty meal. (Reproduced from Mellinger and Bohorfoush (1966) with permission of authors and publishers of Arch. int. Pharmacodyn)

capacity of the excretion systems is reached. Obviously, the dose-concentration relationship of rifamycin is nonlinear, therefore it is difficult to apply the dosage regimen theory to this drug.

C. Distribution

The dose regimen theory for linear dose-concentration relationships is based on three assumptions:

1. An uniform drug distribution is achieved rapidly as compared with the rate of drug elimination.

2. Drug elimination, comprising biotransformation and excretion, may be sufficiently described as a first-order process.

3. Drug absorption may be described as a first-order process or may be neglected because of its rapidity.

For studying drug distribution separately, assumption (2) should hold as closely as possible and drug absorption should be momentary by usage of intravenous administration. Deviations of assumption (1), underlying the dosage regimen theory, may occur with respect to deviations of the uniformity of the drug distribution.

As early as 1923 SCHADE and MENSCHEL pointed out that body water is the only medium of distribution for many drugs. From a physiologic viewpoint the body water may be subdivided into three compartments: plasma water, interstitial water, and intracellular water, the symbols of which are V_1, V_2, and V_3, respectively. DOMINGUEZ (1950) has collected a body of evidence in favor of this viewpoint (cf. KRÜGER-THIEMER, 1964b). Very recently, however, there has been some evidence presented that the circulating lymph itself may represent an additional compartment that may need to be considered. DEMARCO and LEVINE (1969) have shown that the antibiotic tetracycline is concentrated in lymph shortly after intravenous administration. Drugs with appreciable solubility in lipids may also be distributed throughout the body fat, forming an additional compartment, V_4, which may be connected either directly with the plasma water or with the interstitial water. For drugs entering the fat, not only the lipid volume, V_4, but also their lipid water distribution coefficient has to be taken into account. If elimination of drug from the body is not very fast with respect to distribution over one or more distribution volumes, multicompartment kinetics become necessary. The uniformity of drug distribution may be affected by any reversible process of binding to large dissolved particles or to solid body constituents. The most important binding process is the binding of drug by albumin, which circulates in the blood plasma, and in a smaller concentration in the interstitial fluid, including the lymph (GOLDSTEIN, 1949). In the discussion of experimental data one has to take into account that many drugs will display the combined influence of multicompartmentalization and of protein binding as well. This more complex behavior has not been solved as of yet.

Protein Binding Models

Protein binding as a basic principle in drug behavior in human and animal bodies has been known for more than two decades. In spite of this fact it has been neglected until recently in pharmacokinetic models. Since an excellent review on the pharmacologic implications of protein binding is available (GOLDSTEIN, 1949), it is not necessary to discuss this problem here in detail.

Because the degree of binding is not constant but depends on the drug concentration in plasma, the protein binding, which may be adequately (and with sufficient accuracy) described by the law of mass action (GULDBERG and WAAGE, 1867), is of outstanding importance as a cause of nonlinear dose-concentration relationships. This nonlinearity was recognized in studying the pharmacokinetics of highly bound sulfa drugs (BÜNGER et al., 1961; KRÜGER-THIEMER et al., 1964, 1965a, b; KRÜGER-THIEMER, 1966; e.g., sulformethoxine). The law of mass action is sometimes identified, although not correctly, with the adsorption isotherm of LANGMUIR (1916, 1917). The use of the adsorption isotherm of FREUNDLICH (1907) preferred by some authors, should be avoided, for it may adequately describe the protein binding data only in a medium range of concentration (GOLDSTEIN, 1949) and the parameters of the Freundlich equation do not have any physical meaning. The law of mass action for protein binding may be written in the following form (KRÜGER-THIEMER, 1960b):

$$C = C_f\{W + \beta \cdot p/(K_p + C_f)\} . \tag{24}$$

Here C is the plasma concentration, C_f the plasma water concentration, K_p the dissociation constant characterizing the binding of drug to the plasma proteins, β the binding capacity in microval per gram protein, p the protein concentration in g/l, and W the water content of the plasma (e.g., liter water per liter plasma). The quantity Q_b of drug bound to plasma proteins per liter plasma as function of the plasma water concentration C_f may be given by the following equation:

$$Q_b = \frac{\beta \cdot pC_f}{K_p + C_f} . \tag{25}$$

Obviously Q_b as function of the plasma concentration and C_f as function of the plasma concentration are complicated relations that may be found from Equations (24) and (25). This relationship has been given for a few cases in Figure 8. It may be seen that the plasma water concentration parallels the plasma concentration when the dissociation constant is more than 10^{-3} Molar while large deviations occur as K_p is smaller. A pK_p value of 5 or 6 denotes relative strong protein binding.

The fraction of drug bound to plasma proteins may be derived from Equations 24 and 25:

$$\text{fraction bound} = 1 \bigg/ \left\{1 + \frac{W}{\beta \cdot p}(K_p + C_f)\right\} . \tag{26}$$

It is therefore evident that the fraction bound to plasma proteins is greater for low plasma concentrations (Fig. 8). In analogy the fraction of free drug may be derived (Fig. 8). A few experimental examples have been given in Figure 9. Obvious deviations from the functional behavior according to Equation (24) have

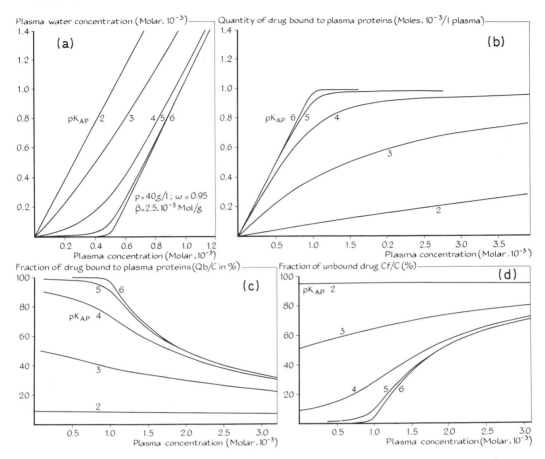

Fig. 8a—d. Relationship between plasma concentration and (a) plasma water concentration, (b) quantity of drug bound to plasma proteins, (c) fraction of drug bound, and (d) fraction of free drug, as calculated with equations 24, 25, and 26 for theoretical drugs with varying affinity pK_{app} to plasma proteins

been explained by the superposition of two terms of the mass action law, suggesting that two different and independent binding processes are involved in the system under study (KRÜGER-THIEMER, 1964a, b, c, 1967a, b; VAN OS, 1966). This complication will be neglected in the following, because Equation (24) is entirely sufficient in the therapeutic range of drug concentrations.

A recently observed type of deviation from the first-order kinetics for drug elimination from the human body is characterized by diminishing steepness of slope of the time-concentration curve in a semilog plot (KRÜGER-THIEMER, 1964c; DILLER, 1964). This type of deviation has been found with many sulfa drugs showing a high degree of binding to the plasma proteins, corresponding to a small value of the dissociation constant K_p, of the drug-protein complex. Several pharmacokinetic models may be used for studying this deviation. Firstly, very high protein binding may be assumed, so that the compound may leave the blood system

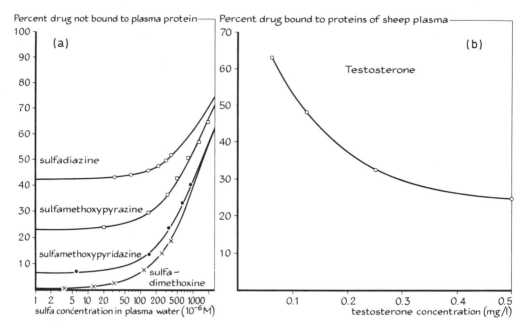

Fig. 9a and b. Relation between plasma concentration and (a) fraction of free sulfa drugs and (b) fraction of testosterone bound to plasma proteins. Compare theoretical curves of Figure 8. [(a) Data from Krüger-Thiemer, 1967b, Year Book Med. Publ.; (b) Data from Lindner, 1964]

only in the smallest amount, e.g., Evans blue used for measurement of plasma volume. Secondly, protein binding may be equal inside and outside the blood vessels. This assumption is ruled out by the facts because the protein concentration in the interstitial fluid is rather low. In addition, strong protein binding of drugs is an exceptional property of serum albumin whose concentration in the interstitial fluid is normally less than half of the albumin concentration in plasma, while albumin is not to be found in the cells. Regarding all these facts, a suitable model that accounts for the distribution behavior of drugs is that drugs are bound solely to albumin in plasma and interstitial fluid and are distributed through the blood plasma, the interstitial fluid, and the intracellular water, while protein binding in the peripheral compartment does not occur.

Experimentally, however, protein binding may occur in the peripheral compartment but other binding parameters are involved. Though the systems of differential equations of these models are nonlinear, because of the involvement of protein binding they may be integrated. But the resulting equations are so complicated that they are of little practical use. For drugs whose renal excretion is much slower than distribution over the entire body of distribution, one may assume that the distribution constants, k_{12} and k_{21} are very large (theoretically infinite). The resulting model is much easier to handle. Already the simplest of these models is helpful in clarifying the influence of protein binding on the relationship between renal clearance and the apparent half-life of elimination (or the apparent rate constant for renal excretion). With this assumption and i.v. administration of the

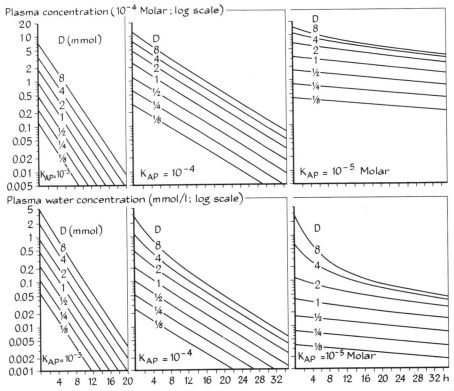

Fig. 10. Theoretical plasma concentration and corresponding plasma water concentration curves of increasing doses of three drugs showing different degree of plasma protein binding. For drugs with strong protein binding ($pK_{AP} = 5$) there is great difference between plasma concentration and plasma water concentration. Nonlinearity occurs

drug, there are two body compartments (plasma water, V_1, and residual body water, V_2), between which drug equilibrium occurs instantaneously. There is protein binding according to the law of mass action only within the plasma water compartment, and the rate of renal excretion (or elimination) is proportional to the concentration of unbound drug in the plasma water. The complete mathematical derivation and discussion of the functional behavior of this model has been published by KRÜGER-THIEMER [1968c, Eqs. (14–16)]. Theoretical plasma-concentration curves using this simplified model are given in Figure 10 for three different values of the dissociation constant K_p. There is a large difference between C and C_f with decreasing values of K_p. If K_p is 10^{-3} molar there is little difference and protein binding is unimportant. Experimental examples are given in Figures 11 and 12.

How one has to account for protein binding in a single-compartment—valid on the assumption that the drug is given intravascularly—has been published by KRÜGER-THIEMER (1961) and KRÜGER-THIEMER et al. (1965a, b). Protein binding within this compartment occurs according to the law of mass action; and the rate of renal excretion (or elimination) is proportional to the concentration of the unbound drug.

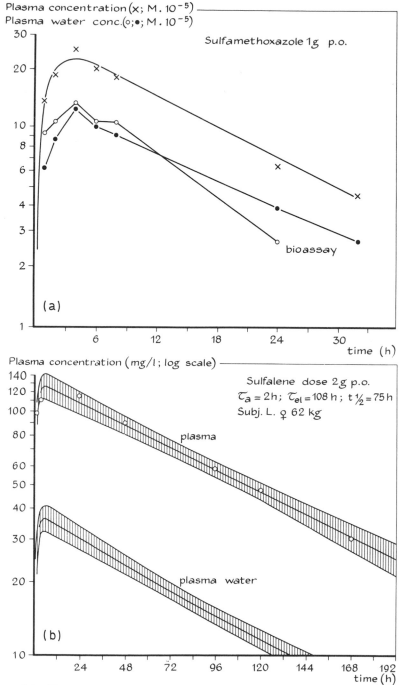

Fig. 11a and b. Plasma concentration and plasma water concentration curves of sulfa drugs: (a) sulfamethoxazole. Plasma water concentration has been determined by chemical means and by bioassay. (Data from Krüger-Thiemer and Bünger (1965/1966a, b) with permission of authors and publishers of Chemotherapia. (b) Sulfalene. Plasma water concentration has been calculated by using in vitro data. (Data from Krüger-Thiemer, 1968c)

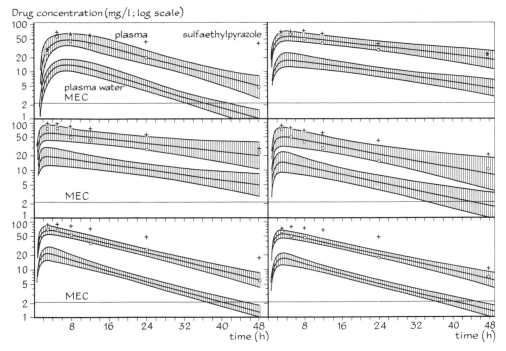

Fig. 12. Experimental plasma concentration curves and calculated plasma water concentration curves of sulfaethylpyrazole in six human subjects. pK_{AP} value of this sulfa is reproduced from KRÜGER-THIEMER (1967b) with permission of author and publishers of Chemotherapia

An important experimental implication of the foregoing is that the estimation of the concentration of strongly protein-bound drug in the whole blood is unnecessary, for such data are difficult to interpret. Since hemoglobin does not bind many drugs which are bound by albumin, the drug concentration in the erythrocyte water will be approximately equal to the concentration in plasma water after achievement of the equilibrium. From the viewpoint of the above-mentioned models, the erythrocytes should be regarded as belonging to the tissue cells. Their membrane is an atypical type 1 membrane (ALBERT, 1960) for they have a carbonic acid dehydration mechanism which permits rapid penetration of anions without the expenditure of energy, whereas only highly lipophilic cations penetrate. If one has estimated the protein binding parameters in an independent in vitro experiment, one may calculate the plasma water concentration of the drug from the measured values of the plasma concentration (KRÜGER-THIEMER and BÜNGER, 1965/66a, b; KRÜGER-THIEMER et al., 1965a, b). There is a good fit between theory and experiment (Figs. 11 and 12). Because of the introduction of the law of mass action, the models of Figures 3 and 13 may be described by a set of nonlinear differential equations, in which Laplace transforms may not be used for the solution (KRÜGER-THIEMER, 1968).

In the case of a two compartment system with protein binding only in the central compartment, renal excretion depends directly on the plasma-water concentration and metabolic elimination depends on the total plasma concentration. The

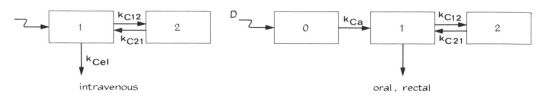

Fig. 13. Block diagrams representing kinetics of elimination of drugs if body is regarded as two compartment system

following equations may be derived:

$$\frac{dQ_1}{dt} = -k_{Cr} \cdot C_f - k_{Cm}C_1 - k_{C12}C_f + k_{C21}C_2, \tag{27}$$

$$\frac{dQ_2}{dt} = k_{C12}C_f - k_{C21}C_2. \tag{28}$$

Under the assumption that the rate of distribution is fast with regard to elimination, Equations (27) and (28) are reduced to the following ones:

$$\frac{dQ_1}{dt} = -k_{Cr} + k_{Cm}\left(W + \frac{\beta \cdot p}{K_p + C_f}\right)C_f. \tag{29}$$

Here Q_1 is the quantity of drug in the central compartment, $(Q_1 = V_1 \cdot C_1)$ and Q_2 the quantity of drug in the peripheral compartment $(Q_2 = V_2 \cdot C_2)$.

Integration leads to an implicit relationship (KRÜGER-THIEMER, 1968b). Obviously, the concentrations in plasma C_1, and in plasma water C_f, are rather complicated functions of the time, t, and the involved parameters. The relationship between the administered dose, D, and the concentrations, C_f and C_1, is not as simple as in a linear dose-concentration relationship, in which the entire curve of the concentration of the drug in plasma water with respect to time would be directly proportional to the administered dose, D.

The model curves show the expected nonlinearity (Fig. 10). The nonlinearity is more pronounced for stronger protein binding (low values of the dissociation constant K_p) and for the higher amounts of the doses. The smaller the dose, the more the concentration curves in plasma and plasma water tend to be parallel in the semilogarithmic plot (Figs. 11 and 12). These latter curves have another interesting feature. The slope of all curves with identical dissociation constants, K_p, and total concentration of binding sites, $p \cdot \beta_1$ is equal at a certain drug concentration C_f or C_1. That means, each set of curves with identical values of K_p and $p \cdot \beta_1$ is congruent or superimposable by a shift parallel to the time axis (KRÜGER-THIEMER, 1968b).

From this it may be concluded that a drug showing substantial protein binding has different apparent values of the half-life of elimination for different concentrations in plasma and plasma water. For dosage regimen estimations one has to use that value of the apparent half-life of elimination, $t_{\frac{1}{2}}$, which has been

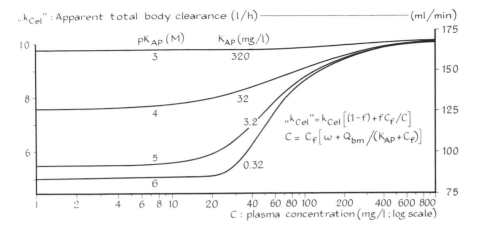

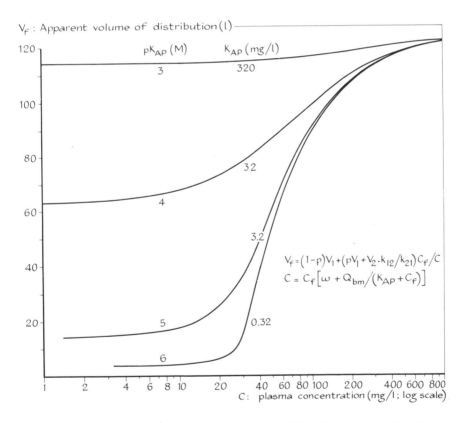

Fig. 14. Total body clearance $\dot{V}_{Cel}$ and apparent volume of distribution as function of plasma concentration for drugs that bind to plasma proteins. Depending on relative routes of elimination, importance of protein binding is more or less pronounced on clearance. In general, the trend is that both clearance and volume of distribution increase with increasing the plasma concentration nonlinearity occurs over concentration traject of factor 10 in range of capacity of protein binding. (From unpublished data by VAN ROSSUM)

calculated from drug concentrations in the therapeutically effective range. The distribution coefficient, d, or volume of distribution, is influenced by protein binding, too (Krüger-Thiemer et al., 1965a, b). As the biological half-life mainly depends on the total body clearance and the volume of distribution, the concentration dependence of the total clearance and the apparent volume of distribution is considered. See in Figure 14. It may be seen that protein binding leads to nonlinearity only in a limited concentration range, provided that only one population of binding sites is involved (Van Rossum, unpublished). A final remark on protein binding might be helpful in studying the literature, where often only insufficient data on the percentage of bound data are given. There is ample evidence that the number of binding sites on the albumin molecules is rather restricted. While some time ago one binding site per molecule of albumin had been calculated (Krüger-Thiemer, 1960b), newer evidence (Nakagaki et al., 1963, 1964) tends to suggest two binding sites per albumin molecule. Assuming this as true, then one may calculate the dissociation constant of protein binding, K_p, from a single measurement, provided the concentration in plasma or in plasma water is given beside the percentage bound.

Goldstein (1949) has warned of a possible misinterpretation of experimental data resulting from a study of the actual antibacterial activity of the protein bound part of the drug concentration in blood plasma. Indeed, this predicted misinterpretation has been made by Madsen et al. (1963) and Madsen (1964). In the series of dilution tests for measuring the drug concentration in serum culture one has used fluids free from serum albumin in order to dilute the serum. Madsen et al. (1963) have used the culture fluid of Adams and Roe (1945) which "is completely dialysable," i.e., it does not contain protein. Both groups of authors have neglected that in their dilution procedure the albumin concentration of the serum progressively decreases according to the dilution titer depending on the sensitivity of the test germs. The dilution of the protein causes a shift of the binding equilibrium. For instance, a serum concentration of 4-sulfanilamido-5, 6-methoxy-pyrimidine of 1.71 µg/ml revealed to be antibacterially active until a 175-fold dilution. In undiluted serum 5% of the drug concentrations were unbound whereas after the 175-fold dilution, 76% were unbound. That explains the erroneous conclusion of Madsen et al. who assumed that the antibacterial activities of equal drug concentrations were equal irrespective of low or high protein binding (cf. Berlin and Krüger-Thiemer, 1964; Krüger-Thiemer, 1967a). The antibacterial activity of the unbound fraction of the drug concentration on blood plasma may be correctly estimated by an ultracentrifugation method (Krüger-Thiemer et al., 1965a).

D. Absorption

All the pharmacokinetic models discussed up to this point were for drugs administered intravascularly or assuming very rapid absorption since the influence of metabolism, excretion, multiple compartments, and protein binding can be studied more easily when the complexities of drug absorption are avoided.

A detailed treatment of the various aspects of drug absorption is unnecessary in the context of this article (cf. reviews by Schanker, 1962, 1964; Levine and Pelikan, 1964). In the following discussion the kinetic aspects will primarily be discussed.

The irregular processes which may complicate the kinetics of absorption can be of pharmaceutic or physiologic origin. When the dosage form (tablet, capsule, etc.) of the drug is administered, the rate of absorption may be affected by the rate of dosage-form disintegration and/or the rate of dissolution of the solid drug (see Sect. III.D.2). For orally administered drugs, the amount of water taken with solid dosage forms not only influences the volume of available solvent and the pH of the gastric contents but also the physiologic process of stomach emptying. In turn, physiologic factors can influence the rate of disintegration, e.g., site of disintegration of pH-dependent enteric coated tablets, or rate of dissolution, e.g., increased with increased gastrointestinal mobility. Many other examples of the influences of the physical state of formulation are provided in recent reviews on biopharmaceutics (DOLUISIO and SWINTOSKY, 1965; BARR, 1969; RIEGELMAN, 1969; and GIBALDI, 1971).

Even when drugs are rapidly dissolved or are administered in solution there are a number of irregular processes involved in absorption. For orally administered drugs the mobility of the gastrointestinal tract, i.e., stomach emptying, peristalsis, rhythmic segmentation, and pendular movement, affect the rate, as well as the site, of absorption. The normal interstitial contents, the "internal milieu" of Claude Bernard, and the "external" environment of the intraintestinal fluids also may markedly affect the concentration or the physico-chemical state of the drug available for absorption.

1. Absorption from Parenteral Sites

The influence of factors such as drug-protein binding, ionization constant, and lipoid solubility is qualitatively the same for absorption from enteral and parenteral sites. In case of extravascular parenteral administration one step in the absorption process is by-passed and this produces the real differences in absorption kinetics. Drug administered by the enteral routes, either orally or rectally, must traverse an epithelial barrier before gaining access to the tissues in direct contact with channels into the general circulation. Drugs given by parenteral routes, either sub-cutaneous or intramuscular, are placed in tissue depots directly in contact with blood and lymph capillaries. The barrier to absorption from parenteral sites is the capillary endothelial membrane.

All substances, whether lipid-soluble, large molecules, lipidinsoluble, or ionized molecules cross the capillary endothelium at rates far in excess of those at which these same materials cross epithelial tissues. The rate of capillary blood flow is the major factor in determining rate of entry into the circulation: the more vascularized the area the greater the rate of absorption.

In general, the rate of absorption for lipid-soluble substances is believed to be roughly parallel to their oil-water partition coefficient, whereas lipid-insoluble substances are absorbed at rates dependent on their diffusion rates in acqueous solution (SCHOU, 1961).

The connective tissue ground substance has some influence on the rate of subcutaneous absorption. This has been demonstrated by hyaluronidase, which increases the rate of subcutaneous absorption by permitting spread of the injected solution through a larger area and consequently allows access to a larger total area of capillary membrane.

Qualitatively, the permeability of capillary walls in muscle hardly differs from that of capillaries in subcutaneous tissues. Therefore, absorption from intramuscular sites is rate-limited merely by blood. Ordinarily, especially in active muscles, the blood flow is greater than through most subcutaneous areas, so there would be higher rates of absorption from muscle than from subcutaneous sites.

The role of lymphatics in absorption from subcutaneous or intramuscular sites is relatively unknown. Even if material were to be removed from site of injection by lymph this would represent only a minor part of the total since the rate of flow of lymph is very slow compared to blood. However, lymphatic absorption may be important in particulate matter removal.

In evaluation of drug absorption data most investigators start with the simple first-order model of drug absorption, assuming that the rate of absorption is proportional to the residual drug amount in the depot. This model holds with sufficient accuracy under certain circumstances, the most important among them being that the drug should be in solution in the depot. A second condition for first-order absorption kinetics is perfect mixing of the drug solution in the depot (e.g., peristaltic movement of the gastrointestinal tract). From the viewpoint of diffusion kinetics the driving force is not the drug amount in the depot, but the drug concentration. However, it is not always possible to predict the relative amounts of a drug that will be absorbed when the same dose is administered in two different concentrations. The lower concentration contained in a larger volume may have access to a larger total area of absorbing surface.

2. Absorption from Enteral Sites

With few exceptions, only dissolved drug molecules may be absorbed from drug depots in the gastrointestinal tract or elsewhere. As indicated earlier, two processes of drug release from dosage form, namely dosage form disintegration and drug dissolution, may have an appreciable effect on time and degree of availability of the administered dose as shown in a series of papers by LEVY and coworkers (LEVY, 1962, 1963; LEVY and PROCKNALL, 1964; LEVY and TANSKI, 1964; LEVY et al., 1964; LEVY and HOLLISTER, 1965). One may try to account for these processes by first- and zero-order models. The law of NOYES and WHITNEY is useful for the description of drug dissolution, since this law relates the rate of dissolution of a solid compound to the drug concentration in the surrounding fluid (C_0), the total drug solubility in the diffusion layer near the surface (C_s), the surface area (A), the thickness of the diffusion layer (h) which depends on fluid convection, and the diffusion constant (D_f), according to FICK's law of diffusion (1855).

$$\frac{dQ_s}{dt} = -\frac{D_f \cdot A \cdot N \cdot W}{h}(C_s - C_0).\tag{30}$$

The NOYES and WHITNEY law (1897) explains why sodium salts of weak acids are absorbed much more rapidly than the acids themselves. Because the surface area usually changes during the dissolution process and the fluid volume, available for dissolution, is presumably variable and difficult to define, no simple time course for the process of dissolution may be expected. Intestinal water circulation, consisting of saliva, gastric, pancreatic, intestinal juice, and bile, lies between 5 and 10 l/day. This is considerable higher than the daily water ingestion of normal adults.

Each dose is contained in and moves along with only a part of the total volume that passes through the intestine. Evidence for incomplete or slow drug dissolution is often to be found in literature (e.g., for sulfaperin Pallidin, KRÜGER-THIEMER and ERIKSEN, 1966; for sulforthomethoxine Fanasil, BÜNGER, 1967). Correlation studies of distribution coefficients d, and half-lives of eliminations, $t_{\frac{1}{2}}$, calculated from drug concentrations in plasma (from experiments of BÜNGER and KRÜGER-THIEMER) have been made for sulfadiazine and sulfamethoxazole (Gantanol). The wide range of scattering of the data points of sulfadiazine may be explained by its slow and incomplete absorption due to low solubility (177 mg/l at pH 6, KRÜGER-THIEMER and BÜNGER, 1965).

3. Transport Through the Gastrointestinal Tract

According to the pH partition theory describing the behavior of the absorption of weak acids and weak bases by passive permeation of the nonionized molecules, all compounds, which are highly ionized in the acid stomach content, will remain largely unabsorbed during their stay in the stomach (SCHANKER, 1962, 1964). Therefore, the beginning of drug absorption depends in these cases on the process of stomach emptying, which has been assumed to be a first-order process (HUNT, 1963). However, NOGAMI et al. (1961, 1962) have questioned this concept. The average time of stomach emptying depends on the food and water taken with the drug and varies ordinarily between 1 and 4 h. Since in many pharmacokinetic experiments, the number of data points obtainable just after drug administration is limited, a proper substitute may be a zero time shift, t_0, which roughly describes the average time for stomach emptying (SCHLENDER and KRÜGER-THIEMER, 1965). The actual value of the zero time shift is rather unimportant, it is needed mainly for getting a close curve fitting of the model curve to experimental data (Figs. 5 and 15).

The stomach emptying is seldom influenced directly by the drug and is mainly an individual property of the test subject. Chloroquine, however, has recently been shown to inhibit gastric emptying in rats in a dose-dependent manner, and to affect its own absorption since it is principally absorbed from the intestine.

Even though the absorption of weak bases takes place mainly in the small intestine, limited absorption of the unionized species may occur in the stomach. One would anticipate for a weak acid such as salicylic acid, on the other hand, that the low normal pH of the gastric contents would favor its absorption and that a major portion of the oral dose would be absorbed in the stomach. However, even when stomach emptying is somewhat delayed, the major portion of a weak acid is absorbed in the small intestine. The ratio of the absorbing area of the small intestine compared with that of the stomach is extremely large and is sufficiently great to overcome the differences in rate of absorption per unit area of absorbing surface. It is also well to bear in mind that there is no abrupt increase in pH of the gastric contents when they are emptied into the intestine. The pH

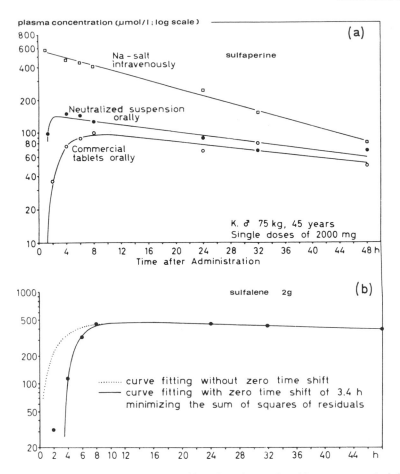

Fig. 15. (a) Plasma concentration curves of sulfaperine after oral and intravenous administration. Tablet dosage form shows largest zero-time-shift, and slowest rate of absorption. (From Krüger-Thiemer and Eriksen, J. Pharm. Sci., 1966. (b) Plasma concentration curve of sulfalene in a patient who collapsed immediately after drug intake. Strong delay in absorption may in part be due to this situation. (Adopted from Krüger-Thiemer, 1968c)

of the contents of the duodenum and the proximal end of the jejunum remains acidic.

Another important problem with respect to dose-concentration relationships is given by the incomplete absorption of several drugs from the gastrointestinal tract. The main reason for such a behavior is that the rate of drug absorption is so slow that the available passage time through the gastrointestinal tract is too short for a nearly complete absorption. Dost (1958) has found an interesting rule, which may be used for the evaluation of the absorbed fraction, F, of the total administered dose, D (Krüger-Thiemer, 1961; Gladtke, 1964; Dost, 1968). The area under the drug concentration curve in plasma water and the time axis from $t = 0$ to $t = \infty$ is proportional to the absorbed dose, $D \cdot F$, and inversely proportional to the clearance constant for elimination, k_{Cel}:

$$A \cdot U \cdot C \equiv \int_0^\infty c_1 dt = \frac{D \cdot F}{k_{Cel}} = 1.44 \frac{D \cdot F \cdot t_{\frac{1}{2}}}{G \cdot d}. \tag{31}$$

This equation is valid for all multicompartment systems, consisting of any number of compartments which are connected by first-order reactions and which have only one exit characterized by the rate constant for elimination, k_{Cel}. It is also valid for nonlinear systems with protein binding. By definition F is equal to unity for intravascular administration. Equating the terms for equal relative doses, D/G, for oral (or) and intravenous (iv) administration results in:

$$F \text{ (or)} = \frac{AUC(\text{or}) \cdot k_{Cel}(\text{or})}{AUC(\text{iv}) \cdot k_{Cel}(\text{iv})}. \tag{32}$$

If the coefficient of distribution, d, and the clearance constant for elimination are assumed to be equal for intravenous and oral administration, F results as the ratio of the areas under the concentration curves for oral and intravenous administration, $AUC(\text{or})/AUC(\text{iv})$. Equation (32) is often used in this sense (LEVY, 1963; GLADTKE, 1964). It is doubtful whether the simple model underlying the previous equation is applicable in the example given in Figure 15, in which the apparent clearance constants for elimination, calculated from drug concentrations in plasma, are obviously unequal. This results from a prolonged absorption phase of the drug whose solubility is very low.

Actually, this model implies that the fraction $(1 - F)$ of the dose, which is supposed to be excreted with the feces, is inert with respect to the absorption kinetics along its way through the gastrointestinal tract. A further discussion on the bioavailability of F will be given in the chapter by VAN ROSSUM and others in this volume.

The time of transit of drugs through the small intestine can present still other problems with respect to dose-concentration relationships of drugs which are transported by specialized and saturable processes. Certain agents, such as some quarternary ammonium compounds (LEVINE and PELIKAN, 1964), are preferentially absorbed by specialized processes in specific areas of the small intestine. The length of time of residence at these special sites can markedly affect the amount of absorption. It has long been appreciated that certain chemical classes of drugs, e.g., proteins, esters, etc., can undergo biotransformation in the gastrointestinal tract. Agents such as these are usually administered by parenteral routes. However, it has been found only recently that the intestinal mucosa is capable of carrying out a number of conjugating processes, and, thereby, inactivating drugs administered orally even before they are absorbed into the general circulation. This intestinal biotransformation is yet one more irregular process in absorption which makes the understanding of absorption kinetics difficult.

4. Absorption from Gastrointestinal Tract

Passive permeation and active absorption.

Many authors have assumed that drug absorption from the gastrointestinal tract may be described by a first-order process. (WIDMARK and TANDBERG, 1924; TEORELL, 1937; DOST, 1953, and others). This assumption may be warranted if disintegration of the dosage form and drug dissolution occur rapidly and drug absorption follows **Fick's** law of diffusion, wherein the intestinal tissue (extra luminal) concentration is kept at a negligible level by blood convection in capillaries of intestinal wall. Drug absorption may then be described by the following differential equations:

$$\frac{dQ_0}{dt} = -k_{Ca} \cdot C_0 \quad \text{and} \quad \frac{dQ_1}{dt} = k_{Ca} \cdot C_0 - k_{Cel} \cdot C_1 \tag{33}$$

where k_{Ca} is the clearance constant for absorption, Q_0 the quantity of drug in the intestinal tract, and C_0 the concentration in the intestinal tract.

A detailed account on absorption problems has been given in reviews by SCHANKER (1962, 1964).

The absorption of certain drugs, e.g., quaternary ammonium compounds, seems to follow a pattern other than that of a passive permeation process as shown by LEVINE and coworkers (LEVINE and PELIKAN, 1964). Because this absorption process is saturable, it may be described by the MICHAELIS and MENTEN (1913) equation resulting in nonlinear differential equations for absorption:

$$\frac{dQ_0}{dt} = -k_{Ca} \frac{1}{1 + C_0/K_0} C_0, \tag{34}$$

$$\frac{dQ_1}{dt} = k_{Ca} \frac{1}{1 + C_0/K_0} C_0 - k_{Cel} \cdot C_1 \tag{35}$$

where k_{Ca} is equal to V_{max}/K_0 and K_0 is the dissociation constant for the active absorption process. It is evident that if $C_0 \ll K_0$, absorption is first order although in fact the absorption process still may be active. If $C_0 \gg K_0$, saturation of the concentration dependent absorption occurs and consequently the absorption kinetics is zero-order. In that case absorption resembles infusion.

5. First-Order Absorption Kinetics with Zero-Time Shift

If, between intake of a medicine and the onset of the absorption process, a period "t_0" elapses, then absorption starts t_0 after administration. Integration of Equation (33) leads to the following well-known equation:

$$C = \frac{D}{V} \cdot \frac{\tau_{el}}{(\tau_{el} - \tau_a)} (e^{-t/\tau_{el}} - e^{-t/\tau_a}). \tag{36}$$

The plasma concentration for a drug following oral, rectal, or other ways of administration may well be described by Equation (36). This equation is often written with rate constants for absorption and elimination instead of time-constants ($k_a = 1/\tau_a$ and $k_{el} = 1/\tau_{el}$) (DOST, 1953). The rate constant for absorption bears the following relation to the clearance constant of absorption and the time-constant for absorption:

$$r_a = k_a/V_0 ; \qquad \tau_a = V_0/k_a . \tag{37}$$

A few examples of oral absorption are given in Figures 5 and 15. From these figures it is clear that the time constant of absorption can be calculated from the ascending part of the plasma curve of, e.g., paracetamol (substraction method).

It is further evident that there is lag-time between drug administration and the onset of absorption.

In this case the zero time shift is 12 min when a tablet is ingested while the elixer of paracetamol starts absorption immediately (VAN GINNEKEN, 1976).

It must be emphasized that the half-life for absorption or the rate constant for absorption as well as the zero time-shift can often be determined with insufficient accuracy because of insufficient plasma concentration data during the first hours after administration. Drug absorption and elimination may also be studied from urinary excretion data (WAGNER, 1971; NELSON, 1961). From such curves only very little information on absorption may be obtained but the half-life of elimination may be reasonably calculated.

6. Nonfirst-Order Models of Absorption

Taking into account all known facts on drug absorption from the gastrointestinal tract it is rather improbable that a simple first-order model will describe carefully registered data on drug absorption with sufficient accuracy. The simple first-order model of absorption assumes that the rate of absorption at zero time (or at the end of the lag time, t_0) should immediately have its highest value. DOMINGUEZ (1950) has shown that this is not the case. BÜNGER (1967) has measured plasma concentration data of a long-acting sulfa drug, sulforthomethoxine (Fanasil), suggesting a zero-order absorption for several hours, presumably caused by the low solubility of the drug.

WAGNER (1961, 1971) has studied several more complicated models of drug absorption. These models are especially useful for the study of different dosage forms for immediate and sustained release of the drug. This area of biopharmaceutics is developing rapidly. A detailed treatment of it lies outside of the scope of this article. Analog-computer-simulations may help in analyzing the dose-concentration relationships of sustained release preparations (TAYLOR and WIEGAND, 1962; KRÜGER-THIEMER and ERIKSEN, 1966).

When plasma protein binding plays a significant role, absorption and elimination is essentially nonlinear. From Figures 11 and 12 and many other similar experiments it may be concluded that irrespective of protein binding, the plasma concentration curve may reasonably well be described by the first-order equations.

The influence of the drug absorption on dosage regimens is small if the rate constant for absorption does not assume especially low values. For this reason the nonfirst-order models of drug absorption will be neglected in the following sections.

E. Multicompartment Kinetics

The study of multicompartment systems has developed, mainly under the influence of radioactive tracer experiments, in the fields of physiology and pharmacology. *Multicompartment analysis* is closely related to the study of electrical networks. Therefore the mathematical methods used in this area may likewise be successfully used in the multicompartment analysis. Among these methods the Laplace transforms are of outstanding importance. RESCIGNO and SEGRE (1961, 1966) have made important theoretic contributions in this field. The most advanced practical approaches have been given by BERMAN and co-workers (1962a, b) who have developed a digital computer program for the analysis of systems of up to 25 compartments, characterized by up to 250 points of measurement in any of the compartments.

A historic approach to the study of multicompartment systems is the hydrokinetic model (BRUNTON, 1899). Of great importance is the use of analog computers (see SCHLENDER and KRÜGER-THIEMER, 1965). Analog computer methods have been introduced into pharmacokinetics by GARRETT and co-workers (1960, 1962, 1963).

The multicompartment analysis using previously mentioned methods is limited by the random errors of the experimental results which are seldom lower than 5% in biological experiments. Therefore it is difficult and hazardous to draw conclusions on the drug behavior within several compartments from measurements in only one compartment. This difficulty results mainly from the fact that it is easy to measure the time course of drug concentration in human plasma and urine, but it is much more difficult or even impossible to follow the drug concentrations in other body fluids and tissues of humans. Fortunately, the dose-concentration problem with respect to the body compartments is, for many drugs, much easier than one would expect at first glance.

From the data of DOMINGUEZ (1950) one may deduce that there are three main groups of drugs and other materials foreign to the body, which differ in their distribution behavior throughout the body fluid (KRÜGER-THIEMER, 1964b).

1. Compounds which are unable to leave the capillary system or which are able to leave it only very slowly or to a very small extent, because of a large molecular weight or very high degree of binding to the plasma proteins, may escape from the blood only very slowly or not at all. This leads to a small volume of distribution (order of 3 l).

1.1. Compounds which are completely ionized, may distribute throughout the extracellular water without difficulty, and may not at all or only very slowly penetrate into most of the cells of the body. The volume of distribution may be in the order of 12 l.

1.1.1. All other compounds may distribute throughout the total body water more or less rapidly, according to their molecular weight, percentage of ionization, lipid-water distribution coefficient, and protein binding. If distribution is homogenous the volume of distribution is in the order of 50 l.

This fairly simple distribution pattern of drugs throughout the body fluids is modified not only by binding to the plasma protein but also by any other type of binding or complexation to any body constituent.

Of great importance is the rate of distribution of drugs from the blood plasma to the various fluids and tissues of the body. The rate of distribution depends on the physicochemical properties of the drugs, the degree of vascularization of the tissues, and the morphology of the tissues. This implies that various compartments in the body should be regarded. However, several compartments may be grouped together because of similar features (RIEGELMAN et al., 1968). In many cases it is sufficient to consider only two compartments in the human body; a central compartment, which consists of the bloodplasma and the tissues that are relatively highly vascularized (e.g., liver, kidneys, etc.) and a peripheral compartment, which is less strongly vascularized (muscle, fat, etc.). Obviously these compartments are abstractions which, for certain drugs, bear a relation to real situations. So for bromsulphaleine, which is very strongly bound to plasma proteins, the central compartment is the blood plasma and the peripheral compartment the rest of the body. In this case the peripheral compartment is very small.

1. The Two Compartment Model

TEORELL (1937) has provided, in two important papers, a detailed mathematical model of a two-compartment system consisting of the blood fluid and the extravascular fluid, including metabolism in the extravascular fluid. This model is characterized by three-six parameters, namely the rate constants for absorption, metabolism, and for diffusion into and out of the tissues and the amount of administered dose.

The model is visualized in Figure 13. In accordance with the convention adopted in this volume, clearance or flow constants have been used instead of rate-constants in the differential equations. In case of intravenous administration of the dose D in the central compartment the following equations describe the situation.

$$\frac{dQ_1}{dt} = -(k_{Cel} + k_{C12}) \cdot C_1 + k_{Cel} \cdot C_2, \tag{38}$$

$$\frac{dQ_2}{dt} = k_{C12} \cdot C_1 - k_{C21} \cdot C_2, \tag{39}$$

$$\frac{dQ_{el}}{dt} = k_{Cel} \cdot C_1. \tag{40}$$

dQ_1/dt is the disappearance rate from the central compartment, dQ_2/dt that for the peripheral compartment, dQ_{el}/dt the rate of drug elimination from the body. The constants k_{Cel}, k_{C12}, and k_{C21} are clearance-constants (e.g., in ml/min or l/h). As $Q_1 = V_1 \cdot C_1$ and $Q_2 = V_2 \cdot C_2$ the concentration in the central and peripheral compartment can be found by integration resulting in a two term exponential function.

$$C_1 = A_1 \cdot e^{-t/\tau_1} + A_2 \cdot e^{-t/\tau_2} = A_1 \cdot e^{-k_1 \cdot t} + A_2 \cdot e^{-k_2 \cdot t} \tag{41}$$

and

$$C_2 = B_1 \cdot e^{-t/\tau_1} + B_2 \cdot e^{-t/\tau_2}$$
$$Q_{el} = k_{el}[A_1 \cdot \tau_1(1 - e^{-t/\tau_1}) + A_2 \cdot \tau_2(1 - e^{-t/\tau_2})]$$
$$(42)$$

where A_1, A_2 and B_1, B_2 are coefficients τ_1 and τ_2 time constants and k_1 and k_2 rate constants. The two time constants depend on all clearance constants k_{C12}, k_{C21}, and k_{Cel} as well as the volume of the two compartments. This relation may be seen from the following equations:

$$(k_1 + k_2) = \frac{\tau_1 \cdot \tau_2}{(\tau_1 + \tau_2)} = \left(\frac{k_{C12}}{V_1} + \frac{k_{C21}}{V_2} + \frac{k_{Cel}}{V_1}\right) = (k_{C12} + k_{C21} + k_{Cel})$$

$$k_1 \cdot k_2 = \frac{1}{\tau_1 \cdot \tau_2} = \frac{k_{Cel}}{V_1} \cdot \frac{k_{C21}}{V_2}.$$
$$(43)$$

It is obvious that the various clearance constants bear a relation to the corresponding rate constants by the appropriate volume (e.g., $k_{C12} = k_{12}/V_1$, etc.).

The exponents and the constant factors at each exponential function are rather complicated functions of the model parameters. From the coefficients A_1 and A_2 and the rate or time-constants the total body clearance and the volume of the central compartment can be calculated

$$k_{Cel} = D/(A_1\tau_1 + A_2\tau_2); \quad V_1 = D/(A_1 + A_2).$$
$$(44)$$

The other parameters are more complicated relations of these coefficients (Van Rossum, 1971). The volume of distribution by taking the concentration in the central compartment C_1 as a reference may be found as follows:

$$V_f = V_1(1 + k_{12}/k_{21}).$$
$$(45)$$

A few examples are given in Figure 16.

The behavior of diazepam may be described by a two compartment model (Van der Kleijn et al., 1971). This also holds for many other psychopharmacologic agents, e.g., lithium (Caldwell et al., 1971). Few literature data are available from which estimations of model parameters from actual measurements are made. Nelson (1964) has done this using a slightly simplified model of Wendel (1961) for the evaluation of eight points of measurement of the blood level after intravenous administration of 2.0 g of sulfaethidole, having an acidic pK_a of 5.1 so that 99.6% of the drug is ionized at the pH of the blood. Nelson found a blood volume of 3.7 l and an extravascular compartment for this drug of 12.1 l, the latter of which is not too far from known values of the volume of the interstitial fluid, suggesting that in this experiment of a duration of 8 h, sulfaethidole seems to permeate only in negligible amounts into the cells because of its high degree of ionization. In animal experiments it is easy to show Schade and Menschel's (1923) viewpoint that the body fluids might be subdivided into only three compartments holds for several drugs.

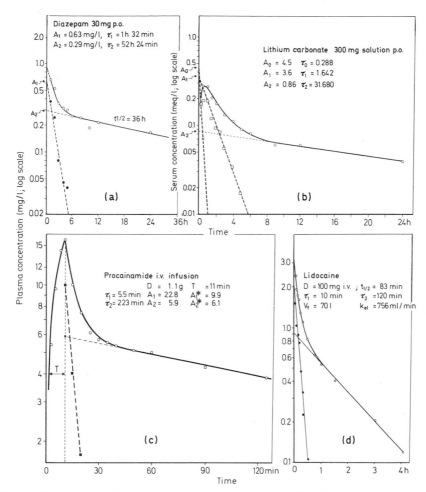

Fig. 16a—d. Serum and plasma concentration curves of a few drugs that are biphasic. (a) Diazepam. (data by VAN DER KLEIJN et al., 1971.) (b) Lithium carbonate (Data by CALDWELL, 1971.) (c) Procainamide (Data by KOCH-WESER, 1971.) (d) Lidocaine (Data by ROWLAND et al., 1971)

LANGECKER (1953) has done this with sulfa drugs using dogs without functioning kidneys. For dogs who do not acetylate the aromatic amino group of sulfa drugs, the concentration curves of these drugs after intravenous administration reflect nothing other than the kinetics of distribution. For sulfamerazine ($pK_a = 7.0$) LANGECKER (1953) found an obvious change in the slope of the declining curve at about 20 min, while the drug equilibrium was reached 60–80 min after intravenous administration.

Since it is possible to measure the volume of plasma water, interstitial fluid, and intracellular water by methods independent from the pharmacokinetic experiments, one may assume that these volumes are known quantities for the purpose of studying drug kinetics.

At first glance one might expect that the distribution of drugs through more than one compartment would cause a deviation from linearity of the dose-concentration relationship. However, this is only the case if elimination is not slow with respect to distribution.

2. The Slope of the Log Concentration-Time Curve

As pointed out earlier, the concentration in the peripheral compartment cannot be accessed experimentally and can not be calculated from that in the central compartment. However, the quantity of drug in the various compartments can be calculated. The drug concentrations C_1 and C_2, in the central and peripheral compartment, follow different patterns in time and are by no means "parallel" to each other in a semilogarithmic plot. Since $Q_1 = V_1 C_1$ and $Q_2 = V_2 C_2$ the quantity-time curves have the same profile as the concentration-time curves. In Figure 16c the quantity of drug is calculated from experiments with procainamide (KOCH-WESER, 1970). It is obvious that concomitantly with the initial fall in the plasma concentration the concentration increases while ultimately both curves (when plotted on a semilogarithmic scale) decline in a parallel fashion. This may be seen from the initial (for $t = 0$) and final slope (for $t = \infty$) of the semilogarithmic curves.

Initially for $t = 0$:

$$\frac{d \ln C_1}{dt} = -(k_{Cel} + k_{C12})/V_1 \quad \text{and} \quad \frac{d \ln C_2}{dt} = k_{C12}/V_1 . \tag{46}$$

So the initial slope of the semilogarithmic concentration curve in the central compartment is negative and that in the peripheral compartment is positive. And ultimately for $t = \infty$

$$\frac{d \ln C_1}{dt} = -k_2 = -1/\tau_2 \quad \text{and also} \quad \frac{d \ln C_2}{dt} = -k_2 = -1/\tau_2 . \tag{47}$$

So the slope is identical for both curves. As a consequence, it is an interesting property of the two-compartment open model that most of the change of the slope from its initial to its final value occurs in a restricted range of time. Therefore the two parts of the curve, separated by this range, may be approximated by straight lines, as has often been done in literature.

3. A Three Compartment Model

A three compartment model may be used to describe the concentration of drug in the plasma, the peripheral tissues, and the brain. A three term exponential equation is obtained. The total body clearance is again a simple relation of the time-constants and coefficients.

$$k_{Cel} = D/(\tau_1 \cdot A_1 + \tau_2 \cdot A_2 + \tau_3 \cdot A_3) . \tag{48}$$

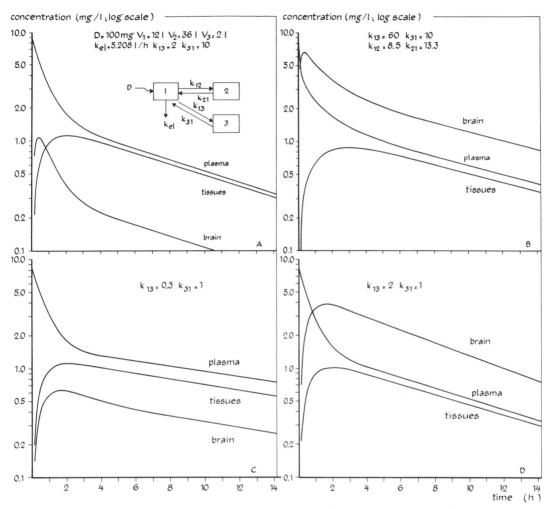

Fig. 17. Theoretical drug concentration curves in blood plasma, brain, and peripheral tissues for drugs which only differ with respect to blood : brain partition ratio (k_{C13}/k_{C31}). Small changes in this ratio evoke large changes in brain concentration curves. Plasma curves, however, remain practically the same, because brain is too small a compartment to influence plasma concentration profile. (Data from VAN ROSSUM, 1973, with permission of publishers of Psychiat. Neurol. Neurochir., Amsterdam)

In Figure 17 a theoretical example is given in which the rate of penetration into the brain is varied while all other parameters are being kept constant. As the brain is a small compartment there is little influence on the plasma curve by the clearance constant characterizing entry in the brain. It may be seen that a small change in this clearance constant has a tremendous influence on the brain concentration. Such clearance constants depend on physicochemical properties of drugs as lipid solubility. It is therefore understandable that in a series of barbiturates a substance such as phenobarbital slowly penetrates into the brain but that one such as thiopentobarbital very rapidly enters the brain.

IV. Multiple Dose Administration

As long as the kinetic processes following a single dose administration may be described by a set of linear differential equations, the plasma concentration is in general a n-term exponential equation:

$$C = \sum_{i=1}^{n} A_i e^{-t/\tau_i} = \sum_{i=1}^{n} A_1 e^{-t \cdot k_i}. \tag{49}$$

If a drug is administered in a fixed dose D, repetitively at fixed time intervals, Δt, the plasma concentration in a particular interval, e.g., the jth interval (the period following the jth dose) may be given by the following general equations (VAN ROSSUM, 1971).

$$C_j = \sum_{i=1}^{n} A_i \frac{1 - e^{-j\Delta t/\tau_i}}{1 - e^{-\Delta t/\tau_i}} e^{-t/\tau_i}. \tag{50}$$

Here t is the time that has the value zero at the moment of administration of the jth dose. It is obvious that following sufficient doses ($j \to \infty$) the plasma concentration reaches a steady state or plateau situation (VAN ROSSUM, 1971) Then:

$$C_j = \sum_{i=1}^{n} A_i e^{-t/\tau_i}/(1 - e^{\Delta t/\tau_i}). \tag{51}$$

This equation is analogous to that derived by DOST (1953). In the steady state the concentration starts to rise from the same initial level with each dose. The concentration at the end of the chronic therapy is described by the same equation, strongly resembling the equation of the single dose. Obviously the same time constants are involved but the coefficients A_i are increased by a factor to A_i^*

$$A_i^* = A_i/(1 - e^{\Delta t/\tau_i}). \tag{52}$$

This factor will be larger as τ_i is larger with respect to the dosage interval Δt. On the other hand, if $\Delta t \gg \tau_i$ the coefficient will be the same. In many cases the number of exponential terms may be reduced to two or three. The consequences of multiple dose-administration will therefore be illustrated first on a two term exponential equation representing absorption and elimination following oral intake.

A. The Therapeutic Purpose

The effect of many drugs is readily reversible if the drug concentration in the body fluids falls under a certain level. This applies to most drugs whose action is a simple function of the drug-receptor complex (ARIËNS, 1964). Only a few drugs have an irreversible action. Among chemotherapeutic agents the reversibly acting drugs are the bacteriostatic ones. For such drugs it is therapeutically desirably to maintain plasma levels above a minimum effective concentration. In other situations, i.e., the bactericide penicillins, it is sufficient to have a few times a day peak levels

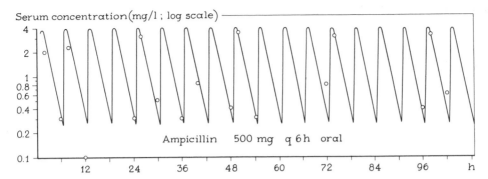

Fig. 18. Plasma concentration curve of ampicilline following repetitive oral administration of 500 mg every 6 h ($= \varDelta t$). Because of short half-life with respect to dosage interval each new dose gives practically same curve as first one. This is example of intermittent therapy. (Composed of data from FOLTZ et al., 1970)

exceeding the minimum effective concentration only for a limited period of time (Fig. 18).

The concept of a therapeutic dosage regimen refers (in the following) to the treatment of such pathologic situations that may not be adequately cured by a single drug administration. Dosage regimens of the type discussed in the following sections are not intended for drugs having an aftereffect, e.g., the bactericidal chemotherapeutic agents penicillin, streptomycin, and isoniazid, for the concentrationtime-activity relationship is not so simple as in the case of reversibly acting drugs.

For achieving the desired therapeutic effect the therapeutically acting concentration level of reversibly acting drugs has to be reached as soon as possible and maintained throughout the whole duration of therapy. It is well known that this level may be attained by an initial dose which is higher than the maintenance doses following repetitive intake at constant dosage intervals. It has been deduced (KRÜGER-THIEMER, 1960b) that the ratio of the initial dose to the maintenance dose, (in the following it is called the dose ratio) is a characteristic quantity important for the understanding of accumulation and other dosage regimen problems.

The duration of the therapy is not a pharmacokinetic problem because it is mainly determined by pathophysiologic conditions or by the host-bacteria interactions. The ratio of the asymptotic maximum and minimum concentrations of a multiple dose curve is of importance to adjust the dose to allow maximum therapeutic and minimum toxic action.

1. Intravascular Administration of Multiple Doses

The first approaches to the multiple dose problem have been made for intravenous injection. To the best of our knowledge WIDMARK and TANDBERG (1924) have been the first to treat this problem. Under the assumption of repeated equal doses, D, administered intravenously with equal dosage intervals, $\varDelta t$, these authors have calculated the mathematical behavior of the accumulation curve. The concentration in the plasma during the jth dosage-interval, that is after the jth intravenous injection, is a reduction of the general Equation (50) (DOST, 1953).

$$C_{(j)} = \frac{D}{V_f} \cdot \frac{1 - e^{-j \cdot \Delta t/\tau_{el}}}{1 - e^{-\Delta t/\tau_{el}}} \cdot e^{-t/\tau_{el}} \tag{53}$$

where $t = 0$ just after injection of the jth dose. After sufficient doses $(j \to \infty)$ a plateau is reached.

$$C_{pl} = \frac{D}{V_f} \frac{1}{(1 - e^{-\Delta t/\tau_{el})}} \cdot e^{-t/\tau_{el}} . \tag{54}$$

The maximum points of the serrated curve lie on a curve given by the following equation obtained just after each injection:

$$C_{max} = \frac{D}{V_f} \bigg/ (1 - e^{-\Delta t/\tau_{el}}) . \tag{55}$$

The corresponding equation for the minimum points of the serrated curve obtained just *before* the injection of each dose, that is the period Δt after each dose, becomes:

$$C_{min} = \frac{D}{V_f} e^{-\Delta t/\tau_{el}} / (1 - e^{-\Delta t/\tau_{el}}) . \tag{56}$$

In Figure 2 such a serratic curve, calculated from data after single dose injections of a sulphonamide, may be seen. From these two equations the asymptotic ratio R_{ext} may be calculated:

$$C_{max}/C_{min} = R_{ext} = e^{\Delta t/\tau_{el}} = 2^{\Delta t/t_{\frac{1}{2}}} . \tag{57}$$

This ratio of extreme concentrations after multiple dosing via the intravascular route of administration is a very simple relation of the dosage interval and the elimination time constant or the biological half-life.

From the concentration at the time period after the first dose:

$$C_{\Delta t} = \frac{D}{V_f} \cdot e^{-\Delta t/\tau_{el}} \tag{58}$$

and the minimum concentration at the plateau [Eq. (56)] the dose ratio, R^*, can be calculated:

$$R^* = 1/(1 - e^{-\Delta t/\tau_{el}}) = 1/(1 - 2^{-\Delta t/t_{\frac{1}{2}}}) . \tag{59}$$

This means that in order to reach the minimum concentration already after the first dose, an initial dose $D \cdot R^*$ should be given.

TEORELL (1937) has given the equations for intravascular administration in the case of a two-compartment system, considering distribution, metabolism in the extravascular compartment, and renal excretion, and WIDMARK and TANDBERG (1924) have developed equations for the description of the behavior of acetone in the human body, at the plateau in a semiempirical form. General asymptotic equations were used by BOXER et al. (1948) for studying the pharmacokinetics of streptomycin.

The ratio of extreme concentrations for a particular drug depends largely on the dosage interval Δt. This implies that by choosing shorter intervals the repetitive injection approaches an intravenous infusion.

2. Continuous Intravenous Infusion

WIDMARK and TANDBERG (1924) have also derived equations for continuous intravascular infusion of a drug (KRÜGER-THIEMER, 1968a). If the amount of drug D is infused during the time T, the drug concentration may be described by the following equation if only a single compartment is considered.

$$C = \frac{D}{V_f} \cdot \frac{\tau_{el}}{T} (1 - e^{-t/\tau_{el}}). \tag{60}$$

If the infusion is continued over sufficient long periods of time $(T \gg \tau_{el})$ the asymptotic value is obtained:

$$C_{pl} = \frac{D}{V_f} \cdot \frac{\tau_{el}}{T} = \frac{D \cdot \tau_{el}}{T \cdot G \cdot d} = \frac{D}{T} \frac{1}{G \cdot d \cdot k} \tag{61}$$

where k is the rate constant of elimination. The maximum (asymptotic) drug concentration for a continuous intravascular administration is proportional to the dose flow, D/T, which is the administered drug amount per time unit, and proportional to the time constant for elimination τ_{el}. The corresponding equations for a model regarding distribution, metabolism in the extravascular compartment, and renal excretion have been given by TEORELL (1937).

3. Extravascular Administration of Multiple Dose Therapy

The next step toward an understanding of the dose-concentration relationship with the goal of a dosage regimen theory is the calculation of accumulation curves corresponding to Equation (36) for extravascular drug administration (DOST, 1953; DRUCKREY and KÜPFMÜLLER, 1949). It may be calculated from the following equation, which is a special form of Equation (50) that:

$$C_{(j)} = \frac{D}{V_f} \cdot \frac{\tau_{el}}{(\tau_{el} - \tau_a)} \left[\frac{1 - e^{-j\Delta t/\tau_{el}}}{1 - e^{-\Delta t/\tau_{el}}} e^{-t/\tau_{el}} - \frac{1 - e^{-j\Delta t/\tau_a}}{1 - e^{-\Delta t/\tau_a}} e^{-t/\tau_a} \right]. \tag{62}$$

The time t is zero at the start of each dose while $\tau_{el} \neq \tau_a$ [Eq. (19)]. In this equation it is again assumed that j is the number of doses, D, including the first one, given until a certain point of time and that the first dose equals all the following ones. From such an equation DOST (1953) has deduced an equation for the asymptotic *minimum* concentration ($t = 0$ and $j \to \infty$):

$$C_{min} = \frac{D}{V_f} \frac{\tau_{el}}{(\tau_{el} - \tau_a)} \left[\frac{1}{1 - e^{-\Delta t/\tau_{el}}} - \frac{1}{1 - e^{-\Delta t/\tau_a}} \right] \tag{63}$$

and corresponding equations for the asymptotic maximum concentration, C_{max}, and for the time, t_{max}, at which this maximum will be reached. Obviously the maximum concentration is less than that obtained in case of intravascular administration. If, however, $\tau_{el} \gg \tau_a$ the equation approaches that for the intravascular injection.

4. Drug Accumulation and the Desired Plateau Effect

A generalization of Dost's equation for accumulation has been derived by WIEGAND et al. (1963) and by KRÜGER-THIEMER (1962) for arbitrary values of the first dose, D^* (see KRÜGER-THIEMER and BÜNGER, 1965/66a, b). WIEGAND et al. have first concluded from this equation that the application of equation for the dose ratio yields the desired plateau effect only if the time constant for absorption, τ_a, is appreciably smaller than the time constant for elimination, τ_{el}. Because this condition $\tau_{el} \gg \tau_a$ is valid, e.g., for sulfa drugs, dose-rate calculations have been successfully used for the dosage regimen estimation of many new sulfa drugs (BÜNGER, et al., 1961; BÜNGER, et al., 1964; BERLIN and KRÜGER-THIEMER, 1964; KRÜGER-THIEMER and BÜNGER, 1965/1966a). A theoretical study (KRÜGER-THIEMER, 1966a) of the general equation of accumulation has proved that equation (61) holds with sufficient accuracy, if τ_{el} is about 5 times τ_a or even higher. This is true for all sulfa drugs as far studied.

B. Dosage Regimens

1. Empirical Rules for Dosage Regimens

It is rather interesting that the clinician, SCHREUS (1926), obviously without knowledge of the article of WIDMARK and TANDBERG (1924), has deduced from clinical observations quite correct ideas on the dosage regimen of arsphenamine having the best therapeutic activity and the least toxic result. Actually, the idea of SCHREUS (1926) was ahead of those of his predecessors and also of TEORELL (1937), BOXER et al. (1948), and DOST (1953), even though he did not use the mathematical language. Figure 19 is taken from the article of SCHREUS (1926, p. 415), commented by him in the following way: after 15 min only about 35% of the initial blood concentration of arsphenamine is left. For restoring the initial situation it is necessary to administer at that moment only 65% of the initial dose. The more rapid the second dose follows the first one, the lower the second dose may be. This may be repeated as long as it is necessary to maintain a certain drug level in the blood.

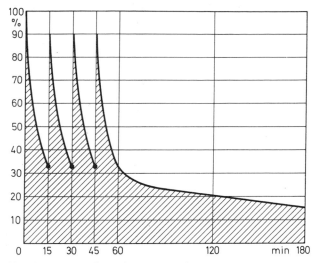

Fig. 19. Relative blood concentration of arsphenamine achieved by an initial dose of 300 mg i.v. followed by 150 mg every 15 min. This curve is probably the first example of rational dosage regimen. (Adopted from SCHREUS, Arch. Dermat. Syph., 1926)

2. Theory of Dosage Regimens

The concentration during the dosage interval. If the plasma concentration of a drug may be described by a set of linear differential equations, the plasma concentration at the time t after administration of a single dose D may be given by the following equation:

$$C = \sum_{i=1}^{n} A_i e^{-t/\tau_i}. \tag{64}$$

The equation of repetitive administration of the same dose D spaced by time-intervals or dosage intervals Δt has been given before, also (see Eq. (50)]. In general the initial dose is R^* times the maintenance dose D so that the plasma concentration in the jth dosage interval, implying that the first dose is the initial dose $R^* \cdot D$ followed by $(j-1)$ doses D, may be described by the following equation:

$$C_j = \sum_{i=1}^{n} A_i^* e^{-t^*/\tau_i} \quad \text{where} \quad t^* = t - (j-1)\Delta t \tag{65}$$

and

$$A_i^* = A_i \left[\frac{1 - e^{-j\Delta t/\tau_{e1}}}{1 - e^{-\Delta t/\tau_{e1}}} + (R^* - 1) e^{-(j-1)\Delta t/\tau_i} \right]. \tag{66}$$

It is obvious that if the initial dose is equal to the maintenance dose the second term in A_i^* is zero and Equation (50) is obtained again (see Figs. 20 and 21).

If t^* is zero at the moment of administration of the jth dose, that is the start of the jth dosage interval. The minimum concentration that is the concentration

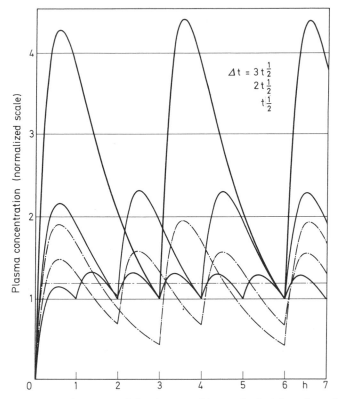

Fig. 20. Plasma concentration curves following repetitive oral administration of a drug in order to achieve a certain average concentration or maintainance of concentration above a minimum value by using dosage intervals equal to half-life, double the half-life, or three times $t\frac{1}{2}$ (Reproduced from Krüger-Thiemer, Proc. 3rd Int. Pharmacol. Meeting, Vol. 7 (1968c)

just before the administration of the jth dose is given by the following equation:

$$C_j^{\min} = \sum_{i=1}^{n} A_i^* \text{ where } A_i^* \text{ is given by Equation (66).}$$

After sufficient doses when $j\Delta t \gg \tau_i$, a plateau is reached.

$$C_{\text{plateau}} = \sum_{i=1}^{n} A_{i_{\text{pl}}}^* e^{-t^*/\tau_i} \tag{67}$$

but now $A_{i_{\text{pl}}}^*$ is given by the following equation:

$$A_{i_{\text{pl}}}^* = A_i/(1 - e^{-\Delta t/\tau_i}). \tag{68}$$

This equation is equal to Equation (52) for the case that the initial dose is equal to the maintenance dose. Consequently, irrespective of the initial dose, the plateau is merely determined by the maintenance dose. This is also the case for the minimum concentration in the plateau situation.

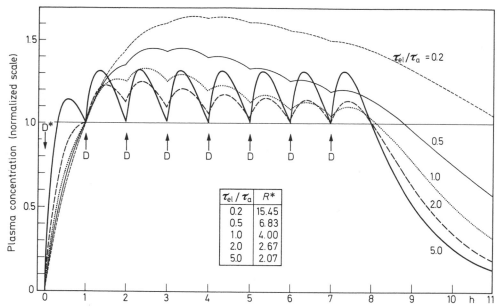

Fig. 21. Plasma concentration curves of five different drugs following repetitive oral administration in order to maintain concentration above minimum value. Dosage interval is equal to elimination half-life. Initial dose is varied and time constant for absorption, too. Curves are normalized by giving at the ordinate the concentration relative to minimum value and time scale in units of half-life. Curves show insufficient plateau concentration for drugs, which are slowly absorbed. Reproduced from KRÜGER-THIEMER, Proc. 3rd Int. Pharmacol. Meeting, Vol. 7 (1968c)

3. Theory of Dosage Regimens: The Average Concentration in the Dosage Interval

During chronic medication it is not easy to obtain sufficient plasma data in order to calculate the serratic plasma curve. If the curve does not oscillate too much it is useful to calculate the average plasma concentration over each dosage interval. The average plasma concentration in the jth interval that is between the jth and the $(j+1)^{th}$ dose is obtained by integration of Equation (65) from 0 till Δt

$$\bar{C}_j = \frac{1}{\Delta t} \int_0^{\Delta t} C_j dt = \frac{1}{\Delta t} \sum_{i=1}^n A_i^* \int_0^{\Delta t} e^{-t^*/\tau_i}\, dt = \sum_{i=1}^n A_i^* \frac{\tau_i}{\Delta t} \cdot (1 - e^{\Delta t/\tau_i}). \qquad (69)$$

Substitution of A_i^* in this equation gives the following equation:

$$\bar{C}_j = \sum_{i=1}^n A_i\, \frac{\tau_i}{\Delta t} \left[(1 - e^{-j\Delta t/\tau_i}) + (R^* - 1)(1 - e^{-\Delta t/\tau_i}) e^{-(j-1)\Delta t/\tau_i} \right]. \qquad (70)$$

When a fixed dose D is used throughout the repetitive medication the equation is simplified because then $R^* = 1$ and the second term disappears. The average concentration, the jth dosage interval, then becomes:

$$\bar{C}_j = \sum_{i=1}^{n} A_i \frac{\tau_i}{\Delta t} (1 - e^{-j\Delta t/\tau_i}). \tag{71}$$

This equation is analogous to that for continuous intravascular infusion. Compare Equation (60) (which is the reduced form of Equations (71). After enough doses the plateau is reached which is obtained by integration of Equation (67).

$$\bar{C}_{plateau} = \sum_{i=1}^{n} \frac{A_i \tau_i}{\Delta t} = \frac{D \cdot F}{k_{Cel} \cdot \Delta t}. \tag{72}$$

So the average plateau concentration merely depends on the maintenance dose, the bioavailability F, and the total body clearance. Provided that the clearance indeed remains constant.

The biological availability F depends directly on the plateau level. This is obvious because the amount Q_{el} eliminated during each dosage interval at the plateau is equal to the amount of DF entering the general circulation.

$$Q_{el} = \int_{0}^{\Delta t} d \cdot Q_{el} = k_{Cel} \int_{0}^{\Delta t} C_{pl} \cdot dt = k_{Cel} \sum_{i=1}^{n} A_i \tau_i = DF. \tag{73}$$

By measuring the plateau concentration the total body clearance may be calculated if F is known. On the other hand, if one knows what the average concentration should be and the kinetic parameters of a drug are known, the maintenance dose can be accessed.

4. Dosage Regimens for Rapidly Absorbed Drugs

The dosage regimen of drugs, which should be given in such a way that the plasma concentration is kept above a minimum effective level, has to be appropriate. This implies that the maintenance dose D given at regular dosage intervals Δt should be so large that at the end of a dosage interval the concentration still exceeds the minimum effective concentration. Therefore, under steady-state conditions that is in the plateau situation:

$$C_{pl} > C_{min} \quad \text{while} \quad C_{pl}(t = \Delta t) = \sum_{i=1}^{n} A_i \frac{e^{-\Delta t/\tau_i}}{1 - e^{-\Delta t/\tau_i}}. \tag{74}$$

For drugs given orally while absorption is rapid with respect to elimination the following equation holds: $(j = \infty; t = \Delta t)$

$$C_{pl\,min} = A \left[\frac{e^{-\Delta t/\tau_{el}}}{(1 - e^{-\Delta t/\tau_{el}})} - \frac{e^{-\Delta t/\tau_a}}{(1 - e^{-\Delta t/\tau_a})} \right] = A \cdot \frac{e^{-\Delta t/\tau_{el}} - e^{-\Delta t/\tau_a}}{(1 - e^{-\Delta t/\tau_{el}})(1 - e^{-\Delta t/\tau_a})} \tag{75}$$

(see Figs. 20 and 21).

At the end of the first dosage interval, that is Δt after administration of the initial dose $(D^* = R^* \cdot D)$, the concentration is as follows: $(j = 1; t = \Delta t)$

$$C_{j=1} = R^* \cdot A(e^{-\Delta t/\tau_{el}} - e^{-\Delta t/\tau_a}). \tag{76}$$

In order to ensure from the first dose on that the plasma concentration remains above the minimum effective concentration the initial dose should be R^* times the maintenance dose while R^* has the following value:

$$R^* = \frac{D^*}{D} = \frac{1}{(1 - e^{-\Delta t/\tau_{el}})(1 - e^{-\Delta t/\tau_a})}. \tag{77}$$

This ratio may be considered as a kind of accumulation factor. Compare Equation (57).

The maintenance dose D should be so large that $C_{pl}(t = \Delta t) > C_{min}$. This implies that the dose should bear the following relation to the kinetic constants.

$$D = V_f \cdot \phi \cdot C_{min} \tag{78}$$

where ϕ is the pharmacokinetic factor (in this case for oral administration) (KRÜGER-THIEMER, 1966a, 1969)

$$\phi = (1 - \tau_a/\tau_{el}) \frac{(1 - e^{-\Delta t/\tau_{el}})(1 - e^{\Delta t/\tau_a})}{(e^{-\Delta t/\tau_{el}} - e^{-\Delta t/\tau_a})}. \tag{79}$$

The volume of distribution relates to a formal capacity factor d for which KRÜGER-THIEMER introduced the term plasma distribution coefficient $(V_f = G \cdot d)$ (KRÜGER-THIEMER, 1964b). The distribution coefficient strongly depends on plasma protein binding, distribution between plasma, and tissues, etc.

So the maintenance dose D should be:

$$D > F \cdot d \cdot \Phi. \tag{80}$$

The correct initial dose may then easily be calculated. The choice of the initial and the maintenance dose, the estimation of the pharmacokinetic factor Φ (in relation to the dosage interval), and the interrelation of the ratio of maximum-minimum concentration may easily be obtained from nomograms. (KRÜGER-THIEMER and BÜNGER, 1965/66a, b). In these nomograms the mutual dependencies of R^*, Φ, and C_{max}/C_{min} from the relative dosage interval $\Delta t/t_{\frac{1}{2}}$ have been calculated only for three cases where the time constant for elimination is 2–5 times or much larger than the time constant for absorption.

5. Dosage Regimens for Slowly Absorbed Drugs

Drug accumulation following repetitive oral administration of doses after constant dosage intervals may follow equation 70. A problem occurs when the time constant for absorption equals the time constant for elimination. Then (KRÜGER-

Table 1. Maintenance dose calculated for an average patient ($G = 70$ kg, $p = 70$ g/l, $w = 0.934$) for various sulpha drugs on basis kinetic parameters and protein binding

Sulfa drug	Mol. w.	MEC (Molar) $\cdot 10^{-6}$	C_{min}^{f} (Molar) $\cdot 10^{-6}$	C_{min}^{f} mg/l	K_p Molar $\cdot 10^{-4}$	β (Mol/g) $\cdot 10^{-6}$	d (mol/g)	d_f (mg/g)	Φ	$t_{\frac{1}{2}}$ (h)	Δt (h)	Maint. dose D (mg) calc.	used
Sulfalene	280	1.6	16	4.48	3.66	18.2	0.21	0.90	0.32	60	24	90	500
Sulfamethoxazole	253	0.9	9	2.28	5.36	26.3	0.22	0.95	1.24	10	12	190	1000
Sulfadiazine	250	1.0	10	2.50	8.92	16.0	0.92	2.01	0.27	17	6	100	1000
									0.61		12	220	
Sulfamethoxypyridazine	280	1.0	10	2.80	1.14	23.2	0.19	2.66	0.60	35	24	320	500
Sulfamerazine	264	0.9	9	2.38	0.72	7.4	0.36	2.64	0.25	23.5	8	110	1000
									0.92		24	410	
Sulfametin	280	2.0	20	5.60	1.19	18.6	0.26	2.68	0.57	37	24	600	500
Sulfamoxole	267	3.4	34	9.08	3.48	27.0	0.25	1.59	1.10	11	12	1110	500
Sulfamethoxine	310	0.8	8	2.48	0.11	20.5	0.17	13.7	0.49	41	24	1170	500
Sulfanilamid	172	128	1280	220	7.0	7.0	0.69	0.83	0.76	9	8	9700	1000

From data of Krüger-Thiemer and Bünger (1965/66a).

Thiemer, 1966a):

$$C_j = \frac{D}{V}\left[\frac{\left(1-\left(\frac{\Delta t}{\tau}\right)^{(j-1)}\cdot e^{-(j-1)\Delta t/\tau}\right)}{\left(1-\frac{\Delta t}{\tau}\cdot e^{-\Delta t/\tau}\right)}+(R-1)\left(\frac{\Delta t}{\tau}\right)^{(j-1)}\cdot e^{-(j-1)\Delta t/\tau}\right]e^{-t*/\tau}$$

(see Fig. 21).

A detailed description of dosage regimen calculations has been given by Krüger-Thiemer (1966a) while also the calculation of the exact plateau effect has been analyzed by Krüger-Thiemer (1969).

V. Conclusion

From pharmacokinetic data obtained after administration of a single dose to humans and, if necessary, relevant data plasmaprotein binding pK_a and the partition coefficient oil : water, adequate therapeutic dosage regimens can be calculated, provided that the requirements for therapy are known. The latter deals with problems as to whether intermittent blood levels are sufficient or whether a continuous level above a threshold is required. See Figure 18 for intermittent therapy and Figure 2 for continuous therapy.

Intermittent therapy in fact is a repitition of single doses at intervals so far apart that practically no drug is left from the previous dose, when the next dose is given (e.g., penicillins).

Continuous therapy makes use of residuals of the previous doses and actually is guided accumulation. Typical examples are the sulphonamides.

Dose schedules in use are often inadequate because they do not take into account the relevant kinetic data. See Table 1. It is obvious that the so-called trisulphas, in which three sulpha drugs with quite different half-lives have been combined, are inadequate because if the dosage regimen for one compartment is right, it will be wrong for the others.

References

Adams, M. A., Roe, A. S.: A partially defined medium for a cultivation of pneumococcus. J. Bact. **49**, 401—409 (1945).

Albert, A.: Selective toxicity. 2nd Ed. New York: J. Wiley, 1960.

Ariëns, E. J.: Affinity and intrinsic activity in the theory of competitive inhibition. Part I. Problems and theory. Arch. int. Pharmacodyn. **99**, 32—50 (1954).

Ariëns, E. J.: Molecular pharmacology, Vol. I. New York: Academic Press Inc., 1964.

Azzolini, F., Gazzaniga, A., Lodola, E., Natangelo, R.: Elimination of chloramphenicol and thiamphenicol in subjects with cirrhosis of the liver. Int. J. Clin. Pharmacol. **6**, 130—134 (1972).

Barr, W. H.: Factors involved in the assessment of systemic or biologic availability of drug products. Drug. Inform. Bull. **3**, 27—45 (1969).

Beckett, A. H., Rowland, M., Turner, P.: Influence of urine pH on excretion of amphetamine. Lancet **I**, 1963, 303.

Berlin, H., Krüger-Thiemer, E.: Sulfonamidernas proteinbinding. Nord. Med. **72**, 1358—1362 (1964).

Berman, M., Shahn, E., Weiss, M. F.: The routine fitting of kinetic data to models. A mathematical formalism for digital computers. Biophys. J. **2**, 275—287 (1962a).

Berman, M., Weiss, M. F., Shahn, E.: Some formal approaches to the analysis of the kinetic data in terms of linear compartmental systems. Biophys. J. **2**, 289—316 (1962b).

Bönicke, R., Lisboa, B. P.: Über die Erbbedingtheit der Intraindividuellen Konstanz der Isoniazidausscheidung beim Menschen. (Untersuchungen an eineiigen und zweieiigen Zwillingen). Naturwissenschaften **44**, 314 (1957).

Boxer, G. E., Jelinek, V. C., Tompsett, R., Dubois, R., Edison, A. O.: Streptomycin in the blood: chemical determination after single and repeated intramuscular injections. J. Pharmacol. exp. Ther. **92**, 226—235 (1948).

Breimer, D. D.: Pharmacokinetics of Hypnotic Drugs. Ph. D. Thesis. Nijmegen: Drukkerij Brakkenstein, 1974.

Brunton, T. L.: Lectures on the action of medicines. Beeing the course of lectures on pharmacology and therapeutics. New York: MacMillan Co., 1899.

Bünger, P.: Praktische Erfahrungen mit der Anwendung neuer Langzeitsulfonamide. Vortr. 26. Fortbildungskursus Regensburg, 12.5.1961. Regensbg. Jb. ärztl. Fortbildung **10** (1962).

Bünger, P.: Die Pharmakokinetik des Fanasils (Sulfaorthodimethoxin). IV. Internat. Kongr. Infektionskrkh. Verhandlungsber., S. 855—868. Mössner, G., Thomssen, R. (Hrsg.) Stuttgart: Schattauer, 1967.

Bünger, P., Diller, W., Führ, J., Krüger-Thiemer, E.: Vergleichende Untersuchungen an neueren Sulfanilamiden. I. Arzneimittel-Forsch. **11**, 247—255 (1961).

Bünger, P., Isebarth, R., Kiessling, J., Voss, G., Witthöft, R.: Zur Sulfanilamidbehandlung schwerer bakterieller Infektionen. Bericht über eine gemeinsame Untersuchung an 13 Kliniken. Dtsch. Arch. klin. Med. **209**, 608—615 (1964).

Caldwell, H. C., Westlake, W. J., Connor, S. M., Flanagan, T.: A Pharmacokinetic analysis of lithium carbonate absorption from several formulations in man. J. Clin. Pharmacol. New Drugs **11**, 349—356 (1971).

Daehne, W. von, Godtfrensen, W. O., Roholt, K., Tybring, L.: Pivampicillin, a new orally active ampicillin ester. Antimicrob. Agents Chemother. **10**, 431—437 (1970).

DeMarco, T. J., Levine, R. R.: Role of the lymphatics in the intestinal absorption and distribution of drugs. J. Pharmacol. exp. Ther. **169**, 142—151 (1969).

Dettli, L., Spring, P.: Der Einfluß des Urin-pH auf die Eliminationsgeschwindigkeit einiger Sulfanilamid-Derivate. IIIrd Internat. Congr. Chemother. Stuttgart (1963), Proc. **1**, 641—644 (1964).

Diller, W.: Eine neue Methode zur Bestimmung der Geschwindigkeitskonstanten der Absorption und Distribution. Antibiot. and Chemother. **12**, 85—94 (1964).

Diller, W., Bünger, P.: Zur Pharmakokinetik der rectalen Applikation. Arzneimittel-Forsch. **15**, 1274—1278 (1965a).

Diller, W., Bünger, P.: Zur Pharmakokinetik der rectalen Applikation. Arzneimittel-Forsch. **15**, 1445—1456 (1965b).

Doluisio, J. T., Swintosky, J. V.: Factors influencing drug distribution in the body. Amer. J. Pharm. **137**, 144—168 (1965).

Dominguez, R.: Kinetics of elimination, absorption and volume of distribution in the organism. Medical Physics, Vol. **2**, Chicago: Yearbook Publ. Inc., pp. 476—489, 1950.

Dost, F. H.: Der Blutspiegel. Kinetik der Konzentrationsabläufe in der Kreislaufflüssigkeit. Leipzig: Thieme, 1953.

Dost, F. H.: Über ein einfaches statistisches Dosis-Umsatz-Gesetz. Klin. Wschr. **36**, 655—657 (1958).

Dost, F. H.: Grundlagen der Pharmakokinetik. Stuttgart: Thieme, 1968.

Druckrey, H., Küpfmüller, K.: Dosis und Wirkung. Beiträge zur theoretischen Pharmakologie. Pharmazie 8, Beiheft 1, Erg. Bd., p. 645. Aulendorf: Editio Cantor KG., 1949.

Fick, A.: Über Diffusion. Poggendorffs Ann. Physik (1855).

Foltz, E. L., West, J. W., Breslow, I. H., Wallick, H.: Clinical pharmacology of Pivampicillin. Antimicrob. Agents Chemother. **10**, 442—454 (1970).

Freundlich, H.: Über die Absorption in Lösungen. Z. Physik. Chem. **57**, 385—470 (1907).

Garrett, E. R., Johnston, R. L., Collins, E. J.: Kinetics of steroid effects on Ca^{47} dynamics in dogs with the analog computer. I. J. Pharm. Sci. **51**, 1050—1057 (1962).

Garrett, E. R., Johnston, R. L., Collins, E. J.: Kinetics of steroid effects on Ca^{47} dynamics in dogs with the analog computer. II. J. Pharm. Sci. **52**, 668—678 (1963).

Garrett, E. R., Thomas, R. C., Wallach, D. P., Alway, C. D.: Psicofuranine: kinetics and metabolism in vivo with the application of the analog computer. J. Pharmacol. exp. Ther. **130**, 106—118 (1960).

Gibaldi, M.: Introduction to biopharmaceutics. Philadelphia: Lea & Febiger, 1971.

Gillette, J. R.: Factors affecting drug metabolism. Ann. N. Y. Acad. Sci. **179**, 43—66 (1971).

Ginneken, C. A. M., van: Pharmacokinetics of Antipyretic and Anti-Inflammatory Analgesics. Ph. D. Thesis. Nijmegen: Stichting Studentenpers, 1976.

Gladtke, E.: Ermittlung der Absorptionsrate von Sulfonamiden bei Dyspepsien nach dem Gesetz der korrespondierenden Flächen. Mschr. Kinderheilk. **112**, 84—86 (1964).

Goldstein, A.: The interactions of drugs and plasma proteins. Pharmacol. Rev. **1**, 102—165 (1949).

Goldstein, A.: Biostatistics. New York: MacMillan Co., 1964.

Guldberg, C. M., Waage, P.: Untersuchungen über die chemische Affinitäten. Christiana (Oslo): Brögger & Christie, 1867.

Hunt, J. N.: Gastric emptying in relation to drug absorption. Amer. J. dig. Dis. **8**, 885—894 (1963).

Jusko, W. J., Levy, G.: Absorption, metabolism and excretion of riboflavin-5′-phosphate in man. J. pharm. Sci. **56**, 58—62 (1967).

Kalow, W.: Pharmacogenetics. Heridity and the response to drugs. Philadelphia-London: W. B. Saunders Co., 1962.

Keberle, H., Krüger-Thiemer, E., Sackman, W., Schmid, K., Seydel, J.: Proc. Vth. Internat. Congr. Chemother. Vol. 4, p. 157. Wien: Verlag der Wiener Medizinischen Akademie, 1967.

Kleijn, E. van der., Rossum, J. M. van, Muskens, E. T. J. M., Rijntjes, N. V. M.: Pharmacokinetics of diazepam in dogs, mice and human. Acta Pharmacol. et Toxicol. **29**, Suppl. 3, 109—127 (1971).

Koch-Weser, J.: Pharmacokinetics of procainamide in man. Ann. N. Y. Acad. Sci. **179**, 370—382 (1971).

Koizumi, T., Arita, T., Kakemi, K.: Absorption and excretion of drugs. XXI. Some pharmacokinetic aspects of absorption and excretion of sulfonamides 3. Excretion from the kidney. Chem Pharmaceut. Bull. **12**, 428—432 (1964).

Kostenbauder, H. B., Portnoff, J. B., Swintosky, J. V.: Control of urine pH and its effect on sulfaethidole excretion in humans. J. pharm. Sci. **51**, 1084—1089 (1962).

Krebs, H. A., Sykes, W. O., Bartley, W. C.: Acetylation and deacetylation of the p-amino group of sulphonamide drugs in animal tissues. Biochem. J. **41**, 622—630 (1947).

Krüger-Thiemer, E.: Dosage schedule and pharmacokinetics in chemotherapy. J. Amer. pharm. Ass. sci. Ed. **49**, 311—313 (1960a).

Krüger-Thiemer, E.: Funktionale Beziehungen zwischen den pharmakokinetischen Eigenschaften und der Dosierung von Chemotherapeutica. Klin. Wschr. **38**, 514—520 (1960b).

Krüger-Thiemer, E.: Theorie der Wirkung bakteriostatischer Chemotherapeutica. Quantitative Beziehungen zwischen Dosierung, in vitro Wirkung, Pharmakokinetik und Distribution. Jber. Borstel **5**, 316—400 (1961).

Krüger-Thiemer, E.: Cause and prevention of drug cumulation. Paper Presented to the Scientific Section of the American Pharmaceutic Association, Las Vegas, Nevada (1962).

Krüger-Thiemer, E.: Die Anwendung programmgesteuerter Ziffernrechenautomaten für die Lösung spezieller chemotherapeutischer Probleme. Antibiot. et Chemother. **12**, 253—269 (1964a).

Krüger-Thiemer, E.: Die Lösung chemotherapeutischer Probleme durch programmgesteuerte Ziffernrechenautomaten. 4. Arzneimittel-Forsch. **14**, 1332—1343 (1964b).

Krüger-Thiemer, E.: Die Auswertung der pharmakokinetischen Grundgleichung nach Teorell und Dost bei ein- und mehrmaliger Applikation mit programmgesteuerten Ziffernrechenautomaten. IIIrd. Intern. Congr. Chemother., Stuttgart (1963), Proc. **2**, 1686—1694 (1964c).

Krüger-Thiemer, E.: Formal theory of drug dosage regimens. I. J. theor. Biol. **13**, 212—235 (1966a).

Krüger-Thiemer, E.: Die Lösung pharmakologischer Probleme durch Rechenautomaten. 6. Arzneimittel-Forsch. **16**, 1431—1442 (1966b).

Krüger-Thiemer, E.: Influence of protein binding on dosage regimens of chemotherapeutic agents. Proc. Vth. Intern. Congr. Chemother., Wien, Proc. **4**, 215—222 (1967a).

Krüger-Thiemer, E.: Application of kinetic analysis in clinical pharmacology. In: Siegler, P. E., Moyer, J. H. (Eds.): Animal and Clinical pharmacological Techniques in Drug Evaluation. Vol. 2, Chicago: Year Book Medical Publ. pp. 217—238, 1967b.

Krüger-Thiemer, E.: Continuous intravenous infusion and multicompartment accumulation. Europ. J. Pharmacol. **4**, 317—324 (1968a).

Krüger-Thiemer, E.: Nonlinear dose-concentration relationships. Farmaco Ed. sci. **23**, 717—756 (1968b).

Krüger-Thiemer, E.: Pharmacokinetics and dose-concentration relationships. In: Ariëns, E. J. (Ed.): Proc. 3rd. Internat. Pharmacol. Meeting, Vol. 7, pp. 63—113, Physico-Chemical Aspects of Drug Actions. Oxford: Pergamon Press, 1968c.

Krüger-Thiemer, E.: Formal theory of drug dosage regimens. II. The exact plateau effect. J. theor. Biol. **23**, 169—190 (1969).

Krüger-Thiemer, E., Bünger, P.: Evaluation of the risk of crystalluria with sulfa drugs. Proc. Europ. Soc. Study Drug Tox. **6**, 185—207 (1965).

Krüger-Thiemer, E., Bünger, P.: The role of the therapeutic regimen in dosage design. Part I. Chemotherapia **10**, 61—73 (1965/66a).

Krüger-Thiemer, E., Bünger, P.: The role of the therapeutic regimen in dosage design. Part II. Chemotherapia **10**, 129—144 (1965/66b).

Krüger-Thiemer, E., Dettli, L., Spring, P., Diller, W.: Mathematical problems in the calculation of protein binding of drugs with digital computers. Paper presented to the third Congr. Internat. Med. Cibernetica, Naples (1964).

Krüger-Thiemer, E., Diller, W., Bünger, P.: Pharmacokinetic models regarding protein binding of drugs. Antimicrob. Agents Chemother. 1965a, 183—191.

Krüger-Thiemer, E., Eriksen, S. P.: Mathematical model of sustained-release preparations and its analysis. J. pharm. Sci. **55**, 1249—1253 (1966).

Krüger-Thiemer, E., Roesch, E., Rohmer, M., Wempe, E.: Dosage regimen calculation of chemotherapeutic agents. Part IV. 5-Sulfanilamido-1-ethyl-pyrazole. Chemotherapia **12**, 321—337 (1967).

Krüger-Thiemer, E., Wempe, E., Töpfer, M.: Die antibakterielle Wirkung des nicht eiweißgebundenen Anteils der Sulfanilamide im menschlichen Plasmawasser. Arzneimittel-Forsch. **15**, 1309—1317 (1965b).

Langecker, H.: Die Verteilung von Sulfanilsäure und Sulfonamiden beim nierenlosen Hund. Ein Beitrag zu den Gesetzmäßigkeiten von Verteilungsvorgängen im Körper. I. Arch. exp. Path. Pharmakol. **218**, 278—285 (1953).

Langmuir, I.: The constituttion and fundamental properties of solids and liquids. I. Solids. J. Amer. chem. Soc. **38**, 2221—2291 (1916).

Langmuir, I.: The constituttion and fundamental properties of solids and liquids. II. Liquids. J. Amer. chem. Soc. **39**, 1848—1906 (1917).

Larsen, J. A.: Elimination of ethanol as a measure of the hepatic blood flow in the cat. II. The significance of the extrahepatic elimination of ethanol. Acta physiol. scand. **57**, 209—223 (1963a).

Larsen, J. A.: Elimination of glycerol as a measure of the hepatic blood flow in the cat. Acta physiol. scand. **57**, 224—234 (1963b).

Levine, R. R., Pelikan, E. W.: Mechanism of drug absorption and excretion. Passage of drugs out of and into the gastrointestinal tract. Ann. Rev. Pharmacol. **4**, 69—84 (1964).

Levy, G.: Availability of spironolactone given by mouth. Lancet **1962 II**, 723.

Levy, G.: Biopharmaceutical considerations in dosage form design and evaluation. In: Sprowls, J. B., (Ed.): Prescription pharmacy. Dosage formulation and pharmaceutical adjuncts, pp. 31—94. Philadelphia-Montreal: J. B. Lippincott, 1963.

Levy, G.: Salicylurate formation—demonstration of Michaëlis-Menten kinetics in man. J. pharm. Sci. **54**, 496 (1965a).

Levy, G.: Apparent potentiating effect of a second dose of drug. Nature (Lond.) **206**, 517—518 (1965b).

Levy, G.: Pharmacokinetics of salicylate elimination in man. J. pharm. Sci. **54**, 959—967 (1965c).

Levy, G., Amsel, L. P.: Kinetics of competitive inhibition of salicylic acid conjugation with glycine in man. Biochem. Pharmacol. **15**, 1033—1038 (1966).

Levy, G., Amsel, L. P., Elliott, H. C.: Kinetics of salicyluric acid elimination in man. J. pharm. Sci. **58**, 827—828 (1969a).

Levy, G., Hall, N. A., Nelson, E.: Studies on Inactive Prednisone Tablets USP XVI. Am. J. Hosp. Pharmacy **21**, 402 (1964).

Levy, G., Hollister, L. E.: Dissolution rate limited absorption in man. Factors influencing drug absorption from prolonged-release dosage form. J. pharm. Sci. **54**, 1121—1125 (1965).

Levy, G., Matsuzawa, T.: Pharmacokinetics of salicylamide elimination in man. J. Pharmacol. exp. Ther. **156**, 285—293 (1967).

Levy, G., Procknal, J. A.: Dissolution rate studies on methylprednisolone polymorphs. J. pharm. Sci. **53**, 656—658 (1964).

Levy, G., Tanski, W. Jr.: Precision apparatus for dissolution rate determinations. J. pharm. Sci. **53**, 679 (1964).

Levy, G., Vogel, A. W., Amsel, L. P.: Capacity-limited salicylurate formation during prolonged administration of aspirin to healthy human subjects. J. pharm. Sci. **58**, 503—504 (1969b).

Lindner, H. R.: Comparative aspects of cortisol transport: Lack of firm binding to plasma proteins in domestic ruminants. J. Endocr. **28**, 301—320 (1964).

Lundquist, F., Wolthers, H.: Kinetics of alcohol elimination in man. Acta Pharmacol. Toxicol. **14**, 265—289 (1958).

Madsen, S. T.: Serum concentration and antibacterial activity of 4-sulfonamido-5,6-dimethoxy-pyrimidine. Amer. J. med. Sci. **247**, 217—222 (1964).

Madsen, S. T., Øvsthus, Ø., Bøe, J.: Antibacterial activity of long-acting sulfonamides. Acta med. scand. **173**, 707—717 (1963).

Meier, H.: Experimental pharmacogenetics. Physiopathology of heredity and pharmacological responses. New York-London: Academic. Press, 1963.

Mellinger, T. J., Bohorfoush, J. G.: Blood levels of dipyridamole (Persantin®) in humans. Arch. int. Pharmacodyn. **163**, 471—480 (1966).

Michaelis, D., Menten, M. L.: Die Kinetik der Invertinwirkung. Biochem. Z. **49**, 333—370 (1913).

Nakagaki, M., Koga, N., Terada, H.: Physicochemical studies on the binding of chemicals with proteins. I. The binding of several sulfonamides with serum albumin. Yakugaki Zasshi **83**, 586—590 (1963).

Nakagaki, M., Koga, N., Terada, H.: Physicochemical studies on the binding of chemicals with proteins. II. The mechanism of binding of several sulfonamides with serum albumin. Yakugaky Zasshi **84**, 516—521 (1964).

Nelson, E.: Kinetics of drug absorption, distribution, metabolism and excretion. J. pharm. Sci. **50**, 181—192 (1961).

Nelson, E.: Kinetics of the acetylation and excretion of sulfonamides and a comparison of two models. Antibiot. et Chemother. **12**, 29—40 (1964).

Nelson, E., Knoechel, E. L., Hamlin, W. E., Wagner, J. G.: Influence of absorption rate of tolbutamide on rate of decline of blood sugar levels in normal humans. J. pharm. Sci. **51**, 509—515 (1962).

Nelson, E., O'Reilly, I.: Kinetics of sulfisoxazole acetylation and excretion in humans. J. Pharmacol. exp. Ther. **129**, 368—372 (1960).

Nelson, E., O'Reilly, I.: Kinetics of sulfamethylthiadiazole acetylation and excretion in humans. J. pharm. Sci. **50**, 417—420 (1961).

Nogami, H., Hanano, M., Watanabe, J.: Studies on absorption and excretion of drugs. III. Kinetics of penetration of sulfonamides through the intestinal barrier in vitro. Chem. pharm. Bull. **10**, 1161—1170 (1962).

Nogami, H., Matsuzawa, T.: Studies on absorption and excretion of drugs. II. Kinetics of penetration of basic drug, aminopyrine, through the intestinal barrier in vitro. Chem. pharm. Bull. **10**, 1055—1060 (1962).

Noyes, A. A., Whitney, W. R.: The rate of solution of solid substances in their own solutions. J. Amer. chem. Soc. **19**, 930—934 (1897).

Os, J. A. G., van: Some remarks on the interaction of macromolecules with other molecules and ions. Arzneimittel-Forsch. **16**, 1428—1430 (1966).

Pitts, R. F.: Physiology of the kidney and body fluids. Chicago: Year Book Medical Publ., 1963.

Portnoff, J. B., Swintosky, J. V., Kostenbauder, H. B.: Control of urine pH and its effect on drug excretion in humans. J. pharm. Sci. **50**, 890 (1961).

Portwich, F., Büttner, H.: Über die Beeinflussung der Tubulusfunktion bei der Nierenausscheidung des 4-Sulfanilamido-2,6-dimethylpyrimidins. Arch. exp. Pathol. Pharmakol. **229**, 513—519 (1956).

Remmer, H.: Der Beschleunigte Abbau von Pharmaka in den Lebermikrosomen unter dem Einfluß von Luminal. Arch. exp. Pathol. **235**, 279—290 (1959).

Rescigno, A., Segre, G.: La Cinetica dei Farmaci e dei Traccianti Radioattivi. Ed. Torino: Bringhieri Soc. per Azione, 1961.

Rescigno, A., Segre, G.: Drug and tracer kinetics. Boston, Mass.: Ginn, 1966.

Riegelman, S.: Clinical evaluation of the effect of formulation variables on therapeutic performance of drugs. Drug. Inform. Bull. **3**, 59—67 (1969).

Riegelman, S., Loo, J. C. K., Rowland, M.: Shortcomings in pharmacokinetic analysis by conceiving the body to exhibit properties of a single compartment. J. pharm. Sci. **57**, 117—123 (1968).

Ritschel, W. A.: Biological half-lives of drugs. Drug Intell. Clin. Pharm. **4**, 332—347 (1970).

Roepke, R. R., Maren, T. H., Mayer, E.: Experimental investigations of sulfamethoxypyridazine. Ann. N.Y. Acad. Sci. **69**, 457—472 (1957).

Rossotti, F. J. C., Rossotti, H.: The determination of stability constants and other equilibrium constants in solution. New York, N.Y.: McGraw-Hill, 1961.

Rossum, J. M., van: Significance of pharmacokinetics for drug design and the planning of dosage regimens. In: Ariëns, E. J. (Ed.): Drug design, Vol. 1, pp. 470—517. New York: Academic Press Inc., 1971.

Rossum, J. M., van: Pharmacokinetics and psychopharmacological research. Psychiat. Neurol. Neurochir. **76**, 217—228 (1973).

Rowland, M., Thomson, A., Guichard, A., Melmon, K. L.: Disposition kinetics of lidocaine in normal subjects. Ann. N.Y. Acad. Sci. **179**, 383—398 (1971).

Schade, H., Menschel, H.: Über die Gesetze der Gewebsquellung und ihre Bedeutung für klinische Fragen (Wasseraustausch im Gewebe, Lymphbildung und Ödementstehung). Z. klin. Med. **96**, 279—327 (1923).

Schanker, L. S.: Passage of drugs across body membranes. Pharmacol. Rev. **14**, 501—530 (1962).

Schanker, L. S.: Physiological transport of drugs. Advanc. Drug Res. **1**, 71—106 (1964).

Schlender, B., Krüger-Thiemer, E.: Rechenautomaten und Pharmakotherapie. Pharmakotherapia **2**, 3—12 (1965).

Schou, J.: Absorption of drugs from subcutaneous connective tissue. Pharmacol. Rev. **13**, 441—464 (1961).

Schreus, H. Th.: Prinzipielles und experimentelles zur Salvarsantherapie. Arch. Derm. Syph. (Berl.) **150**, 402—422 (1926).

Smith, J. N., Williams, R. T.: The metabolism of sulphonamides. V. A study of the oxidation and acetylation of sulphonamide drugs and related compounds in the rabbit. Biochem. J. **42**, 351—356 (1948).

Swintosky, J. V.: Biological half-life and tissue concentrations. Proceedings of Pharmacy Teachers' Seminar, Madison, Wisconsin, July 10—14 (1961).

Taylor, J. D., Wiegand, R. G.: The analog computer and plasma drug kinetics. Clin. Pharmacol. Ther. **3**, 464—472 (1962).

Teorell, T.: Kinetics and distribution of substances administered to the body. I. The extravascular mode of administration. II. The intravascular mode of administration. Arch. int. Pharmacodyn. **57**, 205—225, 226—240 (1937).

Tephly, T. R., Parks, R. E. Jr., Mannering, G. J.: Methanol metabolism in the rat. J. Pharmacol. exp. Ther. **143**, 292—300 (1964).

Wagner, J. G.: Biopharmaceutics: absorption aspects. J. pharm. Sci. **50**, 359—387 (1961).

Wagner, J. G.: Method for estimating rate constants for absorption, metabolism, and elimination from urinary excretion data. J. pharm. Sci. **56**, 489—494 (1967).

Wagner, J. G.: A new generalized nonlinear pharmacokinetic model and its implications. In: Biopharmaceutics and relevant pharmacokinetics. Ist. Ed., Drug. Intell. Publ., Hamilton, Illinois, pp. 302—317 (1971).

Wagner, J. G., Patel, J. A.: Variations in absorption and elimination rates of ethyl alcohol in a single subject. Res. Comm. Chem. Pathol. Pharmacol. **4**, 61—76 (1972).

Walser, M.: Mathematical aspects of renal function: the dependence of solute reabsorption on water reabsorption, and the mechanism of osmotic natriuresis. J. theor. Biol. **10**, 307—326 (1966a).

Walser, M.: Mathematical aspects of renal function: reabsorption of individual solutes as interdependent processes. J. theor. Biol. **10**, 327—335 (1966b).

Wendel, O. W.: The application of hydrodynamics to elucidate the interrelationships of various body compartment volumes. Phys. med. Biol. **5**, 411—430 (1961).

Widmark, E. M. P.: Studies in the concentration of indifferent narcotics in blood and tissues. Acta med. scand. **52**, 87 (1919).

Widmark, E. M. P., Tandberg, J.: Über die Bedingungen für die Akkumulation indifferenter Narkotika. Theoretische Berechnungen. Biochem. Z. **147**, 358—369 (1924).

Wiegand, R. G., Buddenhagen, J. D., Endicott, C. J.: Multiple dose excretion kinetics. J. pharm. Sci. **52**, 268—273 (1963).

Wilbrandt, W. von: Die biologische Halbwertzeit von Medikamenten, ihre Ermittlung und Bedeutung. Schweiz. med. Wschr. **94**, 737—745 (1964).

Woolf, L. I., Goodwin, B. L., Phelps, C. E.: T_m-limited renal tubular reabsorption and the genetics of renal glucosuria. J. theor. Biol. **11**, 10—21 (1966).

CHAPTER 3

Pharmacokinetics of Biotransformation

J. M. van Rossum, C. A. M. van Ginneken, P. Th. Henderson,
H. C. J. Ketelaars and T. B. Vree

I. Introduction

Drugs and other chemical substances are eliminated from the human or animal
body mainly by renal excretion and metabolic degradation in the liver. Substantial
tubular reabsorption occurs, especially with lipophilic substances, so that the
kidney's part in the elimination of unchanged drugs can often be ignored.

A. Elimination of Drugs by a Clearance Process

Chemical substances are eliminated from the body mainly by a clearance process
in the liver, the kidney, and the lungs. Actually a certain fraction of the drug
present in the blood passing through these organs is extracted.

The rate of elimination, i.e., the quantity of drug (dQ) eliminated per unit
of time (dt) is a function of the concentration of the drug in the blood plasma that
passes through the clearance organs:

$$\frac{dQ}{dt} = \dot{V}_{Cel} \cdot C \tag{1}$$

where $\dot{V}_{Cel}$ is the total body clearance (ml/min or l/h). Under ideal conditions the
clearance is a constant independent of the concentration ($\dot{V}_{Cel} = k_{Cel}$). Drug
elimination, then, is a first-order process. The maximum clearance by a clearance
organ is theoretically equal to the blood flow through that organ if extraction is
complete. Since the clearance generally is the plasma clearance (l plasma/h), the
maximum plasma clearance may be greater than the blood flow if, for instance, the
drug concentration in the erythrocytes is larger than that in the plasma.

In general, extraction is only partial, so that the clearance of a drug is only a
fraction of the maximal clearance or effective plasma flow through the clearance
organs. The clearance may, as a matter of fact, also be referred to the blood
concentration or even to the concentration in the plasma water (see Krüger-
Thiemer, this volume). In agreement with the common use of the term in this chapter,
clearance will be referred only to the plasma concentration.

The total body clearance is the sum of the individual clearances:

$$k_{Cel} = k_{Cm} + k_{Cr} + k_{Calv} + \cdots \tag{2}$$

Table 1. Biological half-life and relative contribution of renal excretion and metabolic degradation

Drug	pH	$t\frac{1}{2}$ (h)	k_{Cr}/k_{Cel} (in %)	k_{Cm}/k_{Cel} (in %)	References
Dexamphetamine	5	6	70	30	Vree (1973)
Dexethylamphetamine	5	2– 5	40– 50	50–60	Vree (1973)
Benzphetamine	5	5–10	0	100	Vree (1973)
Ephedrine	5	7	70– 90	10–30	Vree (1973)
Phenmetrazine	5	4	60– 90	10–40	Vree (1973)
Phentermine	5	8– 9	80–100	10–20	Vree (1973)
Chlorphentermine	6	36–40	30– 50	50–70	Vree (1973)
Propylhexedrine	6	3– 5	7	ca. 90	Vree (1973)
Pipradrol	5	12			Vree (1973)
Hexobarbital	—	4	0.3–0.5	99	Breimer (1974)
Heptabarbital	—	7–10	ca. 0.2	99.5	Breimer (1974)
Vinylbital	—	18–25	1– 2	98	Breimer (1974)
Chloralhydrate	—	1	0	100	Breimer (1974)
Diphenhydramine	5	7– 8	8– 15	85–92	Van Ginneken (1972)
Dexchlorphenamine	5	10–12	10– 15	85–90	Van Ginneken (1972)
Orphenadrine	5	10–15	7– 15	85–93	Van Ginneken (1972)
Medrylamine	5	6	9– 10	90–91	Van Ginneken (1972)
4-Methyldiphen- hydramine	5	5– 6	3– 4	96–97	Van Ginneken (1972)

The metabolic clearance and the renal clearance usually make the largest contribution to the total body clearance. The alveolar clearance is only important for gases and vapors. Metabolic clearance is far more important than renal clearance for most drugs, except for highly hydrophilic substances. Table 1 shows the renal and metabolic clearances for a limited number of compounds as fractions of the total body clearance. The hydrophilic substance ephedrine is cleared mainly be the kidney, while benzphetamine, which is lipophilic, is almost completely cleared by metabolic conversion.

The total amount of a drug eliminated after a sufficiently long time is equal to the quantity of the drug that has entered the general circulation. Therefore:

$$\int_0^\infty dQ_{el} = k_{Cel} \int_0^\infty C \cdot dt \quad \text{or} \quad Q_{el} = D \cdot F \tag{3}$$

where F is the bioavailability or the fraction of the dose D that enters the general circulation.

The amount of the drug that has ultimately been metabolized can be calculated from the following equation:

$$\int_0^\infty dQ_m = k_{Cm} \int_0^\infty C \cdot dt \quad \text{or} \quad Q_m = \frac{k_{Cm}}{k_{Cel}} \cdot D \cdot F. \tag{4}$$

Similarly, the amount excreted unchanged is calculated as follows:

$$\int_0^\infty dQ_r = k_{Cr} \int_0^\infty C \cdot dt \quad \text{or} \quad Q_r = \frac{k_{Cr}}{k_{Cel}} \cdot D \cdot F.$$
(5)

The ratio of the metabolic clearance to the renal clearance can be calculated from the drug excreted unchanged by the kidney; provided elimination occurs merely by biotransformation and renal excretion.

$$k_{Cm}/k_{Cr} = DF/Q_r - 1.$$
(6)

Table 1 gives a few examples.

If less than 5% of the dose is excreted unchanged via the kidney, and absorption is practically complete, the contribution of the kidney to elimination can be disregarded. In other words:

$$Q_m \gg Q_r \quad \text{and} \quad Q_m \approx D \cdot F.$$
(7)

In this case the metabolic clearance is mainly responsible for elimination.

B. Flow-Limited Elimination of Drugs

Since the liver is mainly responsible for metabolic clearance of drugs it is evident that metabolic clearance will be limited by hepatic blood flow. In man the metabolic clearance cannot be greater than the effective portal plasma flow, which equals the blood flow (ca. 2 1/min) if the drug concentration in the erythrocytes equals the drug concentration in the plasma, but the metabolic enzymes may have a much greater capacity. Thus, the metabolic clearance may be equal to the blood flow through the liver but is generally less.

The concentration of a drug leaving the liver (C_{out}) is lower than that entering the liver (C_{in}). The blood leaving the liver is mixed with the body pool, so that the concentration entering the liver also progressively decreases due to the elimination process. The concentration leaving the liver depends on the incoming concentration, which in turn is dependent on the ratio of the real metabolic clearance to the blood flow

$$C_{out} = C_{in} e^{-k_{Cm}/k_f}.$$
(8)

Here k_f is the effective plasma flow through the liver. This equation is modified after an equation derived by NAGASHIMA and LEVY (1968). Since the quantity of a drug eliminated equals the difference between the quantity entering and that leaving the liver:

$$dQ_{el} = dQ_{in} - dQ_{out}.$$
(9)

Substitution of Equation (8) in Equation (9) gives:

$$\frac{dQ_{el}}{dt} = k_f(C_{in} - C_{out}) = k_f[1 - e^{-k_{Cm}/k_f}] \cdot C_{in}. \tag{10}$$

The rate of elimination of a drug is also, by definition, directly proportional to the apparent metabolic clearance $k_{Cm\,app.}$. This implies that:

$$k_{Cm\,app.} = k_f(1 - e^{-k_{Cm}/k_f}) \tag{11}$$

where k_{Cm} is the real metabolic clearance determined by the capacity of the enzymes and the binding constant of the drug to the enzyme. Obviously, if k_{Cm} is large with respect to the hepatic blood flow, the apparent metabolic clearance approaches the hepatic blood flow (i.e., the effective hepatic plasma flow). In this case the rate of drug metabolism is largely dependent on the blood flow through the liver. It also implies that rapidly metabolized drugs which are used for liver function tests may only give an indication of the blood flow and not of the functional state of the liver enzymes. The liver enzymes can be substantially impaired even before this can be seen from the apparent metabolic clearance.

If on the other hand the real metabolic clearance is small with respect to the blood flow, the exponential term in Equation (11) is very small, so that this term can be developed in a series of terms according to a McLaurin series (NAGASHIMA and LEVY, 1968). Thus:

$$k_{Cm\,app.} = k_f\left[1 - 1 + \frac{k_{Cm}}{k_f} - \frac{1}{2!}\left(\frac{k_{Cm}}{k_f}\right)^2 + \frac{1}{3!}\left(\frac{k_{Cm}}{k_f}\right)^3 - \cdots\right]. \tag{12}$$

Rearrangement and rupture of the series at the quadratic term gives the following equation:

$$k_{Cm\,app.} = k_{Cm}(1 - k_{Cm}/2k_f). \tag{13}$$

The apparent metabolic clearance is approximately the same as the real metabolic clearance if $k_f \gg k_{Cm}$. It is evident that when this is so, the metabolic clearance is dependent only to a very slight extent on the blood flow through the liver. Liver function tests aimed at the functional integrity of the metabolic enzymes should therefore make use of drugs that are not too rapidly metabolized.

C. Supply-Limited Elimination of Drugs

When elimination is a first-order process the rate of metabolism or excretion is directly proportional to the concentration of the drug in the fluid entering the clearance organs. Since the volume of the fluid in which the drug is dissolved can be considered constant, the rate of elimination is also directly proportional to the quantity entering the clearance organs. If the flow through the clearance organs is not the limiting factor, elimination can be considered to be supply-limited. Supply-limited elimination occurs when the apparent metabolic clearance equals the real metabolic clearance as determined by the enzymes in the liver, and when the renal clearance is also independent of the concentration (tubular excretion non-existent or also directly proportional to the concentration of the drug), or if renal excretion may be neglected to the metabolic clearance.

If the clearance occurs from a single compartmental volume, the rate of disappearance of drug from the body is given by the following equation (clearance constant: $\dot{V}_{Cel} = k_{Cel}$).

$$\frac{dQ}{dt} = -k_{Cel} \cdot C \quad \text{and} \quad C = A \cdot e^{-t/\tau_{el}} = A \cdot 2^{-t/t_{\frac{1}{2}}} \tag{14}$$

where τ_{el} is the elimination time-constant $(\tau_{el} = V_f/k_{Cel})$, V_f the apparent volume of distribution, and $t_{\frac{1}{2}}$ the biological half-life $(t_{\frac{1}{2}} = \tau_{el} \cdot \ln 2)$. Supply-limited elimination leads essentially to first-order kinetics, whether the body is considered as a single or a multicompartment system.

D. Capacity-Limited Elimination of Drugs

Elimination of drugs through biodegradation occurs mainly in the liver microsomal enzymes. At high substrate concentration enzyme systems become saturated, which implies that biodegradation takes place at a constant maximum rate. In such a case drug elimination is limited merely by the capacity of the liver enzymes and independent of the concentration or the supply to the clearance organs. In this situation:

$$\frac{dQ}{dt} = -\dot{Q}_m \quad \text{and} \quad C = A - \frac{\dot{Q}_m}{V_f} \cdot t \tag{15}$$

where $\dot{Q}_m$ is the maximum elimination rate (mg/h) and A the drug concentration in the plasma immediately after administration $(A = D/V_f)$. It is obvious that per unit of time a constant amount is eliminated and the drug concentration decreases linearly with time. The elimination of ethanol after ingestion of a glass of whisky is a typical example of such a capacity-limited elimination (HAGGARD et al., 1941; WAGNER and PATEL, 1972).

For many drugs, elimination proceeds in a first-order fashion, so that the elimination rate is supply- or diffusion-limited [see Eq. (1)]. Obviously, drug elimination can be neither supply-limited nor capacity-limited but governed by an intermediate relation (see next paragraph). Elimination can also be complicated further by diffusion of drug to other compartments and elimination through other diffusion-limited or capacity-limited processes, and also by concentration-dependent destruction of the elimination processes, such as progressive liver damage or enzyme induction. Some implications will be discussed below.

E. The Relationship Between the Metabolic Enzyme Activity and the Metabolic Clearance

Enzymes localized in the smooth endoplasmic reticulum of liver cells are responsible for most routes of biotransformation. Enzymatic conversion can be described by the following elementary equations:

$$E + S \underset{k_2}{\overset{k_1}{\rightleftharpoons}} ES \xrightarrow{k_3} E + \text{products} \tag{16}$$

where E is the enzyme and S the substrate. The rate of disappearance of substrate is proportional to the concentration of the substrate:

$$\frac{dQ_s}{dt} = -k_1 \cdot C_s \cdot Q_e + k_2 \cdot Q_{es}, \tag{17}$$

$$\frac{dQ_{es}}{dt} = k_1 \cdot C_s \cdot Q_e - (k_2 + k_3) Q_{es}, \tag{18}$$

and

$$\frac{dQ_p}{dt} = k_3 \cdot Q_{es} \tag{19}$$

where Q_e is the quantity of free enzyme, Q_{es} is the quantity of occupied enzyme, Q_s is the quantity of substrate, Q_p is the quantity of products formed, and C_s is the substrate concentration. Under steady-state conditions (which in general have not been proved to be fulfilled):

$$\frac{dQ_{es}}{dt} = 0 \quad \text{and} \quad \frac{C_s \cdot Q_e}{Q_{es}} = \frac{k_2 + k_3}{k_1} = K_M. \tag{20}$$

Since the sum of free enzyme Q_e and occupied enzyme Q_{es} may be considered to be constant and equal to the total quantity of enzyme Q_E:

$$Q_{es} = Q_E \cdot \frac{C_s}{K_M + C_s} \tag{21}$$

and consequently

$$\frac{dQ_s}{dt} = -k_3 \cdot Q_{es} = \frac{-k_3 \cdot Q_E \cdot C_s}{(K_M + C_s)} = \frac{-\dot{Q}_m}{(K_M + C_s)} \cdot C_s \tag{22}$$

where $\dot{Q}_m$ is the maximum metabolic conversion rate ($\dot{Q}_m = k_3 \cdot Q_E$) in mg/min when both C_s and K_M are given in mg/liter.

Supposing that the substrate concentration in the clearance tissue is equal to the plasma concentration, the elimination clearance ($\dot{V}_{Cel}$) bears the following relation to $\dot{Q}_m$ and K_M:

$$\dot{V}_{Cel} = \dot{Q}_m/(K_M + C). \tag{23}$$

The metabolic clearance is therefore not constant, but essentially concentration-dependent. This influence is only felt when the plasma concentration is almost as high as, or higher than, K_M. The metabolic clearance then decreases with increasing plasma concentration.

This implies that if the plasma concentration is low with respect to the Michaelis-Menten constant of the enzyme substrate complex, the metabolic clearance is a constant ($\dot{V}_{Cel} = k_{Cm}$):

$$k_{Cm} = \dot{Q}_m/K_M. \tag{24}$$

In these conditions the metabolic clearance is a simple function of the enzymatic constants governing biotransformation.

As the plasma concentration is directly related to the dose administered, increasing doses will ultimately lead to a concentration-dependent metabolic clearance. However, when given in therapeutic doses, most drugs lead to plasma concentrations considerably lower than their K_M value, so that elimination may indeed be a first-order process.

When Equation (24) is valid elimination is supply-limited, and when the concentration of drug approaches K_M it becomes capacity-limited. In case of toxic overdose, however, the elimination may be very much retarded. Consequently the half-life of elimination may appear long.

The biological half-life of cyclobarbital calculated in a case of toxic overdose was 1.5 day (BRILMAYER and LOENNECKEN, 1962). The half-life following administration of a therapeutic dose in healthy subjects appears to be about 12 h. (BREIMER, 1974). The half-life of salicylic acid is also dose-dependent (LEVY, 1965). Following a dose of 1 g the half-life is about 6 h (BRODIE et al., 1959) but it is 19 h after a dose of 10 g (SWINTOSKY, 1956).

Table 2. Dose-dependent biological half-life values

Drug	Dose	Route	Half-life value	References
Salicylic acid	250 mg	I.v. infusion	2.4 h	WURSTER and KRAMER (1961
Salicylic acid	385 mg	Oral	2.3 h	VAN GINNEKEN (1974)
Salicylic acid	1 300 mg	I.v. infusion	6.1 h	BRODIE et al. (1959)
Salicylic acid	10 000 mg	I.v. infusion	19 h	SWINTOSKY (1956)
Cyclobarbital	300 mg	Oral	10 h	BREIMER (1974)
Cyclobarbital	Toxic overdose	Oral	36 h	BRILMAYER and LOENNECKEN (1962)
Ethylbiscoumacetate	240 mg	I.v. injection	0.55 h	VAN DAM (1968)
idem	480 mg	I.v. injection	1.25 h	VAN DAM (1968)
idem	800 mg	I.v. injection	1.8 h	VAN DAM (1968)
Phenytoin	300 mg/d	Oral	18 h	ARNOLD and GERBER (1970)
idem	1 000 mg/d	Oral	69 h	ARNOLD and GERBER (1970)

Following doses of less than 0.5 g the half-life is about 2.5 h (Van Ginneken et al., 1974). Similar dose-dependent half-life values for a number of drugs are given in Table 2. See also Wagner (1973).

F. The Plasma Decay Curve as a Result of Metabolic Clearance

Under the condition that the elimination of a drug proceeds via a single metabolic pathway the clearance may be given by Equation (23). The clearance then is not a constant but it will decrease as the plasma concentration rises. Under the additional supposition that the body may be regarded as a single compartment, the rate of elimination can be described by the following equation:

$$\frac{dQ}{dt} = - \frac{\dot{Q}_m}{(K_M + C)} \cdot C. \tag{25}$$

Only under the special condition that the plasma concentration is very low as compared to the dissociation constant, the clearance becomes a constant as given in Equation (24). Obviously the apparent clearance may be lower as k_{Cm} approaches the blood flow through the liver [see Eq. (13)].

The well-known Equation (14) for the plasma concentration as a function of time holds true, provided that the body may be regarded as a single volume of distribution. The time constant and the biological half-life are simple functions of the capacity of metabolism, the affinity, and the volume of distribution:

$$\tau_{el} = V_f \cdot K_M/\dot{Q}_m \quad \text{and} \quad t_{\frac{1}{2}} = 0.69 \cdot V_f \cdot K_M/\dot{Q}_m. \tag{26}$$

The time constant and therefore the biological half-life under the conditions described is directly proportional to the volume of distribution and the Michaelis constant, and inversely proportional to the maximum metabolic elimination rate. This implies that the biological half-life becomes shorter as the Michaelis-Menten constant falls or as affinity for the enzyme rises. However, as affinity for the enzyme rises, the plasma concentration at which a deviation from first-order elimination is found, declines too. If C is not low with respect to K_M, that is for drugs that are given in high doses or for drugs with a high affinity to the metabolizing enzymes, the half-life decreases with increasing dose because the clearance decreases with increasing dose. Obviously the half-life is then no longer a constant. As a matter of fact also the volume of distribution is of great importance on the magnitude of biological half-life. Compare xylocaine, procainamide, bromsulphaleine, methohexital, and nortriptyline of Table 3. These drugs have approximately the same total body clearance but differ with respect to the biological half-life because of a difference in the volume of distribution. The shorter half-life of hexobarbital in contrast to the long half-life of pentobarbital may be due to a greater affinity of hexobarbital for the microsomal enzymes, although a greater maximum reaction velocity is another possible explanation. If the first suggestion is correct, an overdose of hexobarbital will cause an increase in the biological half-life earlier than the one of pentobarbital.

Table 3. Pharmacokinetic parameters of some drugs

Farmacon	$t\frac{1}{2}$ (d, h, min)		V_f (l)	k_{Cel} ml/min
Dexamfetamine	8	h	250	250
Practolol	13	h	150	140
Methyldopa	1.4	h	160	1600
Digoxine	36	h	100	150
Digitoxine	5	d	37	4.5
Xylocaine	1.5	h	86	785
Procainamide	2.9	h	185	745
Penicilline	0.55	h	21	420
Chloramfemicol	2.3	h	40	200
Tetracycline	10	h	240	260
Rifampicine	1.5	h	200	2000
Acetazolamide	4.1	h	14	315
Bromide	10	d	21	1.1
Bromsulphaleine	5.6	min	2.3	800
Nortriptyline	27	h	1750	760
Desipramine	18	h	3080	1500
Theophylline	4.4	h	32	84
Pentobarbital	42	h	130	36
Hexobarbital	4.2	h	28	280
Methohexital	1.6	h	77	825

On the other hand, under the special condition of very high plasma concentration with regard to K_M the differential is independent of the plasma concentration. Equation (25) reduces to Equation (15). This Equation (15) gives the well-known relationship for zero-order elimination (LEVY, 1965; WAGNER and PATEL, 1973). Also here the possibility exists that the elimination is apparently first-order if the capacity of the liver largely exceeds the supply.

Between the two extreme conditions Equation (25) holds true, which may be integrated to an implicit function:

$$\ln C = \ln A + (A - C)/K_M - t/\tau_{el} \qquad (27)$$

or

$$C = A \cdot e^{(A - C)/K_M} \cdot e^{-t/\tau_{el}} \qquad (28)$$

where τ_{el} is the time constant encountered at low concentrations $(C \ll K_M)$. Equation (28) differs from Equation (14) in a concentration-dependent, exponential term. This term can be ignored when $D/V_f \ll K_M$, i.e., when the initial concentration is much lower than the Michaelis-Menten constant. Equation (30) also shows that if the concentration drops so far that $C \ll D/V_f$, the term is not concentration-dependent but a simple constant $(\exp(A/K_M))$. The influence of the K_M value and the dose on the plasma decay curve is seen most clearly when the concentration is plotted on a logarithmic scale. The influence of the dose and the K_M value on the profile of the plasma decay curve is seen in Figure 1. The significance of the dose-dependent constant in Equations (27) and (28) is shown in Figure 1a and b (VAN GINNEKEN et al., 1974).

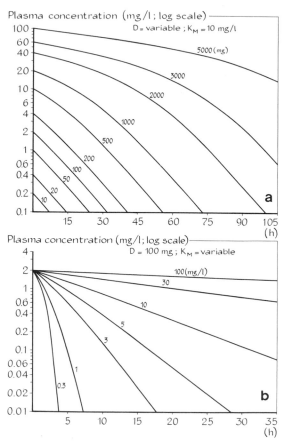

Fig. 1a and b. Plasmaconcentration curves showing nonlinear kinetics of elimination. (a) Dose variation. Plasma curves become flat at higher dose, but they are straight lines with slope determined by τ_{el} at concentrations lower than K_M. (b) K_M variation while dose and $\dot{Q}_m$ are kept constant. Nonlinearity occurs with K_M values lower than 3 mg/l while straight part of curve is steeper as K_M is smaller. (Reproduced from VAN GINNEKEN et al., 1974 with permission of authors and publishers of the J. Pharmacokin. Biopharmac.)

It is clear that with decreasing K_M the rate of elimination increases as the clearance increases but that zero-order elimination occurs earlier. It is also clear that with increasing doses the traject of zero-order elimination in the plasma decay curve rises. In fact, the intercept with the ordinate is given by the first term ($\ln A$) of Equation (27), the shift over the time scale by the second term $(A - C)/K_M$, and the straight line occurring at low concentrations by the third term.

Obviously it is not admissible to calculate a half-life from the flat part of the curve following relatively high doses ($D > V_f \cdot K_M$); the apparent half-lives obtained for high doses, as given in Table 2, bear no relation to the actual half-life. The real half-life can be calculated if the curve is extended to sufficiently low plasma concentrations. Figure 2 gives a few examples of semilogarithmic plasma curves. Both phenytoin (ARNOLD and GERBER, 1970) and ethylbiscoumacetate (VAN DAM,

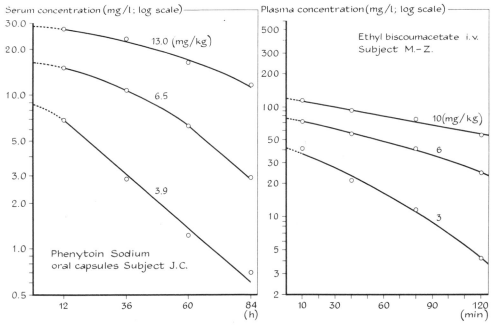

Fig. 2. Serum levels of phenytoin (data from ARNOLD and GERBER) and ethylbiscoumacetate (data from VAN DAM) in human subjects following various doses. Rate of elimination is faster for lower doses than for higher doses analoguous to capacity-limited elimination at higher plasma concentrations. Compare with Figure 1

1968) show dose-dependent elimination suggesting capacity-limited elimination. In these cases it is not certain that it is admissible to regard the body as a single compartment. However, the trend is obvious.

G. Calculation of Enzymatic Constants from the Plasma Decay Curve

When so much drug has been eliminated that the plasma concentration is only a small fraction of the initial concentration ($C \ll D/V_f$), the second term of Equation (31) can be regarded as a constant. Then the semilogarithmic plasma decay curve is a straight line with a slope determined by τ_{el} but the extrapolated intercept is

$$\ln A_{\text{extrap.}} = \ln A + A/K_M. \tag{29}$$

The difference between this extrapolated intercept and the real intercept $\ln A$ is simply A/K_M (see Fig. 3).

This implies that the K_M can be calculated from the difference in real and extrapolated intercepts

$$K_M = A/(\ln A_{\text{extrap.}} - \ln A). \tag{30}$$

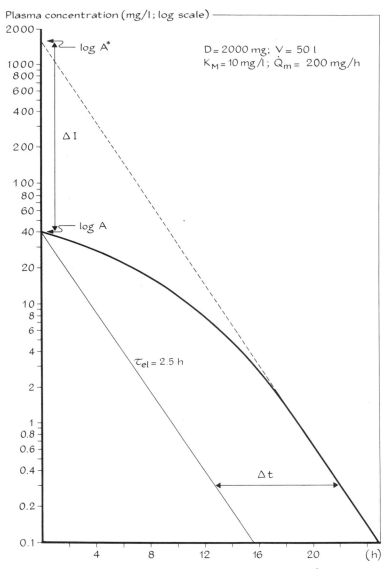

Fig. 3. Outline of procedure for initial estimation of parameters K_M and $\dot{Q}_m$. See text reproduced from van Ginneken et al., 1974 with permission of the authors and publishers of the J. Pharmacokin. Biopharmac.)

The K_M value can also be obtained from the shift in the straight part of the semilogarithmic decay curve. A straight line is drawn parallel to the straight part of the curve seen at low concentrations. The extrapolated curve is shifted by a time period Δt. At $t = \Delta t$ it can be derived from the extrapolated semilogarithmic curve that:

$$K_M = A \cdot \tau_{el}/\Delta t. \tag{31}$$

Table 4. Drug parameters calculated for nonlinear elimination kinetics according to Equation (28). (Data from VAN GINNEKEN et al., 1974)

Drug		Ethanol		Phenytoin
D		48	64	0.25
A^*_{est}	(mg/l)	660000	720000	5.90
A_{est}	(mg/l)	1330	1220	4.55
A_{fit}	(mg/l)	1310	1320	4.66
$\tau_{el, est}$	(h)	0.43	0.68	21
$K_{M, est}$	(mg/l)	210	190	16
$K_{M, fit}$	(mg/l)	200	140	10
V_{est}	(l)	27.1	43.4	54
V_{fit}	(l)	36.7	48.5	53.7
$k_{Cel(calc)}$	(l/h)	64.5	72.3	2.7
$\dot{Q}_{m(calc)}$	(mg/h)	12900	10100	27

Since it is also known that τ_{el} relates to both K_M and $\dot{Q}_m$, $\dot{Q}_m$ can also be calculated. Substitution of Equation (31) in Equation (26) and rearrangement gives:

$$\dot{Q}_m = D/\Delta t . \tag{32}$$

So once either parameter K_M or $\dot{Q}_m$ and τ_{el} has been determined, the other parameter can be calculated. The values of these parameters obtained by the above procedure for ethanol and phenytoin are given in Table 4. It must be realized that the above procedure is only valid with respect to elimination after i.v. administration, when drug distribution ought to be fast, and in the case of oral administration when absorption is rapid. Furthermore, elimination by other routes, as renal clearance, should be very low compared to elimination by means of the enzyme under consideration.

If all these requirements have not been fulfilled, the differential equations are either very complex or insoluble, and extrapolation of the simple equations may introduce grave errors. Values obtained by this method can, however, be used as initial approximations.

H. Simultaneous Supply-Limited and Capacity-Limited Elimination of Drugs

Capacity-limited elimination of a drug, if already existent at the dose administered, is usually accompanied by supply-limited elimination. For instance, one metabolic pathway may be concentration-dependent while other elimination pathways are not or not yet. For instance, renal clearance may occur simultaneously and independently of the plasma concentration. This implies that the clearance is composed of a concentration independent and a concentration dependent component:

$$\dot{V}_{Cel} = k_{Cr} + k_{Cml} + \dot{Q}_m/(K_M + C) \tag{33}$$

where k_{Cr} is the renal clearance constant, k_{Cml} is a clearance constant of the merely supply-limited metabolic pathways and the third term is the capacity-limited clearance component of a particular metabolic pathway. The concentration independent components may be grouped together such that a fraction of the clearance is constant and another fraction is concentration-dependent. So Equation (33) may be rearranged to:

$$\dot{V}_{Cel} = k_{Cel}\{(1-f) + f K_M/(K_M + C)\} \tag{34}$$

where $\dot{Q}_m/K_M = f \cdot k_{Cel}$ and k_{Cel} is the clearance constant at low plasma concentration. Substitution of the clearance function of Equation (34) in Equation (1) leads to the differential equation governing the elimination of a drug from the body, when the body may be regarded as a single compartment (Van Ginneken et al., 1974)

$$\frac{dQ}{dt} = -k_{Cel}\{(1-f) + f K_M/(K_M + C)\} \cdot C. \tag{35}$$

This equation can be integrated, leading to an implicit equation:

$$\ln C = \ln A + \frac{f}{(1-f)} \ln \frac{1 + (1-f)\, A/K_M}{1 + (1-f)\, C/K_M} - \frac{t}{\tau_{el}} \tag{36}$$

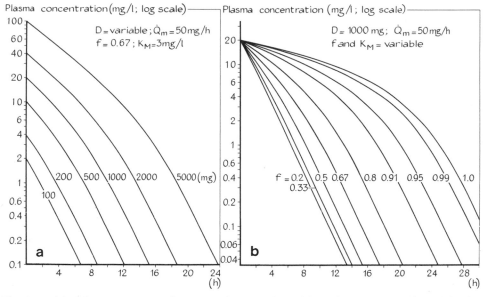

Fig. 4a and b. Plasma concentration curves in case of combined linear and nonlinear kinetics of elimination. (a) Dose variation for theoretical drug that for 67% ($f = 0.67$) is eliminated by potentially capacity-limited pathway. A straight part is observed at low but also at high plasma-concentrations. Nonlinearity occurs at plasma concentrations around K_M value. (b) Variation of the fraction of body clearance that represents elimination via capacity-limited pathway. Nonlinearity is only apparent if capacity-limited pathway accounts for more than 20% of clearance. (Reproduced from Van Ginneken et al., 1974 with permission of authors and publishers of the J. Pharmacokin. Biopharmac.)

where $\tau_{el} = V_f/k_{Cel}$ is the elimination time constant at low plasma concentration $(C \ll K_M)$. The influence of the dose on the plasma concentration profiles is shown in Figure 4. Obviously a straight line is obtained when $f = 0$, while the influence of the concentration becomes more apparent when f increases from zero to unity. If f equals unity the influence is maximal. Then Equation (36) reduces to Equation (27) (VAN GINNEKEN et al., 1974). From Figure 4a it may be seen that at high plasma concentrations straight lines are also obtained although the slope is flatter. It is obvious from Equation (34) that the clearance function becomes concentration-independent not only at low plasma concentrations $(C \ll K_M)$. Under conditions of high plasma concentration $(C \gg K_M)$ the clearance is reduced as follows:

$$k_{Cel}^* = k_{Cel}(1 - f). \tag{37}$$

This implies that under conditions of high plasma concentrations $(C \gg K_M)$ Equation (36) reduces to a linear expression. Then:

$$\ln C = \ln A - t/\tau_{el}^* \tag{38}$$

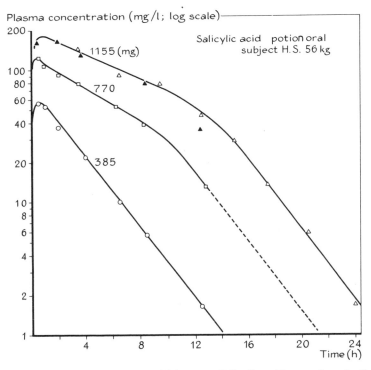

Fig. 5. Nonlinear kinetics of salicylic acid in man. Salicylic acid was given in three doses as potion so that rapid absorption took place. Except for short absorption phase, curves resemble those of Figure 4. A linear part is obtained at low $(t_{\frac{1}{2}} = 2.5\,\text{h})$ and at high plasma concentration $(t_{\frac{1}{2}} = 6\,\text{h})$. (Reproduced from VAN GINNEKEN et al., 1974 with permission of authors and publishers of the J. Pharmacokin. Biopharmac.)

Table 5. Drug parameters calculated for nonlinear elimination kinetics from Equation (36). (Data from VAN GINNEKEN et al., 1974)

D (mg)		Salicylic acid		4-hydroxybutyric acid		
		770	1155	2900	4000	4500
A_{est}^*	(mg/l)	600	2500	1170	9900	900
A_{est}	(mg/l)	125	200	220	250	230
A_{fit}	(mg/l)	129	191	201	244	238
$\tau_{el, est}^*$	(h)	7.2	9.7	1.3	2.7	2.1
$\tau_{el, est}$	(h)	3.3	3.3	0.62	0.83	0.61
$\tau_{el, fit}$	(h)	2.8	2.5	0.44	0.46	0.56
f_{est}	g	0.54	0.66	0.48	0.70	0.71
f_{fit}		0.79	0.91	0.85	0.88	0.85
$K_{M, est}$	(mg/l)	21	25	25	14	36
$K_{M, fit}$	(mg/l)	26	27	31	10	15
V_{est}	(l)	6.0	6.0	14	16	19
V_{fit}''	(l)g	5.98	6.0	14.4	16.4	18.9
$k_{Cel, (calc)}$	(l/h)	2.1	2.4	31.8	34.8	33.9
$\dot{Q}_{m, (calc)}$	(mg/h)	44	59	840	310	430

where τ_{el}^* equals $\tau_{el}/(1-f)$. Therefore it is possible to calculate f from the ratio of the slopes of the straight lines at high and at low plasma concentration (VAN GINNEKEN et al., 1974a). Once f has been calculated it is possible to calculate K_M from the real intercept and the extrapolated intercept analogous to the method illustrated in Figure 3. The extrapolated intercept, $\ln A^*$, is obtained by extrapolating the straight line seen at low plasma concentration:

$$\ln A^* = \ln A + \frac{f}{1-f} \ln\{1 + (1-f) A/K_M\}. \tag{39}$$

In addition the metabolic capacity $\dot{Q}_m$ can be calculated from k_{Cel}, f and K_M since:

$$\dot{Q}_m = f \cdot K_M \cdot k_{Cel}. \tag{40}$$

In a recent paper VAN GINNEKEN et al. (1974) have calculated these kinetic parameters for salicylic acid and 4-hydroxybutyric acid. See Figure 5 and Table 5. These drugs are, to a considerable fraction, metabolized via a concentration-dependent pathway. It may be seen from the theoretical curves of Figure 4 that when f is less than 0.2, nonlinear kinetics may easily be overlooked. However, such minor metabolic pathways may have a strong influence on elimination of other drugs.

I. Dissociation Constants Obtained from Microsomal Enzymes

Enzymes localized in the smooth endoplasmic reticulum of liver cells are mainly responsible for biotransformation of drugs and other foreign substances (FOUTS, 1971). These enzymes can be separated from other cell constituents present in liver tissue homogenates as microsomes (DALLNER and ERNSTER, 1968). The so-called cytochrome P450 plays an important part in the microsomal oxidation process (ESTABROOK, 1971). Binding of drugs to cytochrome P450 appears to be an important step in the sequence of reactions, leading to bio-oxidation (SCHENKMAN, 1970).

In many cases binding constants of drugs to cytochrome P450 may give a reasonable estimate of the binding constant or Michaelis-Menten constant governing

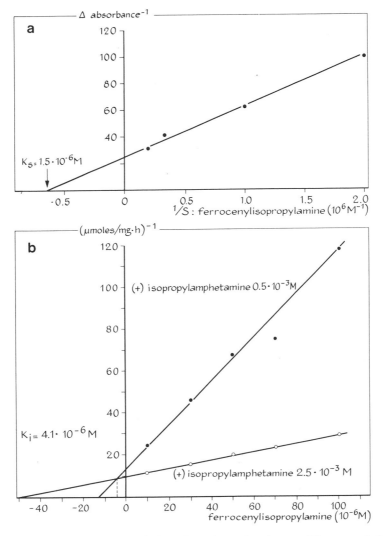

Fig. 6. (a) Lineweaver—burk plot of dose-dependent absorbance difference of ferrocenyl-isopropylamine and rat liver cytochrome P450 from which binding constant of this drug to cytochrome P450 has been calculated. (b) Dixon plot of inhibiting effect of ferrocenyl-isopropylamphetamine on N-dealkylation of isopropylamphetamine by rat liver microsomes. Inhibition constant corresponds to binding constant of inhibitor to cytochrome P450. (Data from VREE et al., 1973 with permission of authors and publishers of Xenobiotica)

drug metabolism in vivo. These binding constants are easily determined from a difference-spectrum of a solution of enzyme against a solution of enzyme plus substrate (Remmer et al., 1966, 1969). Two types of binding have been classified as type I and type II. The spectral difference as a function of the concentration leads to a relation from which the dissociation constant, K_s, governing the binding to the cytochrome, can be calculated (see Fig. 6). K_s values have been determined for a number of drugs and foreign substances (Vree et al., 1973, Henderson et al., 1974). Table 6 shows a selection of these. Even in the same class of drugs, e.g., the barbiturates (Jansson et al., 1972) or the amphetamines (Vree et al., 1973), there are considerable differences in binding to cytochrome P450. Imipramine and amitriptyline bind strongly to cytochrome P450, so that one would expect capacity-limited elimination were it not that the plasma concentration is very low with a normal dosage regimen.

The K_s values determined for the binding of drugs to microsomal cytochrome P450 obtained from rat liver may be similar to those for the same enzymes in the liver of man, in which case these K_s values can be used for initial screening of

Table 6

Drug	pK_s (molar)	Species	Type	References
Hexobarbital	4.1	Rat	I	Jansson et al., 1972
Pentobarbital	4.2	Rat	I	Jansson et al., 1972
Phenobarbital	3.8	Rat	I	Jansson et al., 1972
Butobarbital	4.0	Rat	I	Jansson et al., 1972
Cyclobarbital	4.2	Rat	I	Jansson et al., 1972
Heptabarbital	4.4	Rat	I	Jansson et al., 1972
Amobarbital	4.2	Rat	I	Jansson et al., 1972
Secobarbital	4.2	Rat	I	Jansson et al., 1972
SKF 525A	6.2	Rat	I	Topham, 1970
Propranolol				Topham, 1970
Tremorine	3.4	Mouse	I	Topham, 1970
Aminophenazon	3.5	Rat	I	Schenkman et al., 1967
Imipramine	5.6	Rat	I	von Bahr, 1972
Desipramine	5.6	Rat	I	von Bahr, 1972
Amitriptyline	5.6	Rat	I	von Bahr, 1972
Orphenadrine	5.7	Rat	I	Vree, 1973
Chlorpromazine	4.5	Rat	I	Topham, 1970
Amphetamine	2.3	Rat	II	Vree, 1973
N-Methylamphetamine	2.3	Rat	I	Vree, 1973
N-Ethylamphetamine	2.3	Rat	I	Vree, 1973
Norephedrine	2.4	Rat	I	Vree, 1973
N-isopropylamphetamine	2.1	Rat	I	Vree et al., 1973
Ferrocenylisopropylamine	5.8	Rat	II	Vree et al., 1973
Biphenylamine	5.2	Mouse	II	Temple, 1971
Testosterone	5.1	Rat	I	Orrenius et al., 1970
Ethylmorphine	3.6	Rat	I	Davies et al., 1969
Metyrapone	6.2	Rat	II	Leibman et al., 1969
1–6 Tetrahydrocannabinol	4.9	Rat	I	Kupfer et al., 1972
Cannabinol	4.9	Rat	I	Kupfer et al., 1972

drugs that may show capacity-limited metabolic clearance in man. Obviously, these K_s values, with all restrictions that should be taken into account, have to be compared with the expected concentration in the intracellular fluid. If there is only a small difference between the therapeutic concentration and the K_s value, difficulties can be anticipated in case of suicide or accidental overdose.

For drugs that bind substantially to plasma proteins the concentration in the intracellular fluid may be relatively low, so that protein binding can have a corrective influence on capacity-limited elimination. On the other hand, a drug with strong protein binding may replace another drug from plasma protein and thereby enforce capacity-limited elimination.

J. Inhibition of Drug Metabolism by Other Drugs

It is well-known from enzymologic studies that the enzymatic conversion of a substrate can be inhibited by the presence of another substance which is also converted, and therefore is a substrate, or by a drug that is merely an inhibitor. The following differential equations can be used to describe the situation when a drug or a substrate S is eliminated in the presence of an inhibitor I:

$$\frac{dQ_S}{dt} = -k_1 C_S \cdot Q_E + k_2 Q_{ES} + k_2 Q_{EI}, \tag{41}$$

$$\frac{dQ_I}{dt} = -k_1 C_I \cdot Q_E + k_2 Q_{EI} + k_2 Q_{ES}, \tag{42}$$

$$\frac{dQ_{ES}}{dt} = k_1 C_S \cdot Q_E - (k_2 + k_3) Q_{ES}, \tag{43}$$

$$\frac{dQ_{EI}}{dt} = k_1 C_I \cdot Q_E - (k_2^* + k_3^*) Q_{EI} \tag{44}$$

with a constant inhibitor concentration (k_3^* is small) and under steady-state conditions dQ_{ES}/dt and $dQ_{EI}/dt = 0$, so that if the sum of occupied and free enzyme is known to be constant the following relationship can be found:

$$\frac{dQ_S}{dt} = -k_3 \cdot Q_{ES} = \frac{-k_3 \cdot Q_E \cdot C_S}{K_M(1 + I/K_I) + C_S} = \frac{-\dot{Q}_m}{K_M(1 + I/K_I) + C_S} \cdot C_S. \tag{45}$$

For many drugs, when administered in the therapeutic dose range $K_M > C_S$, the metabolic clearance of drugs will be decreased when an inhibitor is present. At a given constant inhibitor concentration, the metabolic clearance is decreased according to the following equation:

$$k_{Cm(I)} = \frac{\dot{Q}_m}{K_M(1 + I/K_I)}. \tag{46}$$

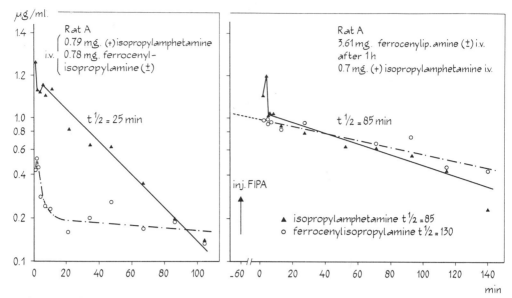

Fig. 7. In vivo inhibition of elimination of isopropylamphetamine in a rat by ferrocenyl isopropylamine. Half-life of isopropylamphetamine increases from 25 min to 85 min. Assuming a constant inhibitor concentration (in blood) of 0.9 mg/l, inhibitor constant is estimated as 0.4 mg/l. This value approaches binding constant of this drug to cytochrome P450. Compare with Figure 6. (Data from Vree et al., 1973 with permission of authors and publishers of Xenobiotica)

From this relationship it is evident that inhibition of elimination and therefore the retardation of elimination occurs only if the inhibitor concentration approaches or exceeds the value of its dissociation constant K_I.

When the body can be regarded as a single compartment the biological half-life bears a simple relation to the total body clearance, so that the biological half-life increases with enzyme inhibition to a proportion given by the change in metabolic clearance (see Figs. 7 and 8).

In formula:

$$t_{\frac{1}{2}} = t_{\frac{1}{2}}(1 + I/K_I) \,. \tag{47}$$

This implies that the dissociation constant of the inhibitor, K_I, can be found from the change in the biological half-life, provided the concentration of inhibitor is kept constant during the experiment and that renal clearance can be neglected (see Fig. 7). The first requirement may be fulfilled when the drug is more rapidly eliminated than the inhibitor. For instance, in the case of the inhibition of metabolic elimination of phenazone by phenobarbital, the dissociation constant of the inhibitor phenobarbital can be calculated from the increase in the half-life. Figure 7 shows that the half-life of isopropylamphetamine is increased by its ferrocenyl analogue. The binding constant K_I (obtained from such data) is consistent with the value obtained for binding to cytochrome P450 (see previous paragraph). It is known that salicylic acid and salicylamide are both subject to capacity-limited elimination when

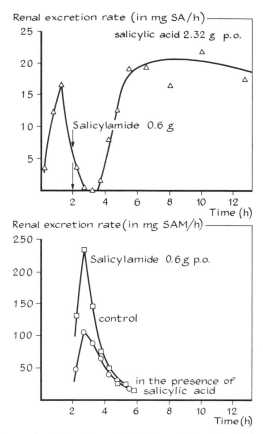

Fig. 8. Mutual inhibition of elimination of salicylic acid and salicylamide in man. Renal excretion rate of salicylic acid is greatly reduced by short-acting salicylamide. Renal excretion of salicylamide is also reduced by salicylic acid. (Reproduced from LEVY, 1971 with permission of author and publishers of Ann. N.Y. Acad. Sci.)

given in therapeutic doses (LEVY, 1971). Combination of these two drugs causes a mutual interference in the metabolic degradation (LEVY, 1971) (see Fig. 8).

It should be realized that if a drug inhibits metabolism of another drug the concentration of the first should be high enough for its elimination to be capacity-limited for at least one metabolic pathway. Consequently, drugs for which the clearance is not dose-dependent will not interfere with the elimination of other drugs. Capacity-limited elimination may easily be overlooked, however, if it occurs for a minor metabolic pathway. Obviously, drugs given in doses high enough for the elimination of them to be dose-dependent may only interfere with the elimination of other drugs if the *same* enzyme is involved.

K. Induction of Microsomal Enzymes and the Liver Clearance

Exposure to phenobarbital, chlordane, and several other chemicals causes an increase of enzyme protein in the smooth endoplasmic reticulum, referred to as enzyme induction (REMMER, 1964; CONNEY, 1967). In vitro enzyme studies have revealed that the metabolic capacity is increased and that in many cases the K_M value does not change (CONNEY, 1967; RUBIN et al., 1964). The enzyme capacity in vitro, however, depends strongly on the addition of co-factors, ions, etc., so that an in vitro value as such cannot be directly transferred to an in vivo situation in animals or even in man.

It is, nevertheless, logical to conclude from the increased amount of organelles containing the drug-metabolizing enzymes, that increased enzyme capacity is the result of enzyme induction. Consequently, the metabolic clearance will be increased and therefore, if the body is regarded as a single compartment the biological half-life will be decreased.

$$k_{Cm(ind)} = \frac{\dot{Q}_{m(ind)}}{K_M} \quad \text{and} \quad t_{\frac{1}{2}(ind)} = \frac{0.69 \, V_f \cdot K_M}{\dot{Q}_{m(ind)}}. \tag{48}$$

It should be realized that if phenobarbital treatment, for instance, causes enzyme induction leading to an increased rate of biotransformation of phenazone, the rate of metabolism of other drugs metabolized by the same enzyme will also be increased to the same extent if the conditions stated are valid. A deviation may occur when the rate of metabolism is dependent on hepatic blood flow, because in this case further increase of $\dot{Q}_m$ will not lead to an increase in the apparent metabolic clearance. A second deviation is possible when K_M also changes due to induction; for instance, drug transport in the liver cells may increase, leading to a reduction in apparent K_M. A reduction of this type in the apparent K_M may vary for different drugs.

L. The Liver Clearance Under Pathologic Conditions

In patients with diseases of the liver, such as hepatitis, liver cirrhosis, etc., several enzyme systems may be impaired, including those responsible for biotransformation of foreign compounds. Consequently, the elimination of drugs may be retarded. For instance, in patients with liver cirrhosis the biological half-life of meprobamate (HELD and von OLDERSHAUSEN, 1969), indocyanine green (COOKE et al., 1963) is prolonged (Fig. 9). Under the conditions of single-compartment kinetics and first order elimination, the biological half-life is directly proportional to the metabolic capacity of the liver enzymes. It seems likely that this capacity $\dot{Q}_m$ is decreased by liver function impairment. Theoretically, however, K_M might be increased at the same time. In pathologic conditions the biological half-life is:

$$t_{\frac{1}{2}} = 0.69 V_f \cdot K_M^* / \dot{Q}_m^* \tag{49}$$

when K_M^* and $\dot{Q}_m^*$ are the dissociation constant and metabolic capacity under pathologic conditions. Since the apparent volume of distribution (V_f) depends on plasma protein binding, body weight, etc., changes in V_f can also cause a change in half-life in pathologic conditions, but a change (decrease) in the metabolic capacity, $\dot{Q}_m$, is most likely. If the biological half-life is doubled, this may therefore imply a

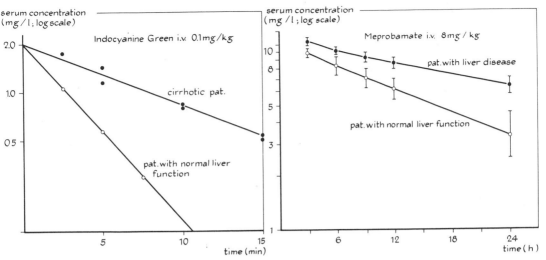

Fig. 9. Decrease in elimination of indocyanine green and meprobamate in patients with liver disease. See text. (Data reproduced from: a) COOKE et al., 1963, with permission of authors and publishers of the Am. J. Digest. Dis. N. Series. b) HELD and VON OLDERSHAUSEN, 1969, with permission of authors and the Klin. Wschr.)

reduction of metabolic capacity by one-half if elimination is merely by bio-transformation.

As pointed out above, a change in the metabolic clearance becomes manifest only if the blood flow through the liver is not the limiting factor. Consequently, for drugs with a high value for the metabolic clearance such that $\dot{Q}_m/K_M \gg k_f$, the half-life will not be increased when $\dot{Q}_m$ decreases, unless this decrease is very pronounced.

M. Drug-Dependent Destruction of Metabolic Clearance Processes

Toxic overdose of several drugs and other chemicals can damage the liver or kidney and thereby further retard their own elimination. The following differential equation describes the elimination process when both capacity-limited elimination and dose-dependent destruction of metabolism occur. The elimination clearance then may be described by the following:

$$\dot{V}_{Cel} = k_{Cel}\left[(1-f) + f\frac{K_M}{(K_M+C)}\cdot\frac{K_d}{(K_d+C)}\right] \tag{50}$$

where K_d is a kind of dissociation constant characterizing enzyme destruction.

If the body is regarded as a single compartment and f equals one, integration of the differential Equation (1) in which for $\dot{V}_{Cel}$ Equation (50) is substituted, then an implicit equation results:

$$\ln C = \ln A + (A-C)/K_M + (A-C)/K_d + (A^2-C^2)/2K_M\cdot K_d - t/\tau_{el}. \tag{51}$$

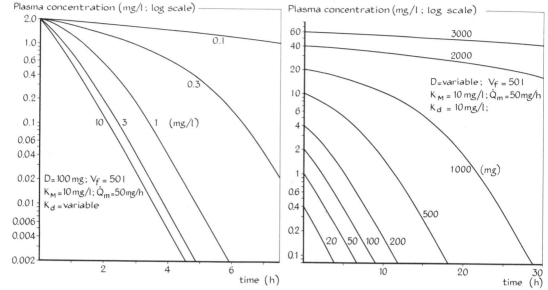

Fig. 10. Plasma curves showing nonlinear kinetics of elimination when both capacity-limited pathway and concentration-dependent enzyme inactivation takes place. Dose-dependency is stronger than in Figure 1

This equation is an extension of Equation (27) such that the concentration influence is stronger.

The influence of variation of the destruction constant is seen in Figure 10. According to Equation (50), increasing doses cause a very progressive retardation of drug elimination. Compare Figure 10 with Figure 1. When the value of K_d is low, the enzyme destruction occurs even at low drug concentrations. Such drugs are very toxic to the liver. Obviously there may be several mechanisms of destruction of metabolic enzymes.

N. Elimination of Parent Drug and its Metabolite

Biotransformation in the body of man or animals results in the occurrence of biologically inactive or active metabolites which in turn are removed from the body by excretion or further metabolism. As pointed out in Section A, the fraction of parent drug metabolized is given by the quotient of the metabolism and total elimination clearance constants. However, only a fraction of the total amount metabolized is converted into any particular metabolite. Therefore the following equations are valid when a drug is given intravenously, when a fraction of the drug is converted to a particular metabolite and the elimination of this metabolite is characterized by a clearance constant k_{Cmel}.

$$\frac{dQ}{dt} = -\{k_{Cr} + f_m \cdot k_{Cm} + (1 - f) k_{Cm}\} C, \tag{52}$$

$$\frac{dQ_m}{dt} = f_m \cdot k_{Cm} \cdot C - k_{Cmel} \cdot C_m \tag{53}$$

where f_m is the fraction of total metabolism directed to the particular metabolite under consideration. C_m is the concentration of that metabolite and k_{Cmel} is the total body clearance constant of that metabolite. When elimination of parent drug and metabolite is merely supply-limited, the time constants for elimination of parent drug and the particular metabolite depend merely on their elimination-clearance constants and their volume of distribution. The concentration of parent drug is described by Equation (14), while that of the particular metabolite is given by the following equation:

$$C_m = \frac{D \cdot f_m \cdot k_{Cm}/k_{Cel}}{V_f} \cdot \frac{\tau_{mel}}{(\tau_{mel} - \tau_{el})} \; (e^{-t/\tau_{mel}} - e^{-t/\tau_{el}}) \tag{54}$$

where τ_{el} and τ_{mel} are the time constants for elimination of parent drug and particular metabolite respectively ($\tau_{mel} = V_{fm}/k_{Cmel}$), and V_{fm} is the apparent volume of distribution of the metabolite. The fraction of the dose injected that is converted in the particular metabolite is $f_m k_{Cm}/k_{Cel}$.

The metabolite may differ from the parent drug in its spectrum of pharmacodynamic actions and also in the main pharmacokinetic aspects, the elimination clearance, the volume of distribution, and the time constant of elimination or biological half-life. Figure 11 gives a few theoretical and experimental examples. When the metabolite is more rapidly eliminated than the parent drug, the two curves are parallel and the biological half-life of the metabolite cannot be calculated from the plasma concentration curve. However, when the metabolite is more slowly eliminated, the plasma curve of the metabolite is less steep than that of the parent drug and both half-life values can be calculated. Obviously the kinetics of the metabolite may be more complicated in formation, elimination, and distribution. However, the clearance constant and the volume of distribution are the important parameters, characterizing parent drug and metabolite. It may be difficult to evaluate these parameters from plasma concentration curves of parent drug and metabolite.

O. Saturation Kinetics of Metabolite Formation and Capacity-Limited Elimination

When the maximum capacity of a clearance system for biotransformation of a drug is reached, the rate of disappearance of parent drug is constant. Consequently, the rate of formation of the metabolite is also constant. Thus:

$$\frac{dQ_m}{dt} = \dot{Q}_m - k_{Cmel} \cdot C_m \tag{55}$$

where Q_m is the quantity of metabolite present, $\dot{Q}_m$ the maximum rate of formation of metabolite, and k_{Cmel} the total body clearance constant of the metabolite. The pattern of concentration of metabolite is similar to what would be produced if the metabolite was introduced by linear infusion:

$$C_m = \frac{\dot{Q}_m}{k_{Cmel}} \; (1 - e^{-t/\tau_{mel}}) = \frac{\dot{Q}_m}{k_{Cmel}} \; (1 - 2^{-t/t_{m1/2}}) \tag{56}$$

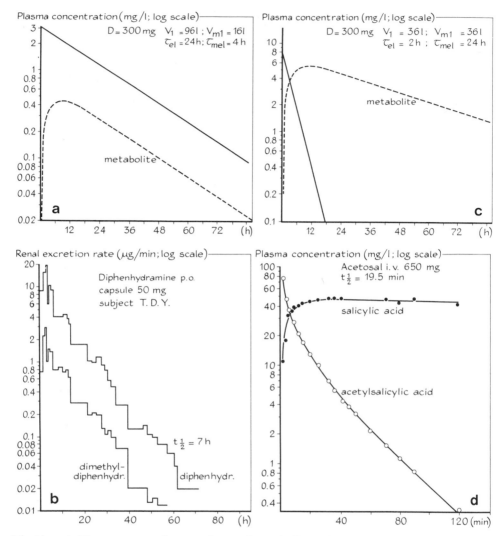

Fig. 11a—d. Plasma curves of parent drug and metabolite under conditions that metabolite is more rapidly cleared than parent drug [(a) theory, (b) Diphenhydramine] and also when metabolite is more slowly eliminated than parent drug [(c) theory, (d) Acetosal]. (Diphenhydramine date from VAN GINNEKEN, unpublished data and Acetosal data from ROWLAND et al., 1967, with permission of authors and publishers of Nature)

where τ_{mel} is the time constant for elimination of the metabolite. It is evident that if the constant rate of metabolite formation proceeds over sufficiently long periods of time ($t > 3t_{m\frac{1}{2}}$), a plateau concentration is obtained.

Where the drug concentration is not high enough to ensure a maximum rate of formation of metabolite, the following differential equation is valid:

$$\frac{dQ_m}{dt} = \frac{\dot{Q}_m}{K_M + C} \cdot C - k_{Cmel} \cdot C_m \, . \tag{57}$$

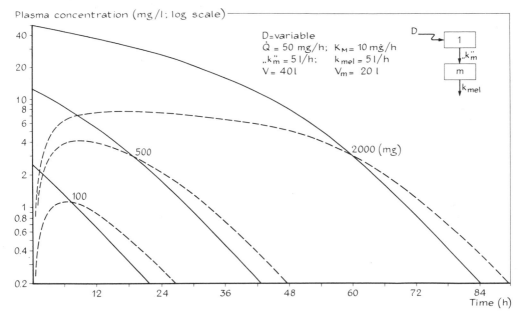

Fig. 12. Plasma curves of parent drug and metabolite in case of capacity-limited elimination of parent drug. By increasing dose, metabolite reaches plateau value. See text

This equation cannot be solved by integration. A numerical solution for C_m is given for chosen values of $\dot{Q}_m, K_M$, and k_{Cmel}, together with the parent drug in Figure 12. The metabolite concentration is seen to approach a plateau if sufficiently high doses of the parent drug have been given.

Often more than one metabolite is formed, and it is possible that more than one metabolic pathway is capacity-limited. Recently LEVY et al. (1972) have given a detailed and brilliant analysis of the complex pattern of salicylic acid elimination in man. A typical example of their results is presented in Figure 13. LEVY et al. concluded that after 3 g salicylic acid the formation of salicyluric acid ($\dot{Q}_m = 60$ mg/h) and salicylphenol glucuronide ($\dot{Q}_m = 32$ mg/h) was concentration-dependent while the formation of salicylacylglucuronide and gentisic acid and the renal excretion of parent drug were controlled by supply-limited clearance processes.

P. Multicompartment Kinetics and Capacity-Limited Elimination

Intravenous administration of a drug is followed by both elimination and distribution over various body compartments. If we assume only a central compartment from which clearance occurs and one peripheral compartment we obtain the following set of nonlinear differential equations (in general it is sufficient to consider the body as a two-compartment system; RIEGELMAN et al., 1968).

$$\frac{dQ_1}{dt} = -k_{Cel}\{(1-f)+f\,K_M/(K_M+C)\}\,C - k_{C12}C + k_{C21}C_2, \qquad (58)$$

$$\frac{dQ_2}{dt} = k_{C12}C - k_{C21}C_2. \qquad (59)$$

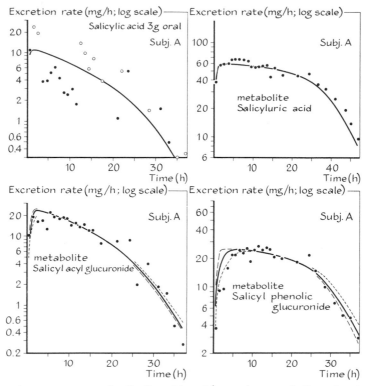

Fig. 13. Excretion rate curves of salicylic acid and its major metabolites showing capacity-limited elimination. (Reproduced from LEVY et al., 1972, with permission of authors and publishers of Clin. Pharmacol. Ther.)

This set of equations cannot be solved analytically. Therefore a digital-computer simulation was performed with values approaching those in the ideal case of Figure 1 for the dose and the enzymatic constants (see Fig. 14). The distribution clearance constants were also varied, which entailed variations in the apparent volume of distribution (see Fig. 14). Obviously, when k_{C12} and k_{C21} are largely relative to the apparent metabolic clearance, distribution is rapid and can therefore be ignored. In this case the body can be regarded as a single compartment. In general, a large peripheral compartment causes a fall in the drug concentration in the central compartment; this lower concentration and consequently higher clearance compensate for the lower clearance at the higher concentration that would occur in case of a smaller volume of distribution.

Figure 15 shows a few examples, one being the plasma curve for gamma-hydroxybutyric acid when injected in anesthetic doses in man (VAN DER POLL et al., 1974). It shows a similar profile to the curves in Figure 14. The distribution phase can be ignored so that the curves fit Equation (36). Figure 15 also shows an apparent, partially capacity-limited elimination of hexobarbital in a patient with hepatitis (BREIMER, 1974). It can be concluded from these figures that capacity-limited elimination can easily be overlooked if the plasma curves are

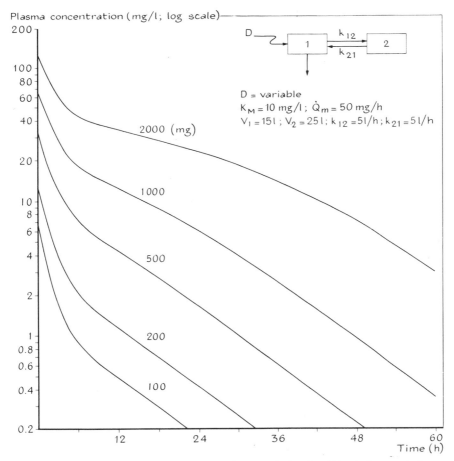

Fig. 14. Theoretical plasma curves for capacity-limited elimination if body is regarded as two-compartment system, obtained by numerical solution with the computer. Except for initial rapid fall, curves are similar to those of Figure 1. At moderate high plasma concentrations, non-linear part in curve may be masked because initial rapid fall may compensate flat part of capacity-limited elimination

not studied after administration of a variety of doses and are not followed over an extensive concentration trajectory; it may appear that the biological half-life is dependent entirely on the dose administered.

Q. Oral Administration and Capacity-Limited Elimination

Most drugs are given by the oral route. The absorption process in the gastro-intestinal tract complicates the kinetic behaviour of drugs so that a capacity-limited elimination may be overshadowed by the absorption. If absorption occurs very rapidly, as is the case for salicylic acid when given as a potion, Equation (1) may be applied (see Fig. 5). In general, the absorption process has to be taken into account. The following equations then are valid, provided that the body may be

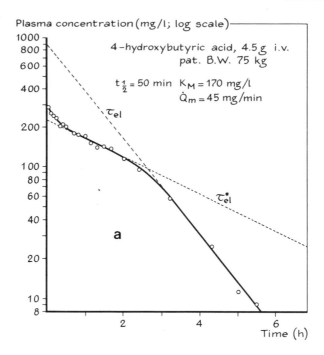

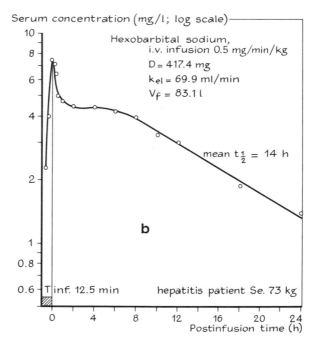

Fig. 15a and b. Plasma curves showing capacity-limited elimination following intravenous infusion of (a) 4-hydroxybutyric acid (data from Van der Poll et al., 1974) and (b) hexobarbital (data from Breimer, 1974). Compare with Figure 14

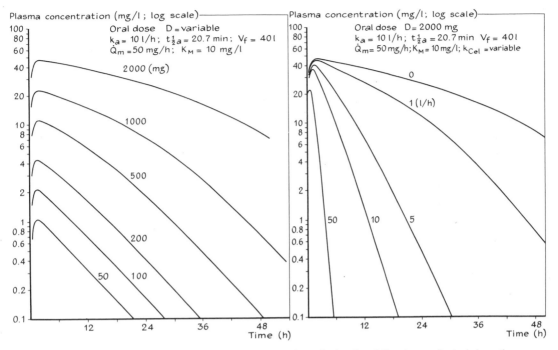

Fig. 16. Theoretical plasma curves for capacity-limited elimination following oral administration obtained by numerical computer method. Except for initial rise, curves are similar to those of Figure 1. At moderate high plasma concentration nonlinear part in curve may be masked by absorption phase

regarded as a single compartment:

$$\frac{dQ_0}{dt} = -k_{Ca} \cdot C_0,$$ (60)

$$\frac{dQ}{dt} = k_{Ca} \cdot C_0 - \dot{V}_{Cel} \cdot C$$ (61)

where k_{Ca} is an absorption clearance constant and C_0 is the concentration in the intestinal tract. If the elimination clearance is not constant but concentration-dependent Equation (61) cannot be integrated. A numerical solution for the case that a single-capacity-limited pathway is involved according to Equation (23), is shown in Figure 16. By comparing Figure 16 with Figure 1 it can be seen that, except for the absorption process, the profile of the curves are very similar. Only if absorption is very slow may it obscure a possible capacity-limited elimination process.

R. Oral Administration and Capacity-Limited Elimination in the Liver

Following oral administration of a drug, absorption in the gastrointestinal tract delivers the drug into the portal system. Consequently, before the drug reaches the general circulation it first passes through the liver. This may imply that only a fraction of the dose administered may reach the general circulation and become subject to distribution and renal excretion. In principle, the bioavailability (the fraction of the dose that reaches the general circulation) of a drug given by the oral route will always be less than one. If drug absorption is rapid, high concentrations may be reached in the liver, so that the metabolic clearance system becomes saturated earlier after oral than after parenteral administration. In this respect the liver should be regarded as a separate compartment (see Fig. 17). In addition, the drug may be transported back to the intestine via the blood stream as well as via the bile. On the other hand, the drug may be transported directly to the general circulation via the lymph. All these transport processes may be characterized by clearance constants (see Fig. 17).

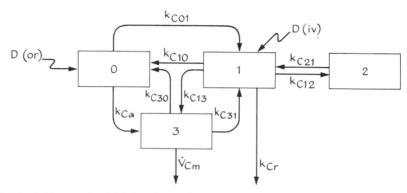

Fig. 17. Block diagram in which liver is considered as separate compartment. A first-pass effect is always in operation but it may be neglected if metabolic clearance is small with respect to total liver flow or if elimination occurs exclusively via kidneys

The following set of differential equations describes the transfer of drug between the various compartments, while the elimination clearance in part occurs via the liver ($\dot{V}_{Cm}$) and via the kidney (k_{Cr}).

$$\frac{dQ_0}{dt} = -(k_{Ca} + k_{C01}) \cdot C_0 + k_{C10} \cdot C + k_{C30} \cdot C_3 , \tag{62}$$

$$\frac{dQ}{dt} = -(k_{Cr} + k_{C10} + k_{C12} + k_{C13}) \cdot C + k_{C01} \cdot C_0 + k_{C31} \cdot C_3 + k_{C21} \cdot C_2 , \tag{63}$$

$$\frac{dQ_2}{dt} = k_{C12} \cdot C - k_{C21} \cdot C_2 , \tag{64}$$

$$\frac{dQ_3}{dt} = k_{Ca} \cdot C_0 + k_{C13} \cdot C - (k_{C30} + k_{C31} + \dot{V}_{Cm}) \cdot C_3 , \tag{65}$$

$$\frac{dQ_{el}}{dt} = \dot{V}_{Cm} \cdot C_3 + k_{Cr} \cdot C \tag{66}$$

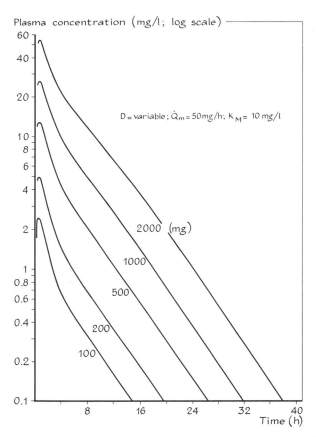

Fig. 18. Plasma curves calculated by numerical computer methods using block scheme of Figure 17 as model ($V_0 = 6\,l$; $V_1 = 12\,l$; $V_3 = 3\,l$; $V_2 = 25\,l$; $k_{Ca} = 12\,l/h$; $k_{C12} = 10\,l/h$; $k_{C21} = 10\,l/h$; $k_{C10} = 12\,l/h$; and $k_{C13} = 60\,l/h$; $k_{C31} = 60\,l/h$; $k_{C30} = 0.1\,l/h$; $k_r = 5\,l/h$). Depending on relative clearance constants in general, the curves closely resemble the more simple situations. Obviously it is not possible to estimate all clearance constants from plasma curve alone

where C_0 is the concentration in the intestinal tract, C_3 the concentration in the liver, C the concentration in the blood plasma, and C_2 the concentration in the peripheral compartment. Again, this set of equations cannot be solved unless the metabolic clearance is a constant.

The various clearance constants influence the fraction of drug excreted unchanged, which would not be so if the liver were regarded as part of the central compartment. A digital-computer simulation has been performed with Equations (59)–(63) for a given set of values for the clearance constants and the enzymatic constants (see Fig. 18).

As the dose increases, the fraction excreted unchanged will also rise because the capacity of the biotransformation is reached when doses are sufficiently high.

In models most frequently used for oral absorption only first-order processes are used, while the liver is considered as part of the central compartment. In these conditions the fraction of drug excreted by the kidney unchanged is independent of the dose and the clearance constant for absorption and distribution. The fraction excreted unchanged, however, becomes dose-dependent when bio-transformation is capacity-limited.

The plasma curves obtained by numerical computer methods for the complicated compartment system of Figure 17 do not essentially differ from the curves calculated from Equation (35), which describes only a single compartment.

S. The Accumulation Plateau Following Repetitive Dosing of a Drug

The average concentration over the dosage interval of a drug following repetitive administration of a constant dose D at a fixed interval is described by the following equation if the kinetic processes are in accordance with linear elimination ($\dot{V}_{Cel} = k_{Cel}$).

$$\bar{C}_j = \frac{1}{\varDelta t} \sum_{j=1}^{n} A_i \tau_i (1 - e^{-j\varDelta t/\tau_i}) \tag{67}$$

where j indicates the jth dose and $\varDelta t$ the fixed dosage interval while τ_i is the ith time constant and A_i the ith dose-dependent coefficient observed after administration of a single dose D.

If sufficient doses have been given, a plateau level is reached. Then $j \cdot \varDelta t \gg \tau_i$ so this equation is reduced to Equation (68):

$$\bar{C}_{pl} = \frac{1}{\varDelta t} \sum_{j=1}^{n} \tau_i A_i = \frac{D \cdot F}{\varDelta t \cdot k_{Cel}} \tag{68}$$

where F is the bioavailability and k_{Cel} the total body clearance constant. $D/\varDelta t$ can be regarded as the average dose flow ($\dot{D}$). A similar equation is obtained when a drug is infused over a sufficiently long period, in which case:

$$C_{pl} = \frac{D}{T} \cdot \frac{1}{k_{Cel}} = \dot{D}/k_{Cel} \tag{69}$$

where D is the dose and T the infusion time so that $D/T = \dot{D}$ is the dosage flow (in this case $F = 1$) because of intravenous administration. The change in the average plasma concentration following repetitive dosing is a discontinuous process with decrements equal to the dosage interval, while after infusion it is a continuous process. This implies that infusion is easier to handle mathematically, while similar conclusions can be drawn from both repetitive dosing and continuous linear infusion. The influence of capacity-limited elimination on the plateau levels following repetitive administration will therefore be analyzed by means of an analysis of the infusion process.

T. The Accumulation Plateau and Capacity-Limited Elimination

Most drugs are administered via the oral route, while the kinetic process can reasonably be described as a two-compartment model. If a drug is "infused" via the oral route with a dosage flow $\dot{D}$, Equation (60) of Section Q is changed into the following equation:

$$\frac{dQ_0}{dt} = \dot{D} - k_{Ca} \cdot C_0 . \tag{70}$$

On the other hand, if intravenous infusion is applied to Equation (61), a dosage flow term is added:

$$\frac{dQ}{dt} = \dot{D} - \dot{V}_{Cel} \cdot C . \tag{71}$$

If infusion is continued over sufficiently long periods a plateau is ultimately reached, provided the dosage flow does not exceed the rate of elimination. In this case the differential equations are zero, so that:

$$\dot{D} = \dot{V}_{Cel} \cdot C_{pl} . \tag{72}$$

Consequently the plateau concentration depends in the following way on the total body clearance k_{Cel} and on the enzyme constants K_M and Q_m, characterizing the one capacity-limited metabolic pathway. Under the conditions that the elimination clearance $\dot{V}_{Cel}$ may be represented by Equation (34), the plateau concentration bears the following relation to the dosage flow, the clearance constant, and the enzyme constants:

$$C_{pl} = \dot{D}/k_{Cel} \cdot [(1-f) + f \cdot K_M/(K_M + C_{pl})] . \tag{73}$$

The concentration dependence of the clearance may be calculated from Equation (34) and consequently the plateau concentration from Equation (73) (Figs. 19 and 20).

Equation (73) shows that the plateau concentration is directly proportional to the dosage flow only if $K_M \gg C_{pl}$. If C_{pl} approaches or exceeds K_M the plateau concentration increases in a much larger proportion. If C_{pl} is very high with respect to K_M, the plateau concentration is again directly proportional to the dosage flow. This relation is visualized in Figure 20.

Obviously C_{pl} is a quadratic expression of the constants present in Equation (73), as may be seen after rearrangement of this equation:

$$C_{pl}^2 + \frac{\dot{Q}_m - f\dot{D}}{f(1-f)k_{Cel}} \cdot C_{pl} - \frac{\dot{D} \cdot \dot{Q}_m}{f(1-f)k_{Cel}^2} = 0 . \tag{73a}$$

It can be seen from this equation that real values can be obtained if $f \cdot \dot{D}$ is smaller than $\dot{Q}_m$. If the value for dosage flow is higher, a plateau will not be reached and the concentration may increase to such a level that the organism is severely damaged.

LEVY has recently predicted that when salicylic acid is given in doses of 2–6 g/day the accumulation plateau will increase sharply if the dose is increased (LEVY and TSUCHIYA, 1972). Actual measurement of the plasma concentration substantiates this prediction (VAN GINNEKEN et al., 1974). VAN GINNEKEN (1976) has studied

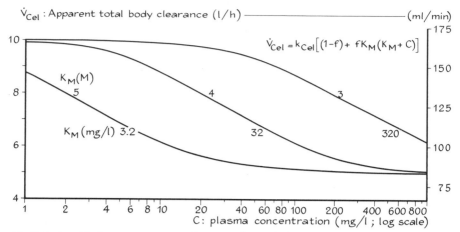

Fig. 19. Relationship between apparent clearance $\dot{V}_{Cel}$ and plasma concentration in case of linear and nonlinear elimination kinetics ($k_{Cel} = 10\,l/h$; $f = 0.5$). With increasing plasma concentration, clearance decreases from 10 to 5 l/h over a concentration range dictated by K_M value. Linear elimination kinetics always occurs at high plasma concentration ($\dot{V}_{Cel} = $ constant)

chronic salicylic acid medication in patients with chronic rheumatic illness. The plasma concentration was measured over one dosage interval when patients were taking 1 g 3 dd. and 0.5 g 3 dd. The average plasma concentration over the intervals differed by a factor of 5–6, which is in agreement with capacity-limited elimination of salicylic acid in the dose range studied (Fig. 21). It must be concluded

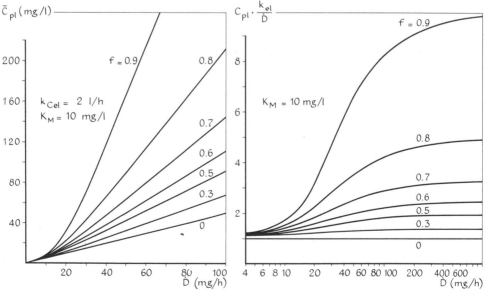

Fig. 20. Relationship between plateau concentration during continuous infusion and dosage flow for various values. Normally plateau is directly proportional to dosage flow ($f = 0$) but in case of capacity-limited elimination, plateau is much higher as expected

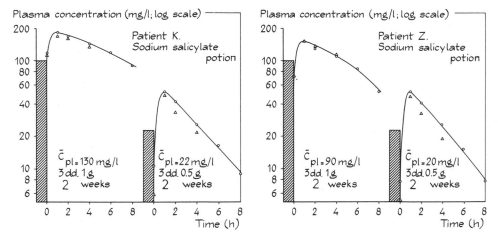

Fig. 21. Plateau concentration of salicylic acid in two patients following repetitive administration of 1 g 3 dd. over 2 weeks, followed by 0.5 g 3 dd. over 2 weeks. Plasma concentration was followed during two corresponding intervals a week apart (first week, second week). Average plateau value following 1 g 3 dd. is about five times larger than value following 0.5 g 3 dd. If capacity-limited elimination was not involved, plateau values should differ only by factor of 2. (Adopted from data by VAN GINNEKEN, 1976).

that the dose of salicylic acid should be increased cautiously in the dose range above 1 g/day, i.e., the range used in the treatment of rheumatic disease.

U. The Accumulation Plateau and Capacity-Limited Elimination in the Liver Compartment

Obviously it is not the concentration in the blood plasma that determines whether the capacity of a metabolic pathway for a drug is reached, but the concentration at the sites where the enzymes are located. The kinetic processes are described by Equations (62)–(66).

In Section T it did not matter whether infusion was direct into the central compartment or via the oral route. When the liver is considered as a separate component it obviously does matter, because substantial metabolism can occur during the first passage through the liver. This so-called first pass effect has been examined by several authors (GIBALDI and FELDMAN, 1972; ROWLAND, 1972). Here we give a general discussion, also allowing absorption via the lymph (k_{C10}) and excretion via the bile (k_{C03}). For a fruitful analysis one may again distinguish and infusion by the oral route and an intravenous infusion. In case of "oral" infusion Equation (62) is changed as follows:

$$\frac{dQ_0}{dt} = \dot{D} - (k_{Ca} + k_{Cel}) \cdot C_0 + k_{C10}C + k_{C30} \cdot C_3 . \tag{74}$$

While in case of intravenous infusion a dosage flow term is added to Equation (63). Then:

$$\frac{dQ}{dt} = \dot{D} - (k_{Cr} + k_{C10} + k_{C12} + k_{C13})\, C + k_{C01} C_0 + k_{C31} C_3 + k_{C21} C_2 . \quad (75)$$

Under the supposition that the dosage flow does not exceed the capacity of elimination a plateau level is reached after a sufficiently long infusion period. From the differential Equation (66) in this case follows that the dosage flow equals the elimination rate:

$$\dot{D} = k_{Cr} C_{pl} + \dot{V}_{Cm} C_{3pl} \quad (76)$$

where $\dot{V}_{Cm}$ is the metabolic clearance which may be a constant at liver concentrations much lower than the dissociation constants of the drug for the metabolizing enzymes. If a plateau is reached there is a fixed relation between the liver concentration C_3 and the plasma concentration. This relationship depends on oral or intravenous infusion.

In case of oral infusion this relation may be found for the steady state from Equations (63), (64), and (65). Then:

$$C_{3pl} = \frac{k_{Ca}(k_{Cr} + k_{C10} + k_{C13}) + k_{C01} k_{C13}}{k_{C01}(k_{C30} + k_{C31} + \dot{V}_{Cm}) + k_{Ca} k_{C31}} \cdot C_{pl} . \quad (77)$$

Consequently, the plateau level in the blood plasma can be computed by substitution of the expression for C_{3pl} in terms of C_{pl} in Equation (76).

In case of intravenous infusion the relationship between the plateau concentration in the liver and in the plasma can be derived from Equations (62), (64), and (65). Then:

$$C_{3pl} = \frac{k_{Ca}(k_{C10} + k_{C13}) + k_{C01} k_{C13}}{(k_{Ca} + k_{C01})(k_{C31} + \dot{V}_{Cm}) + k_{C01} k_{C30}} \cdot C_{pl} . \quad (78)$$

Again by substitution of this expression in Equation (76) the relation between dosage flow and plateau concentration can be computed.

V. The Renal Excretion Rate in Case of Capacity-Limited Elimination

A plateau is also ultimately reached following repetitive administration of a drug according to a fixed dosage interval Δt. However, considerable occillations are possible. In each interval, the amount of drug excreted unchanged with the urine will be constant as long as the renal clearance is not concentration-dependent and urinary flow and urinary pH are kept within limits.

The amount of drug excreted during one dosage interval with the urine remains strictly proportional to the plasma concentration in that interval, since:

$$\frac{dQ_r}{dt} = k_{Cr} C_{pl}, \quad \text{so that} \quad Q_{r(\Delta t)} = k_{Cr} \int_0^{\Delta t} C_{pl}\, dt . \quad (79)$$

This implies that the quantity of drug excreted in the Δt period or in 24 h is also a good indicator of the plateau level in the case of capacity-limited metabolic elimination, provided renal excretion in fact remains directly proportional to the plasma level (constant renal clearance). It is also evident that the 24-h excretion of unchanged drugs will increase by increasing the dose in comparison to that of the metabolite, that is found via a capacity-limited pathway, because the metabolite concentration falls behind when the plasma concentration increases.

W. Metabolite Concentrations Following Chronic Medication

For many drugs active metabolites are formed. Following repetitive intake of drugs according to a fixed interval Δt also ultimately leads to constant metabolite concentration. It is of interest to study the metabolite concentration, which is formed via a capacity-limited pathway. This particular metabolite concentration is represented by Equation (57) under the supposition that only one metabolite is formed. In general, only a fraction f_m is formed.

In the steady-state situation when the plasma concentration of unchanged drug reaches a plateau value, that of the metabolite also reaches a plateau level:

$$C_{mpl} = f_m \frac{k_{Cel}}{k_{Cmel}} \cdot \frac{K_M}{(K_M + C_{pl})} \cdot C_{pl} \tag{80}$$

where f_m is the fraction of the drug that is metabolized to the particular metabolite. This implies that the plateau concentration of the metabolite is directly proportional to the plasma concentration of unchanged drug only when $C_{pl} \ll K_m$. Then:

$$C_{mpl} = f_m \cdot k_{Cel}/k_{Cmel} . \tag{81}$$

It may be noted that the plateau level of the metabolite may exceed that of the parent drug if f_m is large (unity) and the elimination clearance of the parent drug is larger than that of the metabolite.

If, however, C_{pl} approaches or exceeds K_M, the plateau level of the metabolite does not follow the plateau level of unchanged drug. Finally, for a high dosage flow, when $C_{pl} \gg K_M$, Equation (81) reduces to:

$$C_{mpl} = \dot{Q}_m/k_{Cmel} . \tag{82}$$

This implies that the metabolite level does not increase any further when the dosage flow is increased.

Since the metabolite may also be excreted in the urine according to its renal clearance constant k_{Cmr}, the quantity of metabolite excreted during a dosage interval is also constant.

It is obvious that if the dosage flow increases to such a high level that the full capacity of the drug-metabolizing system is reached, the amount of unchanged drug excreted in the urine increases in accordance with the plasma concentration but the amount of metabolites excreted over each dosage interval reaches a limit, which is:

$$Q_{mr(\Delta t)} = \dot{Q}_m \cdot \Delta t k_{Cmr}/k_{Cmel}. \tag{83}$$

X. Bioavailability and Capacity-Limited Elimination

The bioavailability is the proportion of a dose administered in a particular dosage form by a given route that reaches the general circulation. It is generally expressed as the fraction of the dose that enters the general circulation. By this definition the bioavailability of an i.v. dose is one.

Obviously, the bioavailability is always less than one following oral administration because even if the drug is absorbed completely a certain fraction is nevertheless eliminated in the liver before the drug enters the general circulation.

If absorption via the lymphatic route is ignored it can easily be seen from Equation (80) that a fraction is extracted during the first passage of the drug through the liver. This fraction equals:

$$\text{fraction extracted} = \dot{V}_{Cm}/(\dot{V}_{Cm} + k_{C31}). \tag{84}$$

It is obvious that if $\dot{V}_{Cm}$ is concentration-dependent, for instance, according to Equation (23), the fraction extracted during the first passage decreases with increasing the dose. The pharmaceutical dosage form may have a great influence also. It is conceivable if a drug with a high metabolic clearance showing capacity-limited elimination reaches a high liver concentration when given as a potion. If such a drug is given in a slow release form the ultimate levels may be very low. In conclusion, it is not always justified to make sustained release preparation of drugs which are rapidly metabolized.

Even if the drug is completely absorbed in the intestinal tract the biological availability F is less than 1 and may be given by the following equation:

$$F = k_{C31}/(k_{C31} + \dot{V}_{Cm}) \tag{85}$$

where $\dot{V}_{Cm}$ is the metabolic or liver clearance and k_{C31} the clearance of drug from liver to general circulation. The sum of k_{C31} and $\dot{V}_{Cm}$ equals the effective plasma flow through the liver. The effective plasma flow through the liver is roughly equal to the liver blood flow, so that the biological availability under assumption of complete intestinal absorption is practically equal to unity if the liver clearance is less than 100 ml/min. This is the case for many drugs.

Drugs with a high liver clearance may have a low biological availability unless substantial capacity-limited metabolism takes place. This may be seen by substitution of Equation (34) in Equation (85).

$$F = k_{C31}/[k_{C31} + k_{Cm}\{(1 - f) + f K_M/(K_M + C_3)\}]. \tag{86}$$

From this equation it follows that if the capacity-limited pathway(s) largely contribute to the liver clearance ($f \to 1$) and the liver concentration exceeds K_M, that F

approaches unity. So a reasonable biological availability may be obtained, despite of a high metabolic clearance. This is probably the case for imipramine.

A more general expression of the biological availability, under the assumption of complete intestinal absorption, can be found from Equations (76), (77), and (78), as the effective dosage flow following oral infusion is $\dot{D} \cdot F$ and following intravenous infusion $\dot{D}$. The following expression can be obtained:

$$F = \frac{k_{Ca}k_{C31} + k_{C01}(k_{C30} + k_{C31} + \dot{V}_m)}{k_{Ca}(k_{C31} + \dot{V}_m) + k_{C01}(k_{C30} + k_{C31} + \dot{V}_m)}. \tag{87}$$

It is obvious that if absorption via the lymph is important ($k_{Cm} \gg k_{Ca}$), the biological availability will approach unity. If, however, absorption via the lymph can be neglected, the expression is reduced to Equation (85). This also holds in case of rectal administration because then the drug reaches the general circulation by-passing the liver. As a matter of fact absorption efficiency as such may be smaller from the rectum than from the intestine.

II. Conclusion

Capacity-limited biotransformation for at least one metabolic pathway may occur much more often than is generally realized. It may easily be overlooked if it is a minor pathway, when metabolic clearance is flow-limited, or when renal elimination is the major pathway of elimination.

Capacity-limited elimination may become manifest during chronic medication and when several drugs are given simultaneously. With drugs that bind strongly to plasma protein, capacity-limited elimination is less likely because of the relatively low free plasma concentration. A similar situation occurs when a drug accumulates in extravascular tissues (large peripheral compartment). Finally, capacity-limited elimination may be dependent on the route of administration. It may be observed after administration by the oral route even if it does not occur after administration of the same drug by the rectal or intramuscular route.

References

Arnold, K., Gerber, N.: The rate of decline of diphenylhydantoin in human plasma. Clin. Pharmacol. Ther. **11**, 121—134 (1970).

Bahr, C. von: Binding and oxidation of amitriptyline and a series of its oxidized metabolites in liver microsomes from untreated and phenobarbital-treated rats. Xenobiotica **2**, 293 (1972).

Breimer, D. D.: Pharmacokinetics of hypnotic drugs. Section IV, Chapter 1. Nijmegen: Drukkerij Brakkenstein, 1974.

Breimer, D. D., Rossum, J. M. van: Pharmacokinetics of (+)−, (−)− and (±)− hexobarbitone in man after oral administration. J. Pharm. Pharmac. **25**, 762—764 (1973).

Brilmayer, H., Loennecken, S. J.: Die Eliminationsgeschwindigkeit von Barbiturat aus dem Blut akut intoxizierter Patienten. Arch. int. Pharmacodyn. **136**, 137—146 (1962).

Brodie, B. B., Burns, J. J., Weiner, M.: Metabolism of drugs in subjects with Laennecs Cirrhosis. Med. exp. (Basel) **1**, 290—292 (1959).

Conney, A. H.: Pharmacological implications of microsomal enzyme induction. Pharmacol. Rev. **19**, 317—353 (1967).

Cooke, A. R., Harrison, D. D., Skyring, A. P.: Use of indocyanine green as a test of liver function. Amer. J. dig. Dis. (N.S.) **8**, 244—250 (1963).

Dallner, G., Ernster, L.: Subfractionation and composition of microsomal membranes: A review. J. Histochem. Cytochem. **16**, 611—632 (1968).

Dam, F. E. van: De invloed van enkele geneesmiddelen op het effect en de verwerking van ethyl biscoumacetaat. Thesis. Nijmegen: Thoben-Offset, 1968.

Davies, D. S., Gigon, P. L., Gillette, J. R.: Species and sex differences in electron transport systems in the liver microsomes and their relationship to ethyl morphine demethylation. Life Sci. **8**, 85—91 (1969).

Estabrook, R. W.: Cytochroom P-450—Its function in the oxidative metabolism of drugs. In: Handb. exp. Pharmakol., Vol. 28/2, 264—284, Berlin-Heidelberg-New York: Springer 1971.

Fouts, J. R.: Some morphological characteristics of hepatocyte endoplasmic reticulum and some relationship between endoplasmic reticulum, microsomes, and drug metabolism. In: Handb. exp. Pharmacol., Vol. 28/2, pp. 243—250, Berlin-Heidelberg-New York: Springer 1971.

Gibaldi, M., Feldman, S.: Route of administration and drug metabolism. Europ. J. Pharmacol. **19**, 323—329 (1972).

Ginneken, C. A. M. van: Renale excretie van enige antihistaminica bij de mens. 13th Federal Meeting of the Dutch Medical-Biological Societies (1972).

Ginneken, C. A. M. van: Pharmacokinetics of Antipyretic and Anti-inflammatory Analgesics. Ph. D. Thesis. Nijmegen: Stichting Studentenpers, 1976.

Ginneken, C. A. M. van, Rossum, J. M. van, Fleuren, H. L. J. M.: Linear and nonlinear kinetics of drug elimination. Part I. J. Pharmacokin. Biopharmac. **2**, 395—415 (1974).

Haggard, H. W., Greenberg, L. A., Carroll, R. P.: Studies in the absorption, distribution and elimination of alcohol. VIII. The diuresis from alcohol and its influence on the elimination of alcohol in the urine. J. Pharmacol. exp. Ther. **71**, 349—357 (1941).

Held, H., Oldershausen, H. F. von: Zur Pharmakokinetik von Meprobamat bei chronischen Hepatopathien und Arzneimittelsucht. Klin. Wschr. **47**, 78—80 (1969).

Henderson, P. Th., Vree, T. B., Ginneken, C. A. M. van, Rossum, J. M. van: Activation energies of α-C-oxidation and N-oxidation of N-alkyl-substituted amphetamines by rat liver microsomes. Xenobiotica **4**, 121—130 (1974).

Jansson, I., Orrenius, S., Ernster, L., Schenkman, J. B.: A study of the interaction of a series of substituted barbituric acids with the hepatic microsomal mono-oxygenase. Arch. Biochem. **151**, 391 (1972).

Kupfer, D., Jansson, I., Orrenius, S.: Spectral interactions of marihuana-constituents (cannabinoids) with rat liver mono oxygenase system. Chem. biol. Interact. **5**, 201 (1972).

Leibman, K. C., Hildebrandt, A. G., Estabrook, R. W.: Spectrophotometric studies of interactions between varies substrates in their binding to microsomal cytochrome P-450. Biochem. biophys. Res. Commun. **36**, 789—794 (1969).

Levy, G.: Pharmacokinetics of salicylate elimination in man. J. pharm. Sci. **54**, 959—967 (1965).

Levy, G.: Drug biotransformation interactions in man: Nonnarcotic analgesics. Ann. N.Y. Acad. Sci. **179**, 32—43 (1971).

Levy, G., Tsuchiya, T.: Salicylate accumulation kinetics in man. New Engl. J. Med. **287**, 430—432 (1972).

Levy, G., Tsuchiya, T., Amsel, L. P.: Limited capacity for salicyl phenolic glucuronide formation and its effect on the kinetics of salicylate elimination in man. Clin. Pharmacol. Ther. **13**, 258—268 (1972).

Nagashima, R., Levy, G.: Effect of perfusion rate and distribution factors on drug elimination kinetics in a perfused organ system. J. pharm. Sci. **57**, 1991—1993 (1968).

Orrenius, S., Kupfer, D., Ernster, L.: Substrate binding to cytochrome P-450 of liver and adrenal microsomes. FEBS Letters **6**, 249 (1970).

Pol, W. S. van der., Deeleman, R., Kleijn, E. van der, Lauw, M., Schönefeld, H., Rossum, J. M. van, Crul, J. F.: Linear and nonlinear pharmacokinetics of 4-hydroxybutyrate in humans. Cited by van Ginneken J. Pharmacokin. Biopharmac. **2**, 395—415 (1974).

Remmer, H.: Drug-induced formation of smooth endoplasmic reticulum and of drug metabolizing enzymes. In: Proc. Europ. Soc. for the study of drug toxicity. Vol. IV, 57—77 (1964). Excerpta Medica Foundation, Amsterdam.

Remmer, H., Schenkman, J., Estabrook, R. W. et al.: Drug interaction with hepatic microsomal cytochrome. Molec. Pharmacol. **2**, 187—190 (1966).

Remmer, H., Schenkman, J. B., Greim, H.: In: Gilette, A. et al. (Eds.): Microsomes and drug oxidation, p. 371. New York: Academic Press, 1969.

Riegelman, S., Loo, J. C. K., Rowland, M.: Shortcomings in pharmacokinetic analysis by conceiving the body to exhibit properties of a single compartment. J. pharm. Sci. **57**, 117—123 (1968).

Rowland, M.: Influence of route of administration on drug availability. J. pharm. Sci. **61**, 70—74 (1972).

Rowland, M., Riegelman, S., Harris, P. A., Sholkoff, S. D., Eyring, E. J.: Kinetics of acetylsalicylic acid disposition in man. Nature (Lond.) **215**, 413—414 (1967).

Rubin, A., Tephly, T. R., Mannering, G. J.: Kinetics of drug metabolism by hepatic microsomes. Biochem. Pharmacol. **13**, 1007—1016 (1964).

Schenkman, J. B.: Studies on the nature of the type I and type II spectral changes in liver microsomes. Biochemistry **9**, 2081—2091 (1970).

Schenkman, J. B., Remmer, H., Estabrook, R. W.: Spectral studies of drug interaction with hepatic microsomal cytochrome. Molec. Pharmacol. **3**, 113—123 (1967).

Swintosky, J. V.: Illustrations and pharmaceutical interpretations of first order drug elimination rate from the bloodstream. J. Amer. pharm. Ass. **45**, 395—400 (1956).

Temple, D. J.: Binding of nitrogen-containing compounds to microsomal cytochromes. Xenobiotica **1**, 195 (1971).

Topham, J. C.: Relationship between difference spectra and metabolism. Barbiturates, drug interaction and species difference. Biochem. Pharmacol. **19**, 1695—1701 (1970).

Vree, T. B., Henderson, P. Th., Rossum, J. M. van, Doukas, P. H.: In vivo and in vitro inhibition of the metabolism of N-alkyl-substituted amphetamines in rat by ferrocenylisopropylamine. Xenobiotica **3**, 23—35 (1973).

Wagner, J. G.: A modern view of Pharmacokinetics. J. Pharmacokin. Biopharmac. **1**, 363—401 (1973).

Wagner, J. G., Patel, J. A.: Variations in absorption and elimination rates of ethyl alcohol in a single subject. Res. Commun. chem. Path. Pharmacol. **4**, 61—76 (1972).

Wurster, D. E., Kramer, S. F.: Investigation of some factors influencing percutaneous absorption. J. pharm. Sci. **50**, 288—293 (1961).

Handb. Exp. Pharmacol. Vol. 47
"Kinetics of Drug Action", Jacques M. van Rossum,
Editor, Springer-Verlag Berlin Heidelberg New York, 1977

CHAPTER 4

General Theory of Drug-Receptor Interactions
Drug-Receptor Interaction Models. Calculation of Drug Parameters

F. G. VAN DEN BRINK

A theory need not be correct or even visibly sensible; it is sufficient for it to be workable. ERIC FRANC RUSSELL

I. Introduction

A. The Utility of Theoretical Mathematical Models in Molecular Pharmacology

In the study of the interaction between pharmacologically active molecules and different types of receptor-effector systems (often designated as molecular pharmacology) an important role is played by theoretical mathematical models with which these interactions can be described (CLARK, 1926, 1937; GADDUM, 1926, 1937; ARIËNS, 1954; ARIËNS et al., 1956a, b, c, 1964a, b, c; STEPHENSON, 1956; VAN ROSSUM, 1958, 1966; PATON, 1961; PATON and WAUD, 1964; PATON and RANG, 1966; VAN DEN BRINK, 1969c, d, 1973a, b). It should be stressed that these models do not pretend to be exact representations of the enormously complicated chain of events leading from the contact between the molecules of a pharmacologically active substance and a biological entity to the ensuing effect. This they cannot do and it is not their purpose. Even on a theoretical level the equations used only hold fully if quite a number of presuppositions are made (VAN ROSSUM, 1966; VAN DEN BRINK, 1969b). In practice the models cannot be expected to give more than a usable overall description of reality.

Nevertheless, in order to be useful as a scientific working hypothesis a model should meet at least two general conditions. First, it should explain the experimental results obtained so far with a minimum of independent presuppositions (law of parsimony; see e.g., HAMILTON, 1868). Second, it should provoke further research: it should predict the results of new critical experiments with which, subsequently, the model can be put to the test. Occasionally models have been proposed which do not meet this second condition, in that they are so flexible that they cannot be disproved by any experimental result. No matter what characteristics future experimental concentration-effect curves may possess, the theory predicts them if the equations are only supplied with the "right" parameters. Such models will not be discussed in this chapter, since, however ingenious, they do not carry us any further.

This chapter will deal with molecular pharmacologic models in common use and with some recent modifications or refinements in this field; the basic concepts used in these models will be discussed. The various subjects are discussed first on the basis of reasonings, whereas the mathematical calculations which accompany the theory, but which may be not indispensible for an insight into the matter, together with the methods for calculation of numerical expressions of intrinsic activity and affinity, follow next. Models which do not describe equilibrium (or steady state) situations, as well as a discussion of time-effect relations are beyond the scope of this chapter, since these subjects are treated by different authors (see the Chapters by R. E. GOSSELIN and

C. A. M. van Ginneken). The various theories about the mechanisms by which the presence of an agonistic drug in the direct environment of its receptors leads to the formation of a stimulus will be mentioned only in passing, since they are discussed in detail in the chapter written by D. Mackay.

B. The Affinity Between Drug Molecules and Receptors; the Concepts Drug Activity and Receptor

Pharmacology is the branch of natural science engaged in studying the interaction between a biological entity and certain chemical substances, in this connection called pharmaca, or drugs. Originally pharmacology was mainly descriptive, since in most cases the processes underlying the observable effects were utterly untransparent. In the early part of this century, however, a breakthrough was made to some understanding of more fundamental events. Essential in this development is the absolute rejection of vitalistic ideas. It was accepted that, as far as science is concerned, vital phenomena should be explained in terms of the same fundamental processes which occur in inanimate systems, although, of course, the interconnection of these processes in the simplest biological entity is very much more complex than in any non-living system. These notions are pithily reflected in the following statement of Storm van Leeuwen (1925a): "The real site of action [*Angriffspunkt*] of drugs is unknown but it is certain, that each drug before being able to exert an action must enter into a chemical or physico-chemical reaction with substances of unknown origin, possessing definite physico-chemical properties. Without this assumption, specific drug action could not be explained." Yet it took a relatively long time before it was generally appreciated that—since a biological object as well as a pharmacon is composed of molecules—an interaction between a living being and a chemical substance essentially is an interaction between molecules, obeying physical and chemical laws.

Some drugs may cause alterations in the organism as a result of more general properties. In the case of many anesthetics, for instance, the effect seems to be caused by an unspecific physicochemical change in the biological milieu (Pauling, 1961). For many other pharmaca, however, such a mechanism of action is rather improbable. Many pharmaca cause highly specific changes in the body—specific in the sense that the effect in question proves to be dependent on the drug possessing a special molecular structure—when given in relatively low doses. Some substances are even effective when they are administered in doses of micrograms per kilogram body weight. A simple comparison of the number of drug molecules and the number of molecules in the organism shows that in such a case only a very small fraction of the molecules of the organism can participate in the interaction with the drug molecules. Probably this fraction distinguishes itself in some way from other molecules in the organism; it may be assumed that there are molecules in the body to which the molecules of the drug have a special affinity.

These molecules—or perhaps parts of molecules or groups of molecules—with which the molecules of a specific drug interact are called its receptors. The name is relatively young; it was Langley who used the term "receptive substance" for the structure in the motor endplate with which curare combines (Langley, 1905). The concept behind it, however, is very old. Often it is carried back to the view of Ehrlich that "corpora non agunt nisi fixata" (EHRLICH, 1913), but indications of it are present already in the didactic poem *De Rerum Natura*, written by Titus Lucretius Carus in the first century before Christ. Lucretius supposed that all bodily sensations in essence are caused by the fact that certain parts of the body are "touched" by certain "atoms", and that the differences in shape and form of these atoms determine, for instance, whether they can cause the sensation of taste by penetrating into the "pores" of palate and tongue, and whether they cause there one kind of taste or another (Lucretius, circa 50 B.C.).

Thus, if no receptors exist in the body for the molecules of a certain chemical substance, this substance cannot be an active and specific drug in the narrower sense of those words. Placebo effects, of course, are not considered to be pharmacologic actions.

Drug-receptor interactions are determinative for the greater part of drugs in use, and in the following the actions due to nonspecific properties are left out of consideration. With these limitations it may be stated that affinity to receptors is the first condition for activity—though not the only one.

Before going further into this, something more should be said about the concept "drug activity". Very strictly taken, any drug that has affinity to receptors possesses activity, for having affinity to a receptor implies the ability to cause an alteration, however small, in this receptor. In this form, however, the concept has no use: in practice no drug will be considered "active" if its effects are imperceptible. This means that what is called drug activity cannot be an objective concept. It is something partly dependent on the observer; it may be defined as the ability of the drug to cause alterations in the biological system which are perceptible to the investigator.

In this connection the concept "receptor" should also be regarded with more accuracy. In the first place it will be clear that the concept is closely related to that of the "active site" in enzymology. As stated before, the fact that interaction between two molecules takes place means that changes occur in both molecules. In the case of an interaction between a substrate molecule and an active site on an enzyme, the alteration in the former is essential with respect to the effect; in the case of a drug-receptor interaction the alteration in the receptor is the essential phenomenon. Nevertheless both situations have much in common, and in what follows some approaches known from the field of enzymology will be recognized.

Secondly, it is not very probable that the molecules of a specific drug only have affinity to the receptors on which the effect can be induced. The drug may also have affinity to other structures in the body, an interaction with these structures being not effective in the sense of the definition of effect given above. According to some authors these structures should not be called receptors; they prefer to use terms like "binding sites", "acceptors" (CHAGAS, 1962), "sites of loss" (VELDSTRA, 1956; CAVALLITO, 1959; FASTIER, 1962), and such. Another possibility is to distinguish this kind of receptors as "secondary receptors" (STORM VAN LEEUWEN, 1925a, b, c), "silent receptors" (GOLDSTEIN, 1949) or "unspecific receptors" («des récepteurs non spécifiques») (BOVET et al., 1956), and to call the receptors from which an effect can originate "dominant receptors" (STORM VAN LEEUWEN, 1925a, b) or "specific receptors" («des récepteurs spécifiques») (BOVET et al., 1956). This seems preferable, since the difference does not lie in the factor "receptivity". In connection with what was said about drug activity it will be clear that the question whether a site of interaction is a specific or an unspecific receptor only depends on the question whether the consequence of the interaction is regarded as "effect". The distinction, therefore, cannot have absolute value, but it is certainly of practical use. Whenever receptors are mentioned in the following text, specific receptors are meant.

C. Intrinsic Activity; the Concepts Agonism, Competitive Antagonism, and Dualism

The dependence of drug activity on affinity is obvious, but the question arises whether this is the only factor determining activity. This point may be illustrated with the following set of simple experiments.

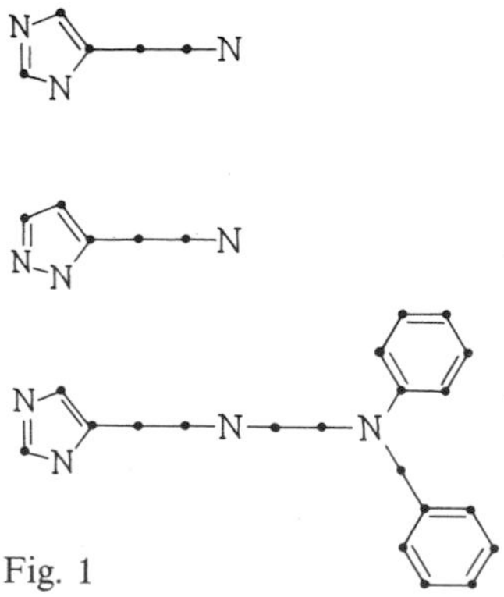

histamine

3-(β-aminoethyl)- pyrazole

N-(N'-phenyl-N'-benzyl-β-aminoethyl)-histamine

Fig. 1

A well-known effect of the drug histamine (Fig. 1) is that it can cause a contraction of smooth muscle fibres. This can be demonstrated on a piece of guinea-pig ileum, used as an isolated organ preparation. The organ is suspended in a bath with a suitable fluid, and if an adequate dose of histamine is added to this fluid, the organ reacts with a certain degree of contraction. Let us suppose that such an amount of histamine is added that a distinct but submaximal contraction of the organ results.

The bath fluid is changed several times, so that all histamine is removed and the organ is relaxed again. Then 3-(β-aminoethyl)-pyrazole, a close structural analogue of histamine (Fig. 1), is added in the same molar amount as the histamine in the first experiment: no contraction of the organ follows. An obvious explanation of this result is, that this analogue has no—or much less—affinity to the histamine receptors in the organ, as a result of its slightly different molecular structure. If this is so, the presence of the 3-(β-aminoethyl)-pyrazole in the medium should have no demonstrable influence. And indeed, if the original dose of histamine is added, without removing the analogue first, a contraction results equal to the original effect of the histamine alone.

So far everything seems clear. Now the experiment is repeated with another derivative of histamine, viz. N-(N'-phenyl-N'-benzyl-β-aminoethyl)-histamine (Fig. 1). Again no contraction results from the addition of an equimolar dose of this compound, and so it could be supposed that it has no affinity to the receptor either. But if the original dose of histamine is added now, the inactive compound still being present in the medium, the effect of the histamine is found to be reduced considerably. Only if higher doses of histamine are added does the original degree of contraction ensue.

Clearly the derivative in the third experiment does have an influence on the organ: it hinders the action of histamine. This fact may suggest that the compound still has affinity to the histamine receptors—a supposition that can be confirmed by other means as will be discussed below. If this is true, why is the substance inactive by itself? Evidently it differs from histamine in a factor distinct from affinity: it interacts with the receptors, but the interaction is not effective in the sense that contraction of the muscle results from it.

In the presence of the derivative a certain fraction of the receptors is not available for interaction with histamine. The interactions should be seen not as static, but as dynamic, reversible processes, and therefore it is also clear that if in the third experiment a larger dose of histamine is added, the percentage of the receptors that is in interaction with it will increase, and the contraction of the organ will become greater.

These experiments illustrate a fact of essential importance. Among the drugs that have affinity to a receptor there may be substances that have the ability to cause a change in the receptor that gives rise to an observable effect and others lacking this ability. Drugs that possess both affinity as well as this ability are called "receptor-activators" (HIGMAN and BARTELS, 1962) or "agonists" (REUSE, 1948) and the ability itself is given the name of "intrinsic activity" (ARIËNS, 1954) or "efficacy" (STEPHENSON, 1956)[1].

From the foregoing it follows that the concept of agonism is different from drug activity, potency, effectivity, or stimulant action. A drug without intrinsic activity but with affinity to the receptors of a certain agonist may show its presence in the organism by clear effects. In the physiologic situation many "receptor-effector systems" are activated to a certain degree as a result of the presence of an endogenous agonist. (By receptor-effector system is meant the whole body of identical receptors plus the structures in which the caused effect, and the chain of events leading to it, take place.) If an endogenous agonistic substance is continually present and interacts with its receptors, administration of a pharmacon that blocks the influence of this agonist causes an alteration in the level of activation.

For instance, if atropine is administered to the eye, the pupil is known to dilate. Atropine causes this effect by blocking the receptors for acetylcholine, a substance secreted by the parasympathetic nerve fibres. Interaction of acetylcholine with its receptors leads to contraction of the constrictor muscle of the pupil. Disappearance of this physiologic constricting action is the cause of the observed dilatation, and though it could be said that atropine stimulates a dilatation of the pupil, yet the drug is not an

---

[1] The differentiation between the two factors which are essential for the action of an agonistic drug is older than the names "intrinsic activity" and "efficacy". In 1937 CLARK had already formulated the hypothesis that the selective action of drugs such as acetylcholine and adrenaline depends firstly on the power to combine with the receptor, and secondly on the power to produce an effect after they have combined, and in this connection he refers to older, corresponding views in enzymology (CLARK, 1937). ÅBERG made the same distinction in a study on the effects of auxins, differentiating between affinity and the "activity of the substance when bound" (ÅBERG, 1952).

As for the name "intrinsic activity", this term had its predecessors in the terms "intrinsic toxicity" and "intrinsic action" (FERGUSON, 1939; DAGLEY et al., 1948), which, however, did not have the same purport as the present-day concept.

agonist itself but a so-called antagonist (counteracting substance) of the normally present agonist acetylcholine.

The kind of antagonism introduced here is named competitive antagonism, and it is only one of the different kinds of antagonism that are usually distinguished. The term speaks for itself: this antagonism is based on a competition between an antagonist and an agonist for receptors to which both have affinity. The agonist, having intrinsic activity, causes its effect by interaction with the receptors as such; the competitive antagonist, which does not possess intrinsic activity, cannot cause an effect except in the presence of the agonist. On "empty" receptors it is inactive.

Among the pharmaca which have affinity to a receptor the choice is not merely between substances with a certain intrinsic activity and others without; theoretically the intrinsic activity can have all values between maximal and zero. In fact it has been shown that many substances by themselves act as agonists but at the same time are competitive antagonists with regard to agonists possessing higher intrinsic activities (ARIËNS, 1954; ARIËNS and DE GROOT, 1954; ARIËNS and SIMONIS, 1954; ARIËNS et al., 1955). Such drugs may be called "partial agonists" (STEPHENSON, 1956), or, with the same right, "partial antagonists"; the name "competitive dualist" is also used.

In practice, actions of drugs on the total organism being in play, it may be very hard to tell whether a drug acts agonisticly or by competitive antagonism, since the situation on the level of the receptor is not known. As will be shown later, the practical classification can be made with greater probability by means of experiments on isolated organs. For the moment one should bear in mind that a drug can be called an agonist only in relation to a certain receptor-effector system, and that the differentiation between agonist and competitive antagonist has sense only on the level of the receptors concerned, and in relation to each other. In other words, when a pharmacon is called a competitive antagonist, this means that it antagonizes a definite type of agonist competitively on a definite kind of receptors.

II. Drugs, Receptors and Effects

A. Different Types of Antagonism

Any drug that counteracts the effect of an agonist can be called an antagonist. Antagonism may occur at different levels, and this is the basis of the following classification. It should be remarked that in general the influence of a second substance with respect to the effect of a certain agonist can be either a reduction of this effect (antagonism) or an augmentation (synergism or, in certain cases, sensitization), so that the different types of antagonism distinguished below should be seen as special forms of more general kinds of interaction, which can be classified in an analogous way.

1. Chemical Antagonism

The antagonist does not cause its effects by virtue of an interaction with molecules of the organism, but it interacts with the agonist itself, which in consequence loses its ability to be effective ("antagonism by neutralization"). The antagonism of protamine against the anticoagulant activity of heparin (CHARGAFF and OLSON, 1937) may serve as an example: protamine, a low-molecular weight protein with a strongly basic character combines with the strongly acidic heparin to form a stable salt, so that the anticoagulant activity of heparin is lost. The antagonism, of course, is mutual. In the guinea-pig heparin as well as protamine sulphate have a strong histaminase-liberating effect on the liver, 5 mg of the latter being as effective as 50 I.U. of the former. When given simultaneously by two different intravenous routes the two substances neutralize each other (with a dose relationship of 1 mg of protamine sulphate to 50 I.U. of heparin) and no histaminase is liberated (HAHN et al., 1966). Another example of chemical interaction is the counteraction of d-tubocurarine by suramine. Here the neutralizing agent reacts with an antagonistic drug; if the latter was blocking the action of an agonistic drug the neutralizing agent now seems to have an action which, in reality, is caused by the unblocking of the original agonist (ARIËNS et al., 1956a). The principle of antagonism by neutralization is used extensively in the treatment of intoxications by heavy metals: the action of dimercaprol against arsenic compounds and of sodium versenate against lead are attributable to it.

2. Competitive Antagonism

In the preceding text it was shown that this kind of antagonism takes place on the level of the receptors of *one* receptor-effector system. Of course it is quite possible that a certain substance may be a competitive antagonist in relation to a certain type of receptor, and also has antagonistic or even agonistic properties with regard to other kinds of receptors (ARIËNS et al., 1956b).

3. Noncompetitive Antagonism

Different kinds of antagonism come under this heading. They have in common that the antagonist interacts with its own receptors, different from those of the agonist. However, the interaction of the noncompetitive antagonist with its receptors does not lead to an independent effect; instead it causes a change in the relation between the agonist concentration in the direct vicinity of the agonistic receptors and the resulting (agonistic) effect. It is worth noticing that this model is older than the formally analogous model of allosteric effects in enzymology (MONOD et al., 1965). Two essentially different possibilities can be distinguished:

a) Metaffinoid Antagonism

The change in the receptors of the antagonist results in a change in the receptors of the agonist. This change causes the affinity between the agonist molecules and their receptors to be reduced (ARIËNS et al., 1956b; VAN DEN BRINK, 1969a). A metaffinoid system has a formal similarity with what in enzymology is indicated as a "pure *K*-system".

b) Metactoid Antagonism

The change in the receptors of the antagonist leads to an interference with the ability of the receptor-effector system of the agonist to respond to the interaction between the agonist and its receptors; in other words: it seems as if the intrinsic activity of the agonist is decreased. This kind of antagonism is generally meant when, in older literature, the term noncompetitive antagonism is used as such. A term for the analogous system in enzymology could be a "pure V_{max}-system" (Van den Brink, 1969a).

It seems not unlikely that the levels on which various metactoid systems interfere with the receptor-effector system of the corresponding agonists may be different. The result of the interaction between the antagonist and its receptors could be that the effector organ of the agonist partially or completely loses its possibility to react on stimulation; on the other hand it could be that the interaction between the agonist and its receptors results in a smaller stimulus, or that the chain of events between stimulus formation and effect is interrupted at some level, again partially or completely. So far these kinds of differences cannot be demonstrated experimentally except in a few cases, so that the metactoid antagonists for the present are classified in one group.

4. Functional Antagonism

Two agonists, interacting with two independent receptor systems, cause effects which counteracts each other, and these effects are realized in the same effector system (Ariëns et al., 1956c, 1964b). The name functional antagonism was originally used for the antagonistic relation between a sympathetic and a parasympathetic nerve impulse on one effector organ, for instance, in connection with the antagonism between the effects of acetylcholine and noradrenaline on the smooth muscle fibres of the gut. The applicability of the model, however, is much wider.

During a number of years the position of the model of functional interactions remained somewhat ambiguous, due to the fact that two verbal definitions were used which were not necessarily equivalent, and that some of the experimental results obtained in clear cases of functional interaction were not covered by the equations originally proposed by Ariëns et al. (Van den Brink, 1969a). Recently a revised version of the model of functional interaction has been published, to which these objections do not apply any longer (Van den Brink, 1973a, b). In this chapter, therefore, the model of functional interaction will be presented in this revised version.

5. Physical Antagonism

Two drugs activate two completely independent receptor-effector systems and the resulting effects counteract each other. The pupil of the eye may again serve as an example. The parasympathetic nerves secrete acetylcholine, which causes contraction of the musculi constrictores pupillae: the pupil narrows. But at the endings of the sympathetic nerve fibres noradrenaline is secreted and this causes a contraction of the musculi dilatatores pupillae, resulting in widening of the pupil. Both substances are agonists for their own receptor-effector systems, but in view of the ultimate effect they are antagonists of each other. Another example of physical antagonism is the antagonism between a substance which causes an increase in blood pressure stimulating the heart action and another substance which causes a decrease in blood pressure by vasodilatation. There are many other examples.

It should be stressed that formally the models of functional and physical antagonism are not essentially different. In the case of physical antagonism the opposite effects are realized in separate effector organs; in the case of functional antagonism they are realized in one effector. However, an effector organ that is considered a unit may yet be composed of separate subunits, one being responsible for the positive effect, another for the negative one. The distinction between physical and functional antagonism, therefore, is of a different order than that between physical antagonism and, e.g., competitive antagonism.

B. Classification of Drugs in Families

For many purposes it is useful to classify drugs in pharmacologic families. Such a family includes all drugs which can interact with the receptors of a certain type of receptor-effector system, and which, by doing so, can cause the same kind of effect. By determining to which family a new drug belongs—information which often can be easily obtained by means of experiments on isolated organs—some predictions about its overall effect in the organism become possible. Moreover it is a prerequisite for the study of structure-activity relations. Here this kind of classification is especially serviceable for agonists.

Agonists and competitive antagonists with affinity to the same receptors are considered to belong to different families, since they have quite different effects. Yet the members of two such groups may be structurally related, which explains their affinity to the same receptors (e.g., the families of β-adrenoceptor stimulants and of β-adrenoceptor blocking drugs). The relationship of agonists and corresponding antagonists is stressed by the fact that often a gradual transition from one group to the other may be found via compounds with intermediate properties, the previously mentioned dualists.

On the other hand groups of competitive antagonists exist which seem to have little or no structural relationship to the members of the corresponding family of agonists, nor to each other. This situation, which at first sight seems rather paradoxical, is explained by the hypothesis that these competitive antagonists block the receptor of the agonist by screening only a small (but essential) part of this receptor. The competitive antagonist hardly interacts with the receptor proper, but is mainly bound to additional receptor areas, i.e., structures directly adjacent to the original receptor.

According to this hypothesis, which is supported by experimental data, a close structural relationship between agonistic drugs and their competitive antagonists is not necessary (ARIËNS and SIMONIS, 1960, 1964; SIMONIS, 1965; ARIËNS, 1966; STUBBINS et al., 1968; VAN DEN BRINK, 1969e). It is not necessary either that all competitive antagonists of a certain agonist would interact with the same additional receptor area, so that it is not difficult to give a possible explanation for a lack in structural relationship within the group. From the foregoing it follows that in structure-activity studies the existing classification of competitive antagonists in pharmacologic families should be used with caution.

The families are often named after some typical member; a family of antagonists may also derive its name from a typical member of the corresponding family of agonists. For families with agonistic properties there are such names as, for instance, "histamine-like drugs" or "histaminomimetics", "β-adrenergic drugs" or "β-adrenoceptor stimulants", etc.; for antagonists names like "atropine-like drugs" or "anticholinergic drugs", "antihistamines" or "histaminolytics", etc.

In the case of noncompetitive antagonists a proper division is often very difficult, since in a number of cases it is not known whether all drugs that counteract a certain effect do so via the same receptors. For reasons of convenience investigators may indicate drugs as being, e.g., "papaverine-like" or having "papaverine-like action", but this does not necessarily mean that these drugs belong to one family, as defined above.

In practice the limits are not always as sharp as in theory. There are two reasons for this. First, the molecules of a drug may have affinity to more than one kind of receptors. If this is so, the affinity to one kind is usually far the greater, so that the interactions with other kinds of receptors do not play a role, unless the drug is administered in an unusual way or in doses much higher than customary. It may be stressed that this holds for many of the drugs in use. The expression "any effect can be caused by any drug, if only the dose is high enough" reflects, with some exaggeration, a general experience. A drug is classified in accordance with its highest (or "specific") affinity, but where the difference between the affinities to the different receptors is not too large, such a drug is considered to belong to different families at the same time. Examples are the α- and β-action of adrenaline (Ahlquist, 1948), the muscarinic and nicotinic action of acetylcholine (Dale, 1914), etc.

Second, not all receptors and effectors of one kind are completely identical. For instance, the interaction of histamine with its receptors may cause contraction of smooth muscle fibres. The receptors and the contractile elements in question may be situated in a number of different organs and the different organs may belong to different kinds of animals. It is hardly probable that in all cases the receptor-effector systems would be absolutely identical. Nevertheless they are equal to a very high degree, enough to consider them one kind when classifying pharmaca. But then it is not surprising when the ratio of the affinities of two members of one family to the common receptor appears somewhat different in different organ systems. It may even happen that a drug has a low but distinct affinity to the receptors in one case and so belongs to the family, but in another case—the affinity being still lower—is considered inactive; of course the line between "low affinity" and "no affinity" is arbitrary. Yet another possibility is that a drug is agonistic in one animal species, but belongs to the corresponding family of competitive antagonists if tested in another species. Such phenomena may complicate things but do not obscure the overall image.

C. From Drug Administration to Effect; Drug-Receptor Interaction Models; Experiments on Isolated Organs

As mentioned above, the family to which a certain drug belongs may be determined with a comparatively easy pharmacologic technique: that of establishing the relation between the concentration of the drug and its effect—in other words, the making of concentration-effect curves—with the aid of simple isolated organs. This kind of experiment is also quite valuable in obtaining data about affinity ratios and intrinsic activity ratios within a family.

The attraction of using isolated organs lies, of course, in the reduction of the amount of variables which have to be taken into account. The question that has to be answered may be which relation exists between the concentration of the drug in the direct vicinity of the receptors and the change caused in these receptors, but what is learned from experiments is something quite different, namely the relation between the dose administered and some measured effect. Is it possible to deduce the first relation from the second?

When a dose of a certain pharmacon is administered to a patient or an experimental animal, the chain of events leading to the final effect consists of three main parts with different characteristics (Fig. 2).

1. The administration results in a certain concentration in the so-called biophase (FERGUSON, 1939; FASTIER and REID, 1948; FASTIER and HAWKINS, 1951; FURCHGOTT, 1955), i.e., the direct vicinity of the receptors, or, more exactly, that compartment of the system in which interaction with the receptors takes place. This concentration depends on the amount of drug given but also on many other factors, partly unknown. These are, among others, the way of administration, the location of the receptors in the organism and the amount of silent receptors for this drug, properties of the drug such as water- or fat-solubility, surface tension and the ratio of dissociated and undissociated molecules at the existing pH, and also the possible influence of the metabolism on the drug, an influence that may result in a bioactivation (if the product of metabolism is more active than the original drug) or, more commonly, in an inactivation.

2. The presence of the drug in the biophase leads to interactions between drug molecules and receptors and thus to a change at receptor level. The magnitude of this change depends on the concentration of the drug in the biophase, and further on its affinity to the receptors and its intrinsic activity. The result of the drug-receptor interactions at receptor level is the formation of a so-called stimulus (STEPHENSON, 1956). The stimulus formation should not be seen as a phenomenon that occurs subsequent to the drug-receptor interaction; the stimulus is a purely theoretical magnitude and its formation is simply an aspect of the interaction of an agonist with its receptors.[2]

By definition the stimulus has a linear relationship to the number of "occupied" receptors.[3] In another vision the stimulus is supposed to be directly proportional to the number of drug-receptor interactions taking place per unit of time ("rate model", PATON, 1961; PATON and WAUD, 1962a, b; PATON and RANG, 1966; cf. RENQVIST, 1919; LASAREFF, 1922). Since, in general, it can be assumed that the concentration-effect curves from which the affinity values and the intrinsic activity values are calculated (see pp. 237—249) are based on equilibrium responses, and since in a situation of equilibrium the number of drug-receptor interactions taking place per unit of time and the number of receptors which, at any moment, are "occupied", are directly proportional, the difference between the two models has no consequence with regard to the subjects to be discussed in this chapter.

Originally the "rate model" was set against the "occupation model", but this does not seem justified; both models give a physicochemical interpretation of the concepts

---

[2] This was overlooked by CHANGEUX when he stated that in his model of drug-receptor interactions "the introduction of an 'intrinsic activity' of the drug is no longer necessary" (CHANGEUX et al., 1967).

[3] STEPHENSON introduced the stimulus S as a relative magnitude, and thus defined it as having a linear relationship to the *proportion* of the receptors which are occupied, whereas the definition given here applies for the absolute stimulus. Stephenson's S equals the quotient $S_A/S_{P_{max}}$, in which S_A represents the stimulus caused by a certain concentration of the drug A and $S_{P_{max}}$ the stimulus which causes the effect $\frac{1}{2}E_{max}$ in the same receptor-effector system (see p. 187).

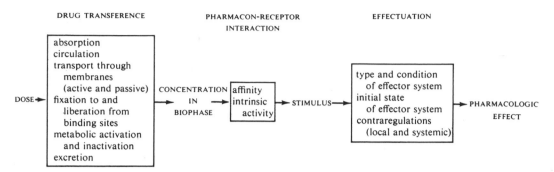

Fig. 2. Schematic representation of chain of events leading from administration of drug to pharmacologic effect. Three consecutive steps with different characters can be distinguished

intrinsic activity and stimulus formation, which may have its counterpart in reality. Many authors have published more or less detailed models for particular cases of drug-receptor interaction; or for agonist-receptor interaction, stimulus formation, and competitive interaction in general. Among these are the occupation theory in its original version (CLARK, 1926a, b, 1933, 1937; GADDUM, 1926, 1937, 1943, 1955) and later modifications and extensions of it (ARIËNS, 1954; ARIËNS and DE GROOT, 1954; ARIËNS and VAN ROSSUM, 1957; ARIËNS et al., 1955, 1956a, 1957, 1964a; VAN ROSSUM, 1966a, b; STEPHENSON, 1956); the theory of CROXATTO and HUIDOBRO, who suppose that the adsorption of a drug onto the receptor is a process analogous to the incorporation of a molecule into a crystal lattice (CROXATTO and HUIDOBRO, 1956; CANEPA, 1962); the theory of DEL CASTILLO and KATZ, who suppose that an agonist may produce its effect in two steps, the first being the formation of an inactive, intermediate combination product of drug and receptor, the second the conversion of the intermediate into an active form, whereas the rate of this conversion determines the final effect (DEL CASTILLO and KATZ, 1957; KATZ and THESLEFF, 1957); the earlier mentioned rate theory and the dissociation theory (PATON, 1961; PATON and WAUD, 1962a, b, 1964; PATON and RANG, 1966, cf. THRON and WAUD, 1968); the flux-carrier hypothesis of MACKAY (1963), in which the response is supposed to result from a carrier-mediated influx of the agonist through the cell membrane (see Chapter 5, this volume); the theory of induced conformational perturbation (BELLEAU, 1964, 1965, 1966; BELLEAU and LAVOIE, 1968) which is patterned in part after the induced fit theory of enzyme action (KOSHLAND, 1963) and in which the receptor has the character of an enzyme; some related theories like that of WATKINS in connection with membrane permeability (WATKINS, 1965) and the dynamic receptor hypothesis of BLOOM and GOLDMAN, in which the adrenergic receptors are not regarded as enzymes but as enzyme-substrate complexes (BLOOM and GOLDMAN, 1966); the allosteric receptor model of KARLIN (1967; cf. THRON, 1963) and the theory of the cooperativity of biological membranes of CHANGEUX et al. (1967, 1968), which are patterned after the model for allosteric oligomers in enzymology (MONOD et al., 1965) and are related to BELLEAU's model; the receptor inactivation model of GOSSELIN (see Chapter 6, this volume); the ion exchange model (TAYLOR et al., 1970); and the charnière theory of competitive antagonism, with which ROCHA E SILVA explains tissue recovery phenomena (Rocha e Silva, 1969, 1970). Many other contributions to this field deserve attention, like those of Rocha e Silva (1957), Beidler (1962), Mackay (1966) and Homer (1967). For a detailed discussion of most of these theories and models the reader may be referred to the chapters of Mackay and Gosselin in this volume. It is important, however, to bear in mind that the basal concepts discussed in this chapter can be handled without any definition of the physicochemical processes which find expression in them. Although here the occupation model is used in order to illustrate the concepts in question, these concepts are by no means dependent on the model used.

3. The stimulus results in the measured effect. However, there may be many steps in between, and all kinds of relations between them are conceivable: linear, all-or-none, or other kinds of nonlinear relations. The character of the stimulus-effect relation may depend on the question which phenomenon is chosen as "effect": in the case of a spasmogen, for instance, the "effect" can be the contraction of a muscle, the depolarization of a membrane, the flux of potassium and sodium ions, etc. Anyhow, when the stimulus formation is accomplished, the process is no longer drug-dependent: a certain stimulus always gives a certain effect, if, at least, the effector system itself remains constant.

The situation now is the following: phase 2 is the object of study, but the known magnitudes that can be controlled or measured are at the beginning of phase 1 (the dose) and at the end of phase 3 (the effect). The only possible way out is either to keep phase 1 and phase 3 constant, or to eliminate them. As for phase 1, keeping this phase constant over some time in the total animal is extremely difficult. Factors such as redistribution and breakdown cause the drug concentration in the biophase to change from moment to moment; not only the maximal concentration reached but also the time in which this concentration is reached may vary from occasion to occasion, so that the making of comparable quantitative measurements is nearly impossible. Administration of the drug by means of an intravenous infusion of longer duration may result in an equilibrium in the biophase for some time, but even then the situation remains difficult.

In the light of the foregoing, experiments on isolated organs become very attractive. The only determining factor in phase 1 now is the concentration of the pharmacon in the bath fluid, the influence of factors like metabolism being considerably reduced, and generally a situation of equilibrium is reached easily and rapidly. Also, but in smaller measure, phase 3 will be less disturbing, since usually simpler effects can be studied than in the total animal. All facts considered and in spite of its limitations, the isolated organ experiment is an indispensable tool of molecular pharmacology, although not the only one.

III. Agonistic Interaction

A. The Model of Agonism

The technique of making concentration-effect curves with the use of isolated organs will not be discussed here; the reader is referred to the literature (e.g., Van Rossum and Van den Brink, 1963; Van Rossum, 1963). In order to elucidate the conclusions drawn from the characteristics of these curves, however, further consideration of the hypothesis of the drug-receptor interaction is necessary.

With a few assumptions the calculation of theoretical graphs of agonist concentration and effect becomes possible, and also the prediction of the influence of different concentrations of an antagonist, and of different types of antagonists, on the position on the concentration axis and on the shapes of these curves. The curves found in experiments tally surprisingly well with these theoretical predictions.

The hypothesis starts with the supposition that pharmacon molecule and receptor interact in the way of an uncomplicated reversible bimolecular reaction:

$$R + A \leftrightharpoons RA$$

in which A is a drug molecule, R the free receptor, and RA their interaction product. It is assumed that in this system the law of mass action holds:

$$\frac{[R][A]}{[RA]} = K_A \tag{1}$$

[A] being the concentration of the drug molecules in the biophase, [R] the concentration of the free receptors, [RA] the concentration of the occupied ones, and K_A the dissociation constant of the pharmacon-receptor complex. K_A is inversely proportional to the affinity of A to R, so that $1/K_A$ can be used as a measure for the affinity (affinity constant) (CLARK, 1937; CLARK and RAVENTÓS, 1937).

The concentration of the free receptors plus that of the occupied ones is equal to the total receptor concentration [r]:

$$[R] + [RA] = [r] . \tag{2}$$

Now the question arises: in what way does the concentration of the occupied receptors [RA] depend on [A]? However, [RA] not only depends on [A], but as appears from the foregoing, also on the total amount of receptors present, therefore on [r]. This factor being unknown the question can better be formulated as follows: In what way does the fraction of the receptors which is occupied, [RA]/[r], depend on the pharmacon concentration [A]? According to (2)

$$\frac{[RA]}{[r]} = \frac{[RA]}{[RA] + [R]}$$

$$\frac{[RA]}{[r]} = \frac{1}{1 + \dfrac{[R]}{[RA]}}$$

and since according to (1)

$$\frac{[R]}{[RA]} = \frac{K_A}{[A]}$$

it follows that

$$\frac{[RA]}{[r]} = \frac{1}{1 + \dfrac{K_A}{[A]}}. \tag{3}$$

In the experiment with simple isolated organs it is assumed that the concentration in the biophase is equal to, or at least directly proportional to the concentration in the bath fluid. This is a permissible assumption if the system is given time to reach an equilibrium. It is further assumed that the concentration in the bath fluid is directly proportional to the dose given. This is true only if the concentration of the drug molecules is very high in comparison with the total amount of receptors in the organ, both specific and silent, so that the concentration does not change notably by the formation of the pharmacon-receptor complexes. Within the usual dose ranges this is actually the case, so that for [A] the concentration in the bath fluid, as calculated from the dose added, can be taken.

The other unknown in Equation (3) is the receptor occupation. From the definition of the stimulus given before, it follows that the stimulus generated is directly proportional to the concentration [RA]:

$$S_A = g[RA] \tag{4}$$

in which S_A is the stimulus caused by a certain concentration of drug A. The maximal stimulus that possibly can be caused by drug A on the receptors in question ($S_{A_{max}}$), will be reached when [RA] has its maximal value. This is the case when all receptors are occupied, thus when [RA] equals [r]. From this follows that

$$S_{A_{max}} = g[r] \tag{5}$$

and combination of the Equations (4) and (5) gives

$$\frac{S_A}{S_{A_{max}}} = \frac{[RA]}{[r]}. \tag{6}$$

Combination of this equation with Equation (3) results in

$$\frac{S_A}{S_{A_{max}}} = \frac{1}{1 + \dfrac{K_A}{[A]}}. \tag{7}$$

It would be possible to calculate the affinity constant from this formula if the stimuli could be measured directly, but this is not the case. Only the effects resulting from the stimuli can be determined; the relation between stimulus and effect, however, is unknown and in many cases it surely is a nonlinear function. (The stimulus-effect relation characterizes the receptor-effector system.)

In the simplest case, a linear relationship between stimulus and effect, the following equations hold:

$$E_A = hS_A \tag{8}$$

and

$$E_{A_{max}} = hS_{A_{max}} \tag{9}$$

in which E_A is the effect caused by a certain concentration of A, and $E_{A_{max}}$ is the maximal effect that can be reached with this drug in the receptor-effector system in question. Equations (8) and (9) may be combined to give:

$$\frac{E_A}{E_{A_{max}}} = \frac{S_A}{S_{A_{max}}}$$

so that in this case the Equations (6) and (7) may be changed into:

$$\frac{E_A}{E_{A_{max}}} = \frac{[RA]}{[r]} \tag{10}$$

and

$$\frac{E_A}{E_{A_{max}}} = \frac{1}{1 + \dfrac{K_A}{[A]}}. \tag{11}$$

In Equation (11) the only variables are the drug concentration and the relative effect, and since these are measurable values, theory and practice can be compared. As will be discussed later (pp. 238—239), Equation (11) is the basis for the calculation of the so-called pD_2 value, a frequently used (but rather inexact) measure for the affinity of an agonistic drug.

B. Intrinsic Activity in the Agonistic Formula

In Equation (11), which gives the relation between drug concentration and relative effect, the factor intrinsic activity is not found. The constant g in Equation (4), however, which gives the relation of $[RA]$ and S_A, contains this factor. Yet g does not represent the intrinsic activity itself. The intrinsic activity of a pharmacon determines to which extent the interaction between this pharmacon and its receptors results in a stimulus. The stimulus S_A, however, is not a relative magnitude (cf. p. 179). Each pharmacon-receptor interaction in the test organ contributes to it; consequently S_A is directly proportional to the number of interaction products—in an absolute sense—in the organ. If this number is called Q_{RA}, the relation may be formulated as

$$S_A = aQ_{RA} \tag{12}$$

and this proportionality constant a actually represents the intrinsic activity.

The concentration of RA in the biophase is [RA], and if this term is multiplied by the volume V of the biophase in the organ used, the product is Q_{RA}. Equation (12) therefore can be written as

$$S_A = aV[RA]. \tag{13}$$

It follows that the factor g in Equation (4) represents the intrinsic activity multiplied by the volume of the biophase in the organ.

Since the volume V and the concentration [RA] are unknown and also the stimulus S_A cannot be measured directly, the absolute value of the intrinsic activity a cannot be determined. If, however, two agonists A_1 and A_2 belonging to one family are tested on the same preparation, the ratio of their intrinsic activities, a_1/a_2, is independent of the volume of the biophase and the receptor concentration. Substitute g in Equation 5 by aV:

$$S_{A_1 max} = a_1 V[r]$$

$$S_{A_2 max} = a_2 V[r]$$

therefore

$$\frac{a_1}{a_2} = \frac{S_{A_1 max}}{S_{A_2 max}}. \tag{14}$$

It will be demonstrated that a practical estimation of the value of such a quotient is possible (see pp. 239—243).

If the intrinsic activities of the members of an agonistic family are all expressed in relation to the intrinsic activity of one reference compound from the same family, the relative intrinsic activity values thus obtained are a suitable basis for comparing the intrinsic activities within the family in question. In principle it is immaterial which drug serves as a reference; the choice only determines the scale on which the relative intrinsic activities of the members of a family are expressed and has no influence on their mutual ratio. Theoretically, however, it seems preferable to express the intrinsic activity of a drug in relation to the highest intrinsic activity in the family. The relative intrinsic activity of a drug A, expressed in this way, is indicated as α. It follows that α may be defined as

$$\alpha = \frac{a}{a_{max}} \tag{15}$$

in which a is the (absolute) intrinsic activity of drug A and a_{max} the highest (absolute) intrinsic activity in the family.

A drug with intrinsic activity a_{max} is able to cause the maximal stimulus that can be brought about via the receptor system in question. If this absolutely maximal stimulus is called S_{max}, the Equations 14 and 15 can be combined to give

$$\alpha = \frac{S_{A max}}{S_{max}}. \tag{16}$$

The advantage of the definition of the (relative) intrinsic activity constant given above is that the intrinsic activities of all agonistic families would uniformly range from 0 to 1, so that a given value of α holds a direct information about the position of drug A within its family. On the other hand the practical difficulty arises that it is generally not yet known which drug has the highest intrinsic activity in a family (especially since a maximal effect does not necessarily mean a maximal stimulus; see pp. 204—207). Moreover, only effects and not stimuli can be measured directly. In view of these limitations the use of other, practical expressions of the intrinsic activity is necessary.

At present three practical expressions of the intrinsic activity are in use, each having its own field of application. The value β^P is only used for functional antagonists and will be discussed in the section relating to functional interaction (see p. 233). Of the other two, the older one, introduced by ARIËNS (1954), may be defined as

$$\alpha^E = \frac{E_{A_{max}}}{E_{max}} . \tag{17}$$

This magnitude was introduced as α,—under the assumption, however, that stimulus and effect are directly proportional[4]. If this is really the case it follows that

$$\frac{S_{A_{max}}}{S_{max}} = \frac{E_{A_{max}}}{E_{max}}$$

and thus that α^E equals α indeed. If, however, the stimulus-effect relation is not linear, α^E is a value with an unknown relation to the α defined above.

If the stimulus-effect relation is linear, Equation (11) was shown to apply (p. 184). Under the same supposition Equation (17) can be transformed into

$$\frac{E_{A_{max}}}{E_{max}} = \alpha$$

and combination of this equation with Equation (11) gives a formula in which the affinity as well as the (relative) intrinsic activity is represented:

$$\frac{E_A}{E_{max}} = \frac{\alpha}{1 + \dfrac{K_A}{[A]}} . \tag{18}$$

---

[4] In his earliest publications (ARIËNS, 1954; ARIËNS and DE GROOT, 1954; ARIËNS et al., 1955, 1956a, 1957; ARIËNS and VAN ROSSUM, 1957) ARIËNS defined the intrinsic activity of a pharmacon as "the contribution to the effect per unit of drug-receptor complex" and identified it with the proportionality constant α in the relation $E_A = \alpha[RA]$. Formally this α is the product of the factors g and h in the Equations (4) and (8), and thus represents the intrinsic activity of the drug—in an absolute sense—multiplied by some factors which are not drug-dependent. From the practical applications of the formula, however, it is evident that the intrinsic activity constant α was considered a dimensionless relative magnitude from the beginning: E_A is always expressed as a percentage of E_{max} and [RA] as a percentage of [r]. Thus the "unit of drug-receptor complex" in the definition should not be understood as an amount of drug-receptor complex with a defined magnitude but as a defined fraction of the total amount of receptors in the organ used, and the definition itself has reference to the relative intrinsic activity and not to the intrinsic activity in an absolute sense.

The determination of α^E is relatively easy. Theoretically there is one problem: Is it acceptable to take the maximal effect of a drug which, at the moment, is known as the most effective member of a family, as E_{max} with respect to the receptor-effector system in question? Suppose that in the future a new substance would be discovered which belongs to the same family but has a larger maximal effect: All intrinsic activity values within this family would have to be changed. In practice, however, this danger is small. In most families of agonists the number of substances tested is considerabl$\digamma$. Only a few of these are partial agonists; the others all have maximal effects of the same magnitude. This strongly suggests that this maximal effect really is the E_{max}-value of the system.

The merit of the α^E is that it indicates directly whether a drug is a full agonist, a partial agonist or a competitive antagonist. The value of α^E ranges from 0 to 1; an α^E with the value 1 designates a drug as a full agonist whereas for a competitive antagonist α^E equals zero. Drugs with an intermediate value of α^E are the earlier mentioned partial agonist or competitive dualists.

In the study of structure-activity relations, however, the α^E has a very limited value. In this kind of study one of the relevant informations would be the ratio of the true intrinsic activities in a family of agonists. If the stimulus-effect relation is not linear, however, the ratio between the respective α^E values is different from the ratio of these true intrinsic activities. Therefore the use of the other intrinsic activity constant, α^S, is indicated for this purpose (VAN ROSSUM, 1966a, b). A method for the calculation of this α^S is discussed on p. 243. The essential difference with α^E is, that under certain general suppositions (cf. pp. 191—192), but without any presuppositions about the character of the stimulus-effect relation, α^S has the same fixed relation to α for all members of a family. Instead of a special supposition concerning the character of the stimulus-effect relation comes the more general assumption that in a certain receptor-effector system the magnitude of the effect only depends on the magnitude of the stimulus and not on the way in which the stimulus was created. (The stimulus-effect relation is „system-dependent" and not "drug-dependent".)

α^S is no approximation of α itself but of α multiplied by a certain factor. It is thus defined that if the general suppositions made agree with reality, the following relation holds:

$$\alpha^S = \frac{S_{A_{max}}}{2 S_{P_{max}}} \tag{19}$$

in which $S_{P_{max}}$ is the maximal stimulus that can be generated by a (hypothetical) partial agonist of the same family, which maximally can cause an effect equal to $\frac{1}{2}E_{max}$. (Since within a family equal effects are supposed to correspond with equal stimuli [see above], $S_{P_{max}}$ indicates the stimulus which corresponds with the effect $\frac{1}{2}E_{max}$, no matter by which agonist this effect is caused.) Comparison of Equation (19) with Equation (16) shows that

$$\alpha^S = \frac{1}{2}\varphi\alpha$$

in which φ is a family constant representing the ratio of S_{max} and $S_{P_{max}}$ and thus dependent on the stimulus-effect relation in the receptor-effector system in question. It follows that every family of drugs has its own scale for the α^S-values; an isolated α^S does not indicate whether the drug in question has a high or low intrinsic activity, but the ratio of the α^S-values within the family is the same as the ratio of the corresponding true values of α, again if the general suppositions made are true.

If the relation between stimulus and effect is linear, $2S_{P_{max}}$ equals S_{max}, so that $\varphi = 2$ and $\alpha^S = \alpha$.

The α^S is analogous to the constant e ("efficacy") introduced by Stephenson (1956). From the convention adopted by this author that "a drug which occupies all receptors to produce an effect which is only 50% of the true maximum has an efficacy $e = 1$", it follows that $e = 2\alpha^S$.

C. Theoretical Concentration-Effect Curves. Sets of Curves Characterized by Parallel Shifting or by a Change in Slope

The relation between the concentration of an agonist in the biophase and the resulting stimulus—or the resulting effect, supposing that stimulus and effect are linearly related—depends on the two magnitudes affinity and intrinsic activity, and on these two magnitudes only. By substituting different values for [A] in Equation (18), with given values of α and K_A, a theoretical concentration-effect curve can be calculated. Another curve will be obtained if the same value for α but different K_A are filled in and if then again a series of different values for [A] are substituted in the formula. Repeating this procedure a number of times, a set of curves representing the concentration-effect relations for a hypothetical family of drugs differing only in affinity will be acquired. The same may be done with a constant value of K_A and different values for α; another set of curves will be produced, this time for a hypothetical family of drugs differing only in intrinsic activity. The two sets of curves show essentially different characteristics, so that it may be expected that the two possibilities, a change in affinity and a change in intrinsic activity, will be discernible also in practice.

When the curves are plotted, it is recommendable to use a linear scale for the relative effect but a logarithmic one for the concentration of the pharmacon. This procedure has a practical advantage, since a linear scale does not enable one to draw a whole set of curves on a single graph, unless it is made awkwardly long; however, its chief merit is that it shows very clearly the characteristic difference between a set of curves made with different values for K_A, and one made with different values for α (Fig. 3).

If the affinity is kept constant but different values are substituted for the intrinsic activity, the curves occupy the same part of the concentration axis but are different in shape. They differ in their maximal heights and, consequently, in their slopes. Suppose that equal concentrations are used of a drug A_1 and a drug A_2, which have the same K_A but different intrinsic activities:

$$\frac{E_{A_1}}{E_{max}} = \frac{\alpha_1}{1 + \dfrac{K_{A_1}}{[A_1]}}, \quad \frac{E_{A_2}}{E_{max}} = \frac{\alpha_2}{1 + \dfrac{K_{A_2}}{[A_2]}}.$$

Since $K_{A_1} = K_{A_2}$ and $[A_1] = [A_2]$ it follows that

$$\frac{E_{A_1}}{E_{A_2}} = \frac{\alpha_1}{\alpha_2}.$$

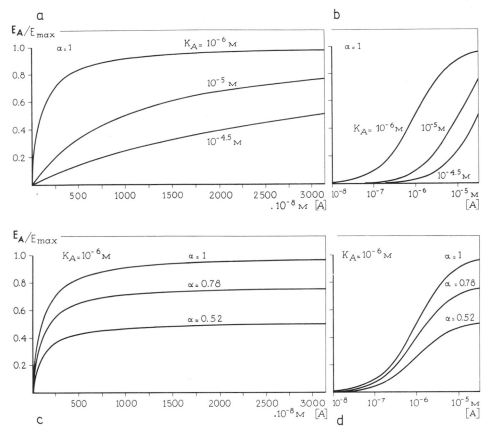

Fig. 3a—d. Theoretical concentration-effect curves based on Equation (18). Path of curves given from $[A] = 10^{-8}$ M to $[A] = 10^{-4.5}$ M $(= 3162 \cdot 10^{-8}$ M). Figure 3a and b: sets of curves made with different values for K_A and same value for α; Figure 3c and d: sets of curves made with different values for α and same value for K_A. In Figure 3a and c, the curves are plotted on a linear concentration axis, in Figure 3b and d on a logarithmic concentration axis

The ratio of the effects of equal concentrations is constant; in other words the concentrations corresponding with the beginning, middle and end of the curves, respectively (i.e., in practice 1%-, 50%- and 99%-points), are equal. Of course this holds regardless of the character of the concentration axis (Fig. 3c, d).

If, however, the intrinsic activity is kept constant and only the affinity differs, the curves are all identical in shape; the only difference is their respective position on the concentration axis. This phenomenon of parallel shifting, as it is called, is observed only if a logarithmic concentration scale is used (Fig. 3a, b). Suppose that the concentrations $[A_1]$ and $[A_2]$ of the drugs A_1 and A_2 cause effects of equal magnitude:

$$\frac{E_{A_1}}{E_{max}} = \frac{E_{A_2}}{E_{max}}$$

and thus, according to Equation (19):

$$\frac{\alpha_1}{1 + \dfrac{K_{A_1}}{[A_1]}} = \frac{\alpha_2}{1 + \dfrac{K_{A_2}}{[A_2]}}.$$

Since the drugs have the same intrinsic activity, it follows that

$$\frac{K_{A_1}}{[A_1]} = \frac{K_{A_2}}{[A_2]} \quad \text{or} \quad \frac{[A_2]}{[A_1]} = \frac{K_{A_2}}{K_{A_1}}. \tag{20}$$

This means that the ratio of equieffective concentrations of the two drugs has a constant value. Thus, if the curves are plotted on a linear concentration scale, they will not be identical in shape. From Equation (20), however, it follows that

$$\log[A_2] - \log[A_1] = \log\frac{K_{A_2}}{K_{A_1}}$$

in other words, the difference between the logarithms of the equieffective concentrations is constant and independent of the concentrations. Thus, if the data are plotted on a logarithmic concentration scale, graphs with identical shapes will result.

In this connection attention may be called to the following point. Suppose that an experimental concentration-effect curve of an agonist is obtained in absence and another one in presence of a certain concentration of an antagonist. The two phenomena mentioned above, viz. a parallel shift of the agonist curve or a reduction of the maximal height of the curve and thus a change in its slope, are among the effects that can be caused by the presence of an antagonist. Would it be correct to suppose, that in the first case the affinity of the agonist to its receptors and in the second case the intrinsic activity of the agonist was reduced? If this is intended as a description of the true mechanism behind the observed phenomena, it usually will be wrong, and even if it is only intended as a formal description ("the influence of the antagonist, whatever its true mechanism, amounts to the same thing as a change in the affinity or the intrinsic activity of the agonist"), it is not necessarily correct.

This observation is made for the following reason. Some authors will indicate the phenomenon of parallel shifting as "competitive antagonism" and that of the change in slope as "noncompetitive antagonism", probably since competitive antagonism and noncompetitive metactoid antagonism, respectively, are the best-known causes of the two phenomena. This is a bad practice. As for a shift of the concentration-effect curve, even if it is perfectly parallel (and in practice it is often very difficult to be sure that a shift is perfectly parallel), it does not necessarily mean that the interaction is based on a competition for receptors which completely or partially coincide. Metaffinoid antagonism (pp. 207—222) and functional antagonism (pp. 222—234) may also result in a perfectly parallel shifting of the agonist curve, whereas a nearly parallel shifting over a certain distance may, for instance, result from a metactoid antagonism, if the system has a threshold[5] ,and a large receptor reserve (see pp. 205—207).

On the other hand it is true that the pure "noncompetitive picture" of a change in slope of the curve without shifting generally will be the result of a noncompetitive metactoid antagonism, but also here some caution is necessary: the same picture can be obtained with irreversible competitive antagonists in a system without receptor reserve. As very properly observed by KIMELBERG et al. (1965), it is undesirable to indicate such substances, which are covalently bound to the specific receptors of an agonist, as noncompetitive: "Terminology which does not consider the chemical interactions at the receptor level is neither satisfactory nor correct."

In conclusion: The fact that an antagonist causes a parallel shift of the agonist curve or a reduction of its maximal height, at best may give an indication about the interaction mechanism involved. Additional information is necessary in order to make certain about this mechanism.

D. Discussion of the Presuppositions in the Agonistic Model

A few words should be devoted to the presuppositions made so far in the model of agonistic action and to the conditions for their validity. A number of general suppositions and a few special assumptions with respect to experiments on isolated organs were made:

1. The specific effect of a drug is caused by the interaction of the drug molecules with their receptors.

2. The same extent of interaction between the receptors and a certain agonist always results in an effect of the same magnitude. This may be not absolutely true, since as a result of growth, illness, involution, and such, the properties of the receptor-effector system may change, but in any case there should be a recognizable regularity in this relationship, otherwise a scientific approach of pharmacologic problems would be impossible. Anyhow, in well-executed experiments on isolated organs, lasting a relatively short time, such factors need not be disturbing.

3. The drug concentration in the biophase is equal to, or at least linearly related to that in the bath fluid. Since simple isolated organs are used, this supposition is not too improbable; it should be taken into account, however, that in certain cases the relation may be less simple.

4. For practical reasons only, the concentration in the bath fluid is supposed to be calculable directly from the volume of the bath fluid and the dose given. This is made acceptable by the condition that drugs should be used which are stable is aqueous solution for some time and that the number of drug molecules should be very large compared with that of the receptors (specific and silent receptors together), so that the formation of drug-receptor combinations does not influence the concentration of the free drug molecules appreciably. If need be, the concentration in the bath fluid may be determined directly.

5. The interaction between drug molecule and receptor can be described as a reversible, bimolecular reaction.

---

[5] This means that the stimulus has to exceed a certain value (the threshold stimulus) before any observable effect ensues (ARIËNS et al., 1960).

6. If equilibrium is established, the relation between the concentration of the drug in the biophase and the percentage of the receptors which are in interaction with the drug is governed by the law of mass action. This will be perfectly true only if the reaction between drug molecules and receptors is reversible and if all drug molecules on the one hand, and all receptors on the other have equal chance and equal ability for interaction. The drug molecules may be homogeneously distributed in the biophase but it does not seem very probable that this holds also for the receptors; there may be cases where the receptors are concentrated on the surface of a membrane, or are grouped in another way deviating from the regular. So long as all receptors have more or less equal ability and chance for interaction, however,—and the condition that the amount of drug molecules should be large in comparison with the amount of receptors gives a greater probability to this supposition—the law of mass action will give a usable description of the system. The Langmuir isotherm that describes the relation of the concentration of a chemical substance and the amount of it absorbed on a surface formally answers to the mass action law, which may describe the situation only approximately, but apparently well enough for most practical purposes. Likewise the supposition that the law of mass action gives a usable description of the situation in the biophase cannot be rejected on theoretical grounds.

7. The relation between stimulus and effect is supposed to be dependent only on the nature of the receptor-effector system and not on the agonist by which the stimulus is generated. If separate values for affinity and intrinsic activity should be derived from the experimental concentration-effect curves this is the minimal supposition about the stimulus-effect relation that has to be made. It may be recalled here that the stimulus is linearly related to the number of "occupied" receptors by definition (see p. 179).

8. In the derivation of Equations (11) and (18) it was assumed that the relation between stimulus and effect is linear. In this more special assumption the preceding one is implied.

In reality, a direct proportionality of stimulus and effect does not seem to be the rule; in a number of cases the experimental results are not explicable on the basis of a direct proportionality of stimulus and effect. If the assumption is maintained that in one kind of receptor-effector system equal effects always originate from equal stimuli, but if the relation between stimulus and effect is not further defined, Equation (18) should be written as

$$\frac{E_A}{E_{max}} = f\left(\frac{\alpha}{1 + \frac{K_A}{[A]}}\right).$$ (21)

The consequences of some kinds of nonlinear relationship between stimulus and effect have been sufficiently discussed elsewhere (Ariëns et al., 1964c) and, with the exception of some aspects of the so-called receptor reserve, will not be dealt with in this chapter.

IV. Competitive Interaction

A. The Model of Competitive Interaction

In the foregoing it was discussed what the hypothesis used predicts about the form of the concentration-effect curves, and how the factors affinity and intrinsic activity are represented in these curves. The next question is: What are the consequences of the hypothesis in the case of competitive interaction? Presume that two drugs A and B with relative intrinsic activities α and β are in interaction with the same receptor-effector system. Then

$$\frac{[R][A]}{[RA]} = K_A, \quad \frac{[R][B]}{[RB]} = K_B, \quad \text{and} \quad [r] = [R] + [RA] + [RB].$$

The combined effect of [A] and [B], E_{AB}, is composed of the effect of [A] in presence of [B], increased by the effect of [B] in presence of [A]:

$$E_{AB} = E_{A(B)} + E_{B(A)}.$$

For the part of the effect caused by [A], according to Equations (10) and (17):

$$\frac{E_{A(B)}}{E_{max}} = \alpha \frac{[RA]}{[r]}.$$

The equation developes as follows:

$$\frac{E_{A(B)}}{E_{max}} = \alpha \frac{[RA]}{[R] + [RA] + [RB]} = \alpha \frac{\dfrac{[R][A]}{K_A}}{[R] + \dfrac{[R][A]}{K_A} + \dfrac{[R][B]}{K_B}}$$

$$= \alpha \frac{1}{\dfrac{K_A}{[A]} + 1 + \dfrac{[B]}{K_B} \cdot \dfrac{K_A}{[A]}} = \frac{\alpha}{1 + \left(1 + \dfrac{[B]}{K_B}\right)\dfrac{K_A}{[A]}}. \tag{22}$$

An analogous reasoning holds for $E_{B(A)}$, so that

$$\frac{E_{AB}}{E_{max}} = \frac{\alpha}{1 + \left(1 + \dfrac{[B]}{K_B}\right)\dfrac{K_A}{[A]}} + \frac{\beta}{1 + \left(1 + \dfrac{[A]}{K_A}\right)\dfrac{K_B}{[B]}}. \tag{23}$$

Comparison of Equation (22) with Equation (18), which refers to the effect of [A] in the absence of a competitor, makes it clear that the influence of B on the receptor occupation of A finds expression only in the factor by which K_A is multiplied. The value of this factor is greater than one; in other words, the presence of B seems to enlarge the dissociation constant K_A. This could be expected, since the competition that A experiences from B reduces its receptor occupation, just as would be caused by a diminution of the affinity of A. In the same way the receptor occupation by B is hindered by the presence of A [Eq. (23)].

B. Implications of the Model of Competitive Interaction

Three types of competitive interaction between an agonist A and a competing drug B are distinguishable, depending on the intrinsic activity of the latter.

a) If β^E is larger than α^E or if it has the same value, B is a competitive synergist of A. A set of theoretical curves based on Equation (23), illustrating competitive synergism of two full agonists, is given in Figure 4.

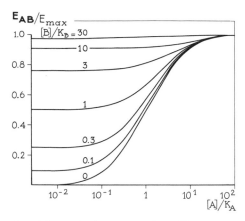

Fig. 4. Competitive synergism. Theoretical concentration-effect curves of full agonist A ($\alpha = 1$) in presence of increasing concentrations of full agonist B ($\beta = 1$). A and B interact with same kind of receptors [Eq. 23)]

b) If the value of β^E lies between that of α^E and 0, B is called a competitive dualist, since, depending on the concentration of A, the action of B will be either synergistic or antagonistic. Sets of theoretical curves illustrating these two aspects of competitive dualism are given in Figure 5; they also were obtained on basis of Equation (23).

c) If β^E equals 0, B behaves as a competitive antagonist of A. In this case Equation (23) becomes

$$\frac{E_{AB}}{E_{max}} = \frac{\alpha}{1 + \left(1 + \dfrac{[B]}{K_B}\right)\dfrac{K_A}{[A]}} . \tag{24}$$

The only result of the presence of the antagonist is an apparent diminution of the affinity of the agonist. As shown before, this will cause a shift of the concentration-effect curve along the logarithmic concentration axis, without influence on the shape and the height of the curve (Fig. 6). But is this true regardless of the nature of the stimulus-effect relation in the concerned receptor-effector system?

Suppose that in absence of B a certain effect is caused by the agonist concentration $[A]_1$, but in its presence the same effect is caused by $[A]_2$:

$$\frac{E_{A_1}}{E_{max}} = \frac{E_{A_2B}}{E_{max}} .$$

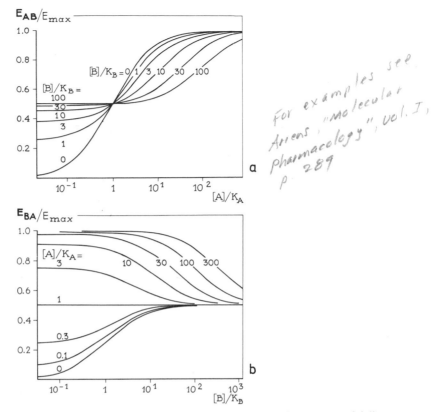

For examples see.
Ariens "molecular
pharmacology", vol. I,
p. 289

Fig. 5a and b. Competitive dualism. Figure 5a: theoretical concentration-effect curves of full agonist A ($\alpha = 1$) in presence of increasing concentrations of partial agonist B ($\beta = 0.5$). A and B interact with same kind of receptors [Eq. (23)]. In presence of lower concentrations of A, drug B acts as synergist (cf. Fig. 4), in presence of higher concentrations of A, as antagonist (cf. Fig. 6). Figure 5b: theoretical concentration-effect curves of partial agonist B ($\beta = 0.5$) in presence of increasing concentrations of full agonist A ($\alpha = 1$). B and A interact with same kind of receptors [Eq. (23)]

Application of the Equations (18) and (24) gives

$$\frac{\alpha}{1 + \dfrac{K_A}{[A]_1}} = \frac{\alpha}{1 + \left(1 + \dfrac{[B]}{K_B}\right)\dfrac{K_A}{[A]_2}} \cdot$$

It follows that

$$\frac{[A]_2}{[A]_1} = 1 + \frac{[B]}{K_B}. \tag{25}$$

Since the axis along which the curve is shifted is logarithmic for the concentrations, it is linear for the logarithms of the concentrations. The unit of this axis is the distance

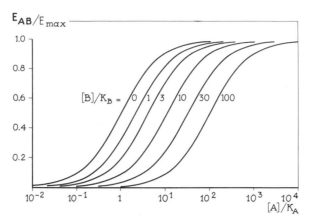

Fig. 6. Competitive antagonism. Theoretical concentration-effect curves of agonist A ($\alpha = 1$) in presence of increasing concentrations of competitive antagonist B ($\beta = 0$). A and B interact with same kind of receptors [Eq. (23) or (24)]. The concentration-effect curve is shifted along concentration axis to higher concentrations, without a change in shape and height of curve

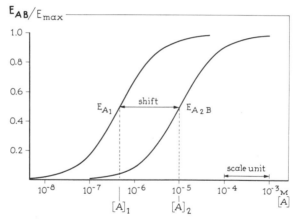

Fig. 7. Theoretical concentration-effect curves of agonist A in absence and in presence of certain concentration of competitive antagonist B. Shift is 1.33 units. Since it is measured in the scale unit, it equals $\log [A]_2 - \log [A]_1$ and this equals $\log (1 + [B]/K_B)$ [Eq. (25)]. It follows that the relation between stimulus and effect has no influence on magnitude of the shift

between two successive degrees of ten, and if the shift is measured in this unit, the result s equals $\log [A]_2 - \log [A]_1$ (Fig. 7). It follows that

$$s = \log \frac{[A]_2}{[A]_1} \quad \text{and thus} \quad s = \log \left(1 + \frac{[B]}{K_B}\right)$$

from which can be seen that the magnitude of the shift depends only on the concentration and the affinity of the antagonist. The relation between stimulus and effect in the receptor-effector system stimulated by the agonist does not play a part.

The model of competitive interaction started with the supposition that the agonist and the competitive antagonist interacted with the same receptors. Formally this is not necessary. As discussed on p. 212, competitive antagonism can be seen as a special case of metaffinoid antagonism. This follows from the fact that Equation (24) can be obtained from Equation (55), but apart from this, it is easily understandable that if the interaction of the antagonist B with its receptor R′ results in a complete disappearance of the affinity between the agonist A and its receptor R, and *vice versa*, the situation will be indistinguishable from a "normal" competitive antagonism.

In principle only equilibrium situations are considered in this chapter, but in connection with preceding sections it is attractive to give a short discussion of a nonequilibrium situation. Suppose a certain concentration of an agonist A is present in the biophase of a receptor system. The fraction of the receptors occupied by A in the equilibrium situation may be indicated as Y_A. If the same concentration of A is present simultaneously with a certain concentration of the competitive antagonist B, a different fraction of the receptors will be occupied by A in the equilibrium situation. This fraction may be indicated as $Y_{A(B)}$. Y_A equals $[RA]/[r]$ in Equation (3), so that

$$Y_A = \frac{1}{1 + \dfrac{K_A}{[A]}} . \tag{26}$$

$Y_{A(B)}$ equals $[RA]/[r]$ in the derivation of Equation (22), so that

$$Y_{A(B)} = \frac{1}{1 + \left(1 + \dfrac{[B]}{K_B}\right) \dfrac{K_A}{[A]}} . \tag{27}$$

It follows that $Y_{A(B)}$ will always be smaller than Y_A.

Further, if the same concentrations of A and B are present simultaneously with a certain concentration of a second competitive antagonist C, a reasoning analogous to the one used to obtain Equation (22) shows that

$$Y_{A(BC)} = \frac{1}{1 + \left(1 + \dfrac{[B]}{K_B} + \dfrac{[C]}{K_C}\right) \dfrac{K_A}{[A]}} \tag{28}$$

in which $Y_{A(BC)}$ again is the fraction of the receptors occupied by A in the equilibrium situation. From this it follows that $Y_{A(BC)}$ will always be smaller than $Y_{A(B)}$. It will be shown, however, that under nonequilibrium conditions a paradoxical situation may arise: with certain quite realistic assumptions the model predicts that the addition of a second competitive antagonist will *enlarge* the receptor occupation by A and thus its effect (STEPHENSON and GINSBORG, 1969; GINSBORG and STEPHENSON, 1974).

First, we will reconsider the competitive interaction of agonist A and competitive antagonist B under equilibrium conditions. Is it possible to express $Y_{A(B)}$ in Y_A and Y_B?

In other words, can the fraction of the receptors which, at equilibrium, is occupied by A in the presence of B, be expressed in the respective fractions which, at equilibrium, are occupied by A and B, if these substances are present alone?

It was shown earlier that, if a certain concentration of A is present alone, the following relation holds:

$$\frac{[A][R]_{(A)}}{[RA]_{(A)}} = K_A.$$

Likewise, if a certain concentration of B is present alone:

$$\frac{[B][R]_{(B)}}{[RB]_{(B)}} = K_B$$

and if these concentrations of A and B are present simultaneously:

$$\frac{[A][R]_{(AB)}}{[RA]_{(AB)}} = K_A \quad \text{and} \quad \frac{[B][R]_{(AB)}}{[RB]_{(AB)}} = K_B.$$

It follows that

$$\frac{[R]_{(AB)}}{[RA]_{(AB)}} = \frac{[R]_{(A)}}{[RA]_{(A)}} \quad \text{and} \quad \frac{[R]_{(AB)}}{[RB]_{(AB)}} = \frac{[R]_{(B)}}{[RB]_{(B)}}. \tag{29, 30}$$

Since in the competitive situation $[r] = [R]_{(AB)} + [RA]_{(AB)} + [RB]_{(AB)}$, it follows that:

$$Y_{A(B)} = \frac{[RA]_{(AB)}}{[r]} = \frac{[RA]_{(AB)}}{[R]_{(AB)} + [RA]_{(AB)} + [RB]_{(AB)}}$$

$$\frac{1}{Y_{A(B)}} = 1 + \frac{[R]_{(AB)}}{[RA]_{(AB)}} + \frac{[RB]_{(AB)}}{[RA]_{(AB)}}$$

$$= 1 + \left(1 + \frac{[RB]_{(AB)}}{[R]_{(AB)}}\right)\frac{[R]_{(AB)}}{[RA]_{(AB)}}. \tag{31}$$

Combining Equations (29), (30), and (31) gives

$$\frac{1}{Y_{A(B)}} = 1 + \left(1 + \frac{[RB]_{(B)}}{[R]_{(B)}}\right)\frac{[R]_{(A)}}{[RA]_{(A)}}. \tag{32}$$

If A is present alone, $[r] = [R]_{(A)} + [RA]_{(A)}$, so that

$$\frac{1}{Y_A} = \frac{[r]}{[RA]_{(A)}} = \frac{[R]_{(A)} + [RA]_{(A)}}{[RA]_{(A)}} = \frac{[R]_{(A)}}{[RA]_{(A)}} + 1$$

$$\frac{[R]_{(A)}}{[RA]_A} = \frac{1 - Y_A}{Y_A}. \tag{33}$$

An analogous reasoning shows that

$$\frac{[R]_{(B)}}{[RB]_{(B)}} = \frac{1 - Y_B}{Y_B}. \tag{34}$$

Substitution of Equations (33) and (34) in Equation (32) gives

$$\frac{1}{Y_{A(B)}} = 1 + \left(1 + \frac{Y_B}{1 - Y_B}\right)\frac{1 - Y_A}{Y_A} = \frac{1 - Y_A Y_B}{Y_A(1 - Y_B)}$$

$$Y_{A(B)} = \frac{Y_A(1 - Y_B)}{1 - Y_A Y_B}. \tag{35}$$

Now, imagine the following situation. A test organ is brought into contact with the competitive antagonist B during a period of time long enough to ensure equilibration, so that the fraction of the receptors occupied by B equals Y_B. Then the agonist A is added and remains for the period of time t. The dissociation rate of RB is relatively low, so that the time t is too short to reach a new equilibrium. For simplicity it may be assumed that during the time t no measurable change in [RB] will occur. The time t is long enough, however, to ensure equilibration in the interaction of A with the fraction of the receptors still available. This fraction is $1 - Y_B$, so that

$$Y^t_{A(B)} = Y_A(1 - Y_B) \tag{36}$$

in which $Y^t_{A(B)}$ is the fraction of the receptors occupied by A at the end of the time t.

Next the agonist is removed and the test organ is incubated simultaneously with the competitive antagonists B and C, again during a period of time which is long enough to reach equilibrium. The fraction of the receptors occupied by B is $Y_{B(C)}$. [$Y_{B(C)}$ is analogous to $Y_{A(B)}$ in Equation (35).] Again A is added and left present during the time t. It is assumed that the dissociation rate of RC is high, so that A will compete with C for the total fraction of the receptors not already occupied by B and this process will reach equilibrium before the end of the time t. It follows that

$$Y^t_{A(BC)} = Y_{A(C)}(1 - Y_{B(C)}) \tag{37}$$

in which $Y^t_{A(BC)}$ again is the fraction of the receptors occupied by A at the end of the time t. By applying Equation (35), Equation (37) can be developed further:

$$Y^t_{A(BC)} = \frac{Y_A(1 - Y_C)}{1 - Y_A Y_C}\left(1 - \frac{Y_B - Y_B Y_C}{1 - Y_B Y_C}\right) = \frac{Y_A(1 - Y_B)(1 - Y_C)}{(1 - Y_A Y_C)(1 - Y_B Y_C)}. \tag{38}$$

Combining Equation (38) and Equation (36) gives

$$\frac{Y^t_{A(BC)}}{Y^t_{A(B)}} = \frac{1 - Y_C}{(1 - Y_A Y_C)(1 - Y_B Y_C)}. \tag{39}$$

It can easily be seen that the value of $Y^t_{A(BC)}/Y^t_{A(B)}$ can be larger than 1. If, for instance, the concentrations of A, B, and C are chosen in such a way that $Y_A = Y_B = Y_C = 0.9$, the value of $Y^t_{A(BC)}/Y^t_{A(B)}$ is 2.77. It is true that this conclusion is based on equations obtained on the assumption that the concentration [RB] does not change at all during the time t, but it will be clear that analogous conclusions can be reached with less extreme assumptions: a certain change of [RB] during the time t may occur without invalidating the general reasoning presented above. We cannot go into further detail here. It may suffice to stress that STEPHENSON and GINSBORG have actually demonstrated the paradoxical potentiation of an agonist by a competitive antagonist in experiments with the so-called single dose technique, and that, as pointed out by these authors, the prediction and demonstration of this paradoxical effect provide strong support for a considerable body of receptor theory.

V. Metactoid Interaction

A. The Model of Metactoid Interaction

The next subject of discussion is the metactoid interaction of drugs (see p. 175). It is supposed that two drugs, A and B, interact with two different kinds of receptors. These receptors, R and R', are independent of each other with regard to their interactions with A and B, respectively, but the receptor-effector systems are interrelated beyond the level of the receptors. B as well as A is an agonist on its own receptors, but the stimulus caused by the interaction of B and R' (indicated as S'_B) does not find expression in a directly measurable effect, but only in a alteration of the effectiveness of the interaction of A and R. This alteration is here supposed to be directly proportional to the stimulus S'_B. If the alteration is a diminution, B may be called a metactoid antagonist, and if it is an enlargement, B may be called a metactoid sensitizer. The latter name is preferable to "metactoid synergist".

If the effect of [A] is called E_A, the effect of [A] under influence of [B] may be called $E_{AB'}$ and the effect of [A] in presence of the maximal stimulus in the metactoid system $E_{AS'_{max}}$. The effect of B can now be seen as the insertion of a multiplication factor between the receptor occupation by A and the effect caused by this interaction. The extreme value $E_{AS'_{max}}$ therefore has a certain fixed relation to the original E_A—the same relation as found between the maximal effect of the agonistic system under the influence of a maximal stimulus from the metactoid system ($E_{maxS'_{max}}$) on one hand, and the original E_{max} of the agonistic system on the other. This relation depends only on the nature of the interrelation between the two systems, and not on the actual value of E_A. This fact is represented in the equation

$$E_{AS'_{max}} = p E_A \tag{40}$$

in which the constant p, or $E_{AS'_{max}}/E_A$, is the value that characterizes the interrelation between the agonistic and the metactoid system.

As for the stimulus formation the noncompetitive drug does not distinguish itself at all from a normal agonist, and therefore the following equation describing the relation between the stimulus on the one side and the concentration, affinity and intrinsic activity of the agonist on the other side is applicable [combination of Equations (7) and (16)]:

$$\frac{S'_B}{S'_{max}} = \frac{\beta'}{1 + \dfrac{K'_B}{[B]}} . \tag{41}$$

Since the alteration caused by the metactoid drug was supposed to be directly proportional to the stimulus, instead of S'_B/S'_{max} may be written the change caused by [B] in the effect of a certain concentration of A, divided by the maximal change in this effect that can be caused via the receptors of the metactoid system in question. The realized change is $E_A - E_{AB'}$ if the metactoid drug is an antagonist, and $E_{AB'} - E_A$ if it is a sensitizer. In the same way the maximal change possible is $E_A - E_{AS'_{max}}$ for the antagonist or $E_{AS'_{max}} - E_A$ for the sensitizer. In the case of a metactoid antagonism

$$\frac{S'_B}{S'_{max}} = \frac{E_A - E_{AB'}}{E_A - E_{AS'_{max}}}$$

and in the case of metactoid sensitization

$$\frac{S'_B}{S'_{max}} = \frac{E_{AB'} - E_A}{E_{AS'_{max}} - E_A} .$$

These two equations are interchangeable, so that for both kinds of metactoid interaction Equation (41) can be written as

$$\frac{E_{AB'} - E_A}{E_{AS'_{max}} - E_A} = \frac{\beta'}{1 + \dfrac{K'_B}{[B]}} . \tag{42}$$

It follows that

$$E_{AB'} = E_A + (E_{AS'_{max}} - E_A) \frac{\beta'}{1 + \dfrac{K'_B}{[B]}}$$

or

$$E_{AB'} = \left\{ 1 + \left(\frac{E_{AS'_{max}}}{E_A} - 1 \right) \frac{\beta'}{1 + \dfrac{K'_B}{[B]}} \right\} E_A .$$

The fraction $E_{AS'_{max}}/E_A$ was introduced before as the constant p:

$$E_{AB'} = \left\{ 1 + (p - 1) \frac{\beta'}{1 + \dfrac{K'_B}{[B]}} \right\} E_A . \tag{43}$$

Division of both terms by E_{max} and application of Equation (18) gives the final formula:

$$\frac{E_{AB'}}{E_{max}} = \left\{ 1 + (p-1)\frac{\beta'}{1 + \dfrac{K'_B}{[B]}} \right\} \frac{\alpha}{1 + \dfrac{K_A}{[A]}}. \tag{44}$$

Attention may be drawn to the fact that β' and K'_B are "drug constants" on which comparison between individual members within one family may be based, but that this does not apply to p. This constant may be called a system constant, since, as mentioned, its value characterizes the interrelation between the agonistic and the metactoid systems. It may also be called a family constant: if the influence of two metactoid drugs on the effect of an agonist is described with different values of p in Equation (44), this implies that the antagonists do not belong to the same pharmacologic family. In this respect the role of p is analogous to that of E_{max} where agonistic drugs are concerned.

The intrinsic activity of a noncompetitive pharmacon can be defined according to

$$\beta' = \frac{S'_{B_{max}}}{S'_{max}} \tag{45}$$

This is the ratio of the maximal stimulus that can be generated by B on R′ to the maximal stimulus that can be provoked via these receptors by any substance. The equation holds for both metactoid and metaffinoid drugs; it is analogous to Equation (16) for the intrinsic activity of agonistic drugs (p. 185) and is subject to the same limitations. For a metactoid drug a derived intrinsic activity constant β'^E can be used. This constant is calculated according to

$$\beta'^E = \frac{E_{AB'_{max}} - E_A}{E_{AS'_{max}} - E_A} \tag{46}$$

in which the numerator represents the maximal change of E_A that can be caused by B, and the denominator the maximal change of E_A that can be caused via the receptors of B by any member of the same family. The constant β'^E equals β' if the relation between stimulus and effect is linear. As may be seen from Equation (46), β'^E only can have values from zero to one, both for sensitizers and antagonists.

The difference between these two possibilities finds expression in the value of p. If this value equals 0 or lies between 0 and 1 the noncompetitive system is an antagonizing one; if p is larger than 1 it is sensitizing. As follows from the definition:

$$p = \frac{E_{AS'_{max}}}{E_A}$$

p cannot have a negative value.

Equation (44) (VAN DEN BRINK, 1969c) differs from the older equations, with which ARIËNS and coworkers described noncompetitive (metactoid) interaction (ARIËNS and VAN ROSSUM, 1957; ARIËNS et al., 1955, 1956b, 1964b). In its latest version ARIËNS' equation runs as follows:

$$\frac{E_{AB'}}{E_{max}} = \left(1 + \frac{\beta'}{1 + \frac{K'_B}{[B]}}\right) \frac{E_A}{E_{max}}. \tag{47}$$

There are two reasons why this equation needed revision. First, strictly taken it only describes metactoid synergism, since β' by definition can only have a positive value. ARIËNS et al. get around this difficulty with the statement that in case of antagonism β' has to be supplied with a negative sign. In fact this means that metactoid antagonism and synergism are described with two different equations. It goes without saying that a single equation covering both aspects of metactoid interaction is preferable (cf. p. 223).

The second reason is more basic: the older equation does not differentiate between metactoid drugs belonging to the same family but differing in intrinsic activity on the

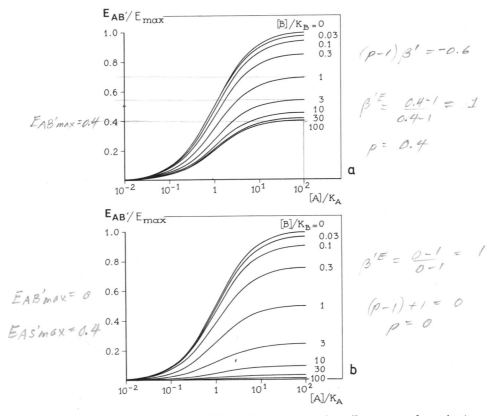

Fig. 8a and b. Metactoid antagonism. Sets of theoretical concentration-effect curves of agonist A ($\alpha = 1$) in presence of increasing concentrations of a metactoid antagonist B [Eq. (44)]. Figure 8a: incomplete metactoid antagonism; $(p-1)\,\beta' = -0.6$. With respect to the metactoid system, B may be a full agonist ($\beta' = 1$, $p = 0.4$) or a partial agonist (e.g., $\beta' = 0.6$, $p = 0$). Figure 8b: complete metactoid antagonism ($\beta' = 1$, $p = 0$). Note that concentration-effect curves are all in same position in relation to concentration axis, but that their maximal heights differ one side, and drugs belonging to different families on the other. This point is especially important if we are dealing with so-called incomplete metactoid antagonism, i.e., the situation that the maximal effect of the antagonist is a reduction of the agonistic effect to a certain fraction of its original value (Fig. 8a, cf. Fig. 25). It is true that the greater part of the metactoid antagonists tested are complete antagonists: they can reduce the effect of the agonist to zero (Fig. 8b). If this is the case, the situation can be described equally well with the older equation as with the new one. Equation (44) represents complete antagonism if $p=0$, meaning that the metactoid system *allows* complete antagonism, and if $\beta'=1$, meaning that the metactoid antagonist B, being a full agonist with respect to its own receptors, is able to realize this possibility. If $p=0$ and $\beta'=1$, Equation (44) can be reduced to

$$\frac{E_{AB'}}{E_{max}} = \frac{\alpha}{\left(1+\dfrac{[B]}{K'_B}\right)\left(1+\dfrac{K_A}{[A]}\right)} \tag{48}$$

Equation (47) represents complete antagonism if the plus sign is replaced with a minus sign (we are dealing with antagonism) and if $\beta'=1$ (B is a full agonist with respect to the metactoid receptors). Under these conditions the equation likewise can be reduced to Equation (48).

It should be noted that the older equation *implies* that complete antagonism via the metactoid system in question is possible. This is not necessarily true. Theoretically a case of incomplete metactoid antagonism can be based on two essentially different mechanisms. The revised equation recognizes both possibilities: a set of curves as given in Figure 8a, where the maximal result of the metactoid antagonism is a reduction of the agonistic effect to 40% of its original value, can be obtained if B is a partial agonist ($\beta'=0.6$) acting via a metactoid system that allows complete antagonism ($p=0$), but also if B is a full agonist ($\beta'=1$) which acts via a metactoid system that only allows an incomplete antagonism ($p=0.4$). In fact there are also intermediate possibilities, the only condition being that $(p-1)\,\beta'=-0.6$. The older equation recognizes only one possibility: it does not describe the set of curves in question unless it is assumed that B has an intrinsic activity value of 0.6. This seems sufficient reason to prefer the revised equation.

B. Implications of the Model of Metactoid Interaction; the Concept Receptor Reserve

Equation (44), derived for the action of an agonist in the presence of a metactoid compound, should be compared with Equation (18) which describes the uncomplicated action of an agonist. Obviously the metactoid interaction finds expression only in a factor with which α is multiplied, so that it seems as if the intrinsic activity of A is changed. According to the conclusions reached earlier (pp. 188—189) this means that the concentration-effect curves of an agonistic drug made in the presence of various concentrations of a metactoid drug are all in the same position with respect to the concentration axis, but that they differ in their maximal heights (Fig. 8a and b).

The foregoing is perfectly true if the relation of stimulus and effect in the system of A is linear and remains so in the presence of B. However, it may not hold if the stimulus-effect relation in the agonistic system is nonlinear. For a more detailed discussion of the consequences of a number of nonlinear stimulus-effect relations the reader may be referred to the literature (see, e.g., ARIËNS et al., 1964c). Here we will restrict ourselves to a situation which is often encountered in practice, viz. that the agonistic system has a so-called receptor reserve.

A receptor reserve (also indicated as "stimulus reserve") is the consequence of a nonlinear stimulus-effect relation with the following characteristic: within certain limits the effect increases with increasing stimulus, but a submaximal stimulus (by definition resulting from a submaximal receptor activation) already corresponds to a maximal effect. If the stimulus increases still further, the effect will remain the same (STEPHENSON, 1956; NICKERSON, 1956, 1957; ARIËNS et al., 1964c).

a) Creation of a receptor reserve by a metactoid sensitizer.

We may start with the supposition that a metactoid sensitizer exerts its influence on an agonistic system with a linear stimulus-effect relation. What will happen depends on the question *where* in the chain of events from receptor activation by the agonist to the ultimate effect the sensitizing stimulus has its influence. If the formation and propagation of the stimulus S_A are unaffected, but the effector organ itself is influenced in such a way as to allow a larger maximal effect, whereas a direct proportionality of stimulus and effect is maintained, the curves remain in the same position with respect to the concentration axis (Fig. 9, curves a, b, c, d). It is obvious that the possible enlargement of the effect must be limited: sooner or later the physiologic properties of the effector organ will set a limit.

If, on the other hand, the sensitization has reference to formation or propagation of S_A, so that the final impulse reaching the effector organ becomes larger, whereas the effector organ cannot react with a larger maximal effect, the direct proportionality between stimulus and effect necessarily is lost when the effect approaches its maximal value. Now a submaximal stimulus will cause a (practically) maximal effect; the stimulus may surpass this value, but the effect cannot increase any further. The interaction of the agonist with only a certain fraction of the receptors suffices to cause E_{max}; in other words, the sensitization has resulted in the creation of a receptor reserve. If formation of a receptor reserve is the only result of the metactoid interaction, the maximal height of the concentration-effect curve does not change but the slope becomes steeper, since the 1%-point of the curve more or less remains in the same position whereas the 99%-point is shifted to the left (Fig. 9, curves a, b', c', d').

b) Disappearance of a receptor reserve under influence of a metactoid antagonist.

It will be evident that if growing concentrations of a metactoid antagonist are added to an agonistic system with a receptor reserve of its own, and if this metactoid antagonist has no influence on the reactivity of the effector organ but causes a diminution of the final stimulus reaching the latter, the reversed phenomenon will be seen. At first the curve will not be depressed, the slope, however, will become less steep—the 99%-point shifting towards higher concentrations—and only when the receptor reserve is exhausted will depression of the curve follow. As discussed above, the metactoid antagonist seemingly causes the intrinsic activity of the agonist to decrease: the contribution of a single interaction of agonist and receptor to the total stimulus

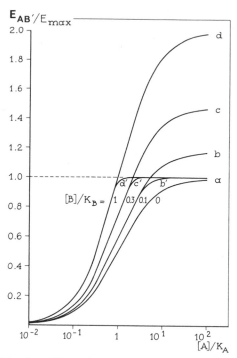

Fig. 9. Metactoid sensitization. Sets of theoretical concentration-effect curves based on Equation (44). Curves a, b, c, d: theoretical concentration-effect curves of agonist A ($\alpha = 1$) in presence of increasing concentrations of a metactoid sensitizer B ($\beta' = 1$, $p = 3$). It was supposed that under influence of metactoid stimulus, effect can become larger than orginal E_{max}, whereas stimulus-effect relation in agonistic system remains linear. Note that concentration-effect curves are all in same position in relation to concentration axis, but that their maximal heights differ. Curves a, b', c', d': ditto, with assumption that effect cannot become larger than original E_{max}; sensitization now results in formation of a receptor reserve (see text). Curves b', c', and d' were calculated with assumption that effect is proportional to stimulus up to about 90% of E_{max}, and with greater values of the stimulus approaches E_{max} asymptotically. Mathematically, this assumption was very closely approximated by using the following equation (Van den Brink, 1973a):

$$E = S - \frac{1}{20}\ln(1 + e^{20(S-1)})$$

in which $E = E_{AB'}/E_{max}$ and $S = S_{AB'}/2S_{P_{max}}$ [cf. Eq. (19); see also p. 229]. The equation is arbitrary; it was chosen only since it is a usable mathematical formulation of assumption made. Note that curves a, b', c', and d' have same maximal height, but that they have different slopes and thus are in different positions in relation to concentration axis

formation seems to become smaller. But, since there is reserve in the system, the loss can be made up by augmenting the agonist concentration, so that the number of interactions increases. As long as the receptor reserve lasts, the original maximal effect can be brought about.

As discussed before (p. 196) the shift of an agonistic concentration-effect curve caused by a competitive antagonist depends only on concentration and affinity of the antagonist. Needless to point out, therefore, that as far as competitive antagonism is

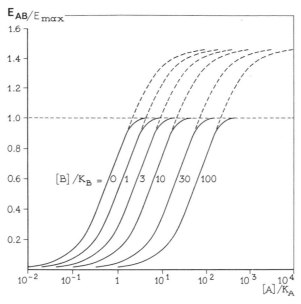

Fig. 10. Competitive antagonism in presence of a receptor reserve. Theoretical concentration-effect curves of agonist A ($\alpha^E = 1$) in presence of increasing concentrations of competitive antagonist B ($\beta = 0$) [Eq. (23) or (24)]. Curves were calculated with assumption that effect is proportional to stimulus up to about 90% of E_{max}, and with greater values of stimulus approaches E_{max} asymptotically. See legend of Fig. 9. Interrupted lines indicate further path of curves for case that stimulus-effect relation would have been directly proportional along whole range. Note that presence of a receptor reserve in agonistic system is of no consequence as for competitive antagonism (cf. Fig. 6)

concerned, the presence or absence of a receptor reserve in the receptor-effector system of the agonist is of no consequence (Fig. 10).

VI. Metaffinoid Interaction

See Ariens in "Molecular Pharmacology" pp. 313-317

A. The Model of Metaffinoid Interaction

In the model of metaffinoid interaction it is assumed that the interaction between substance B and the metaffinoid receptor R' results in a change in the affinity between substance A and the agonistic receptor R. The oldest equation describing this kind of interaction[6] was derived by ARIËNS and coworkers (ARIËNS et al., 1956b, 1964b):

$$\frac{E_{AB'}}{E_{max}} = \frac{\alpha}{1 + f_{AB'} \dfrac{K_A}{[A]}}$$

(49)

---

[6] In order to present the different models discussed in the following sections in corresponding notation, some symbols used in the original publications have been adapted.

in which:

$$f_{AB'} = \frac{1 + \dfrac{[B]}{K'_B}}{1 + \dfrac{[B]}{K'_B} \cdot \dfrac{1}{1 - \kappa_{AB'}}}.$$ (50)

In this model it is supposed that the agonistic receptors R and the metaffinoid receptors R′ occur in interdependent couples RR′. The authors assumed that the "interference of A and B on their respective receptors" is mutual. They further state: "The dissociation constants of the drug-receptor complexes ARR′ and RR′B are K_A and K'_B, respectively. When both interdependent receptors are occupied at the same time, i.e. if ARR′B is formed, the dissociation constants change to $K_A K'_B (1 - \kappa_{AB'})$, in which $\kappa_{AB'}$ represents the mutual interference of the drug molecules on their respective receptors."

The exact meaning of the constant $\kappa_{AB'}$ is not explained in the original publications. Since, however, the authors state that

$$\frac{[ARR'B]}{[RR']} = \frac{[A]}{K_A} \cdot \frac{[B]}{K'_B} \cdot \frac{1}{1 - \kappa_{AB'}}$$ (51)

and since $\dfrac{[RR'B]}{[RR']} = \dfrac{[B]}{K'_B}$ it follows that $\dfrac{[ARR'B]}{[RR'B]} = \dfrac{[A]}{(1 - \kappa_{AB'}) K_A}$. In other words, $(1 - \kappa_{AB'}) K_A$ is the dissociation constant of the agonistic pharmacon-receptor complex when the corresponding metaffinoid receptor is in interaction with B. If this dissociation constant is indicated as $K_{AB'}$, then

$$\kappa_{AB'} = \frac{K_A - K_{AB'}}{K_A}$$

so that $\kappa_{AB'}$ is the proportional change of K_A, caused by the interaction of B and R′. Further it is evident that the authors automatically assumed that the proportional change of K'_B caused by the interaction of A and R has the same value: if $[ARR']/[RR']$ is substituted for $[A]/K_A$ in Equation (51), this equation becomes

$$\frac{[ARR'B]}{[ARR']} = \frac{[B]}{(1 - \kappa_{AB'}) K'_B}$$

so that $(1 - \kappa_{AB'}) K'_B$ is the dissociation constant of the metaffinoid pharmacon-receptor complex when the corresponding agonistic receptor is in interaction with A. If this dissociation constant is indicated as K'_{BA}, then

$$\kappa_{AB'} = \frac{K'_B - K'_{BA}}{K'_B}.$$

Equation (50) therefore can also be written as

$$f_{AB'} = \frac{1 + \dfrac{[B]}{K_B'}}{1 + \dfrac{[B]}{K_{BA}'}}.$$

The original model of ARIËNS et al. has one flaw: since in Equations (49) and (50) the intrinsic activity of B with respect to the metaffinoid system, β', does not occur, the model does not recognize the essential difference between drugs belonging to the same metaffinoid family but differing in intrinsic activity, and drugs belonging to different families. To permit this distinction, and also to accentuate the relationship with the corresponding model of metactoid interaction, a modified version of the model was proposed (VAN DEN BRINK, 1969d).

The basic supposition again is that the interaction between B and R' results in a change in the affinity between A and R. When the metaffinoid stimulus is maximal, the affinity between A and R will acquire its extreme value, $1/K_{AS'_{max}}$. The ratio between $1/K_{AS'_{max}}$ and the original affinity is a constant which depends only on the interrelation between both systems. This is expressed in the following equation, which is analogous to Equation (40) for metactoid interaction:

$$\frac{1}{K_{AS'_{max}}} = q \, \frac{1}{K_A}. \tag{52}$$

The value of the constant q characterizes the interrelation between the metaffinoid system and the system of the agonist.

Furthermore it is again assumed that, if the interaction between B and R' causes a change in the affinity between A and R, the interaction between A and R will also cause a change in the affinity between B and R'. As a matter of fact, a one-way influence will be possible only if energy is supplied to or withdrawn from the total system in a special, directed way; otherwise the influence on the affinity surely will have a mutual character.

As in the original model, for simplicity it is supposed that any receptor for A is coupled to a receptor for B, and *vice versa*. In presence of given concentrations of A and B a situation will result for which holds that

$$[rr'] = [RR'] + [ARR'] + [RR'B] + [ARR'B]$$

and

$$\frac{[A][RR']}{[ARR']} = K_A$$

$$\frac{[A][RR'B]}{[ARR'B]} = K_{AB'}$$

$$\frac{[B][RR']}{[RR'B]} = K_B'$$

$$\frac{[B][ARR']}{[ARR'B]} = K_{BA}'.$$

It follows from these equations that

$$\frac{K_A}{K_{AB'}} = \frac{K'_B}{K'_{BA}}$$

so that the mutuality of the changes in affinity is well established and its character known.

Again the effect of A is supposed to be linearly related to the receptor occupation by A:

$$\frac{E_{AB'}}{E_{max}} = \alpha\frac{[ARR']}{[rr']} + \alpha\frac{[ARR'B]}{[rr']}$$

$$= \frac{\alpha}{\dfrac{K_A}{[A]} + 1 + \dfrac{K_A[B]}{[A]\,K'_B} + \dfrac{K_A[B]}{K_{AB'}K'_B}} + \frac{\alpha}{\dfrac{K_{AB'}K'_B}{[A][B]} + \dfrac{K_{AB'}K'_B}{K_A[B]} + \dfrac{K_{AB'}}{[A]} + 1}$$

$$= \frac{\alpha([A]\,K_{AB'}K'_B + [A][B]\,K_A)}{K_A K_{AB'}K'_B + [A]\,K_{AB'}K'_B + [B]\,K_A K_{AB'} + [A][B]\,K_A}$$

$$= \frac{\alpha}{1 + \dfrac{K_{AB'}K'_B + [B]\,K_{AB'}}{K_{AB'}K'_B + [B]\,K_A}\cdot\dfrac{K_A}{[A]}}$$

$$= \frac{\alpha}{1 + \dfrac{1}{\left(1 + \dfrac{K_A - K_{AB'}}{K_{AB'}}\cdot\dfrac{[B]}{K'_B + [B]}\right)}\cdot\dfrac{K_A}{[A]}} . \tag{53}$$

For the intrinsic activity β' of the metaffinoid drug B Equation (45) holds unaltered:

$$\beta' = \frac{S'_{B_{max}}}{S'_{max}}$$

(although $S'_{B_{max}}$ here could also be indicated as S'_B, since in the system of *one* pair of coupled receptors the stimulus causation by the interaction of B and R' is an all-or-non phenomenon). If the stimulus-effect relation in the metaffinoid system is linear, it follows that

$$\beta' = \frac{1/K_A - 1/K_{AB'}}{1/K_A - 1/K_{AS'_{max}}} = \frac{K_A/K_{AB'} - 1}{K_A/K_{AS'_{max}} - 1} . \tag{54}$$

Combining this equation with Equation (52) gives

$$\frac{K_A - K_{AB'}}{K_{AB'}} = (q - 1)\,\beta'$$

and substituting this relation in Equation (53) leads to the final equation

$$\frac{E_{AB'}}{E_{max}} = \frac{\alpha}{1 + \cfrac{1}{1 + (q-1)\cfrac{\beta'}{1 + \cfrac{K'_B}{[B]}}}} \cdot \frac{K_A}{[A]} \tag{55}$$

It is worth mentioning that the same equation can be derived with quite different suppositions, viz. that the receptors R and R' do *not* occur in interdependent couples and that, although the interaction between B and R' causes a change in the affinity between A and R, the interaction of A and R has *no* influence on the affinity between B and R' (VAN DEN BRINK, 1969d). The relation between the agonistic and the metaffinoid receptors is now supposed to have a more diffuse character: an increasing degree of interaction of B and the metaffinoid receptors causes an increasing, gradual change in the affinity between A and *any* agonistic receptor. From Equation (41), which holds unaltered, together with the supposition that S'_B corresponds linearly with the resulting change in the affinity between A and R, it follows that

$$\frac{\beta'}{1 + \cfrac{K'_B}{[B]}} = \frac{\cfrac{1}{K_A} - \cfrac{1}{K_{AB'}}}{\cfrac{1}{K_A} - \cfrac{1}{K_{AS'_{max}}}} \tag{56}$$

It should be noted, that here S'_B is not identical with $S'_{B_{max}}$, since the stimulus causation by the interaction of B and the metaffinoid receptors is a gradual phenomenon. It follows that $1/K_{AB'}$ in Equation (56) represents the affinity between A and R in the presence of [B], and not the extreme value to which this affinity can change under influence of B.

With application of Equation (52), Equation (56) can be developed into a form analogous to Equation (43):

$$\frac{1}{K_{AB'}} = \left\{ 1 + (q-1)\frac{\beta'}{1 + \cfrac{K'_B}{[B]}} \right\} \frac{1}{K_A} \tag{57}$$

For the effect of [A] in the presence of [B] according to Equation (18) the following holds:

$$\frac{E_{AB'}}{E_{max}} = \frac{\alpha}{1 + \cfrac{K_{AB'}}{[A]}}$$

and substituting Equation (57) in this equation results in Equation (55).

B. Metaffinoid Interaction. Implications of Equation 55

In the next section of this chapter some recent developments of the model of metaffinoid interaction will be discussed. However, the implications of Equation (55) may be considered first.

In the first place it will be clear that what was said about the character of the constant p as a "family constant" (see p. 202) holds also with regard to q: if two metaffinoid drugs have different values for q they do not belong to the same family. If the value of q equals 0 or lies between 0 and 1 the drugs in the group in question are antagonists of the drug A and if q is greater than 1 they are sensitizers; q cannot have a negative value.

Then it may be observed that the only difference between Equation (55) and Equation (18) which describes the effect of an agonist present alone, is the factor with which K_A is multiplied. As discussed before, this means that the presence of B will cause the concentration-effect curve of A to undergo a parallel shift along the logarithmic concentration axis (see pp. 188—191); in this respect the situation resembles a competitive interaction. In the case of the latter, however, an enlargement of the concentration of B always corresponds with an enlargement of the shift [cf. Eq. (25)], whereas in the case of a metaffinoid interaction the maximal shift may be finite (Fig. 11). A reasoning analogous to the one presented on pp. 189—190 but applying the Equations (18) and (55) may show that

$$\frac{[A]_2}{[A]_1} = \frac{1}{1+(q-1)\dfrac{\beta'}{1+\dfrac{K'_B}{[B]}}}. \tag{58}$$

The shift will be maximal if $\beta' = 1$ and $[B]$ is infinitely large. Under these conditions the foregoing formula can be simplified to

$$\frac{[A]_2}{[A]_1} = \frac{1}{q} \tag{59}$$

and it follows that the maximal value of the shift, if measured in the scale unit, equals $-\log q$. The foregoing also implies that formally the maximal shift that can be caused by a metaffinoid antagonist *may* be infinite, viz. if $\beta' = 1$ and q is infinitely small. If the indicated values of β' and q are substituted in Equation (55) the latter becomes identical with Equation (24), so that formally a purely competitive antagonism results (see also p. 197).

A relation like Equation (54), defining the intrinsic activity β' in terms of affinities, is no suitable basis for the calculation of this value in practice. The Equations (58) and (59) are better starting-points. Suppose that in the absence of the metaffinoid drug B a certain effect is caused by the agonist concentration $[A]_1$. The same effect is caused by another agonist concentration, $[A]_2$, if all receptors of B are in interaction with the latter drug, so that the shift of the agonistic curve is the maximal shift that can be caused by B. Still another agonist concentration is needed for the effect in question if all metaffinoid receptors interact with the molecules of a reference compound which

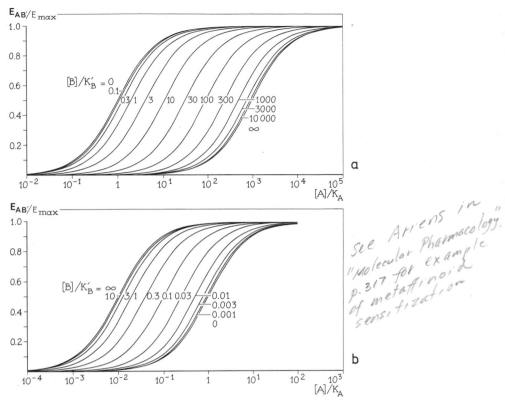

Fig. 11a and b. Metaffinoid interaction. Figure 11a: theoretical concentration-effect curves of agonist A ($\alpha = 1$) in presence of increasing concentrations of a metaffinoid antagonist B. This set of curves is based on Equation (55) with assumption that $\beta' = 1$ and $q = 0.001$; same result is obtained with Equation (83) if it is assumed that $K_{AB'} = 1000\, K_A$ and $K'_{BA} = 1000\, K'_B$ [i.e., $\chi = \phi/(1000 - 999\phi)$ and $\omega = \psi/(1000 - 999\psi)$, see text]. Figure 11b: ditto in presence of increasing concentrations of a metaffinoid sensitizer B. This set of curves is based on Equation (55) with assumption that $\beta' = 1$ and $q = 100$; same result is obtained with Equation (83) if it is assumed that $K_{AB'} = 0.01\, K_A$ and $K'_{BA} = 0.01\, K'_B$ (i.e. $\chi = \varphi/(0.01 + 0.99\,\varphi)$ and $\omega = \psi/(0.01 + 0.99\,\psi)$, see text). Concentration-effect curve is shifted along concentration axis to higher (Fig. 11a) or lower (Fig. 11b) concentrations, without a change in shape of curve; maximal value of shift is finite

possesses a full intrinsic activity ($\beta' = 1$). From Equation (58) it follows that

$$\frac{[A]_2}{[A]_1} = \frac{1}{1 + (q-1)\,\beta'}$$

since in this case [B] can be considered infinitely large. The same holds for the concentration of the reference compound, and since moreover in this case β' equals 1, Equation (59) applies:

$$\frac{[A]_3}{[A]_1} = \frac{1}{q}.$$

On this basis a derived intrinsic activity constant β'^E can be calculated. This constant will equal β' if the stimulus-effect relation in the metaffinoid system is linear (and if the other, general suppositions hold; see pp. 191—192), and it may be defined as

$$\beta'^E = \frac{[A]_1/[A]_2 - 1}{[A]_1/[A]_3 - 1}. \tag{60}$$

Finally it is interesting to compare Equation (55) with the combination of Equations (49) and (50). Since the two formulae represent the same model, they should be interchangeable, and thus it is possible to express $\kappa_{AB'}$ in q and β':

$$\kappa_{AB'} = \frac{(q-1)\beta'}{1 + (q-1)\beta'}.$$

As mentioned earlier, the formula with $\kappa_{AB'}$ does not differentiate between drugs which belong to the same family but have different intrinsic activities on the one hand, and drugs belonging to different families on the other hand. For this reason Equation (55) may be preferable.

C. An Alternative Model for Metaffinoid Interaction

Recently an alternative model for metaffinoid interaction was proposed by Offermeier and Brandt (Brandt, 1973). In the simplest form of this model the following presuppositions were made:

1. In accordance with the assumptions made by Ariëns et al., it is supposed that the agonistic receptors occur in two conformational states. The unchanged receptors are indicated as R_u, the changed receptors as R_c; the dissociation constants of $R_u A$ and $R_c A$ are K_A and $K_{AB'}$, respectively.

2. The stimulus created by the interaction of B with a certain fraction of the metaffinoid receptors leads to a conformational change of the same fraction of the agonistic receptors. This holds also in the model proposed by Ariëns et al., since the agonistic and metaffinoid receptors were supposed to occur in interdependent couples. However, the assumption made here has a more general character: Ariëns' assumption also implies that the numbers of agonistic and metaffinoid receptors are equal, but in the model of Offermeier and Brandt this is not necessarily the case.

3. It is further assumed that the affinity between B and R' is not influenced by the interaction between A and R. In this assumption the model differs essentially from that of Ariëns et al.

The effect produced by the agonist A in the presence of the metaffinoid substance B equals the sum of the effects produced by A on the conformationally changed and the conformationally unchanged agonistic receptors. If the stimulus-effect relation in the agonistic system is linear, it follows that

$$\frac{E_{AB'}}{E_{max}} = \alpha \frac{[R_c A]}{[r_c] + [r_u]} + \alpha \frac{[R_u A]}{[r_c] + [r_u]}.$$

This can also be written as

$$\frac{E_{AB'}}{E_{max}} = \frac{[r_c]}{[r_c]+[r_u]} \cdot \alpha \cdot \frac{[R_c A]}{[r_c]} + \frac{[r_u]}{[r_c]+[r_u]} \cdot \alpha \cdot \frac{[R_u A]}{[r_u]}. \tag{61}$$

The quotient $[r_c]/([r_c]+[r_u])$ is the fraction of the agonistic receptors with a changed conformation, and thus equals the fraction of the metaffinoid receptors occupied by B. Therefore it can be replaced by $1/(1+K'_B/[B])$ [cf. Eq. (3)]. Likewise, the quotient $[r_u]/([r_c]+[r_u])$ is the fraction of the agonistic receptors with unchanged conformation, and thus equals the fraction of the metaffinoid receptors remaining free; it thus can be replaced by $1-1/(1+K'_B/[B])$. The quotient $[R_c A]/[r_c]$, being the fraction of the population of changed agonistic receptors which is occupied by A, equals $1/(1+K_{AB'}/[A])$, and the quotient $[R_u A]/[r_u]$, being the fraction of the population of

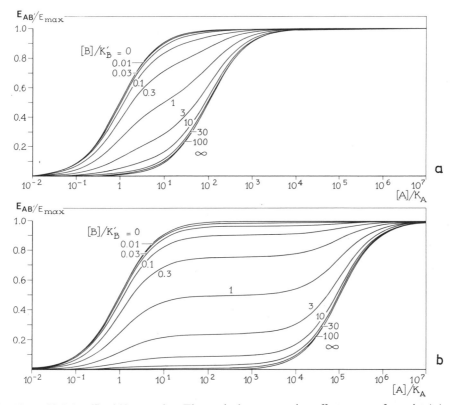

Fig. 12a and b. Metaffinoid interaction. Theoretical concentration-effect curves of agonist A ($\alpha=1$) in presence of increasing concentrations of a metaffinoid antagonist B. Figure 12a: set of curves based on Equation (62) with assumption that $K_{AB'}=100\,K_A$; same result is obtained with Equation (83) if it is assumed that $K_{AB'}=100\,K_A$ and $K'_{BA}=K'_B$ [i.e. $\chi=\varphi/(100-99\,\varphi)$ and $\omega=\psi$, see text]. Figure 12b: set of curves based on Equation (62) with assumption that $K_{AB'} =100\,000\,K_A$; same result is obtained with Equation (83) if it is assumed that $K_{AB'}=100\,000\,K_A$ and $K'_{BA}=K'_B$ [i.e. $\chi=\varphi/(100\,000-99\,999\,\varphi)$ and $\omega=\psi$, see text]. Note difference between these sets of curves and that presented in Figure 11a the unchanged agonistic receptors which is occupied by A, equals $1/(1 + K_A/[A])$. Equation (61) thus can be developed into

$$\frac{E_{AB'}}{E_{max}} = \frac{1}{1 + \dfrac{K'_B}{[B]}} \cdot \frac{\alpha}{1 + \dfrac{K_{AB'}}{[A]}} + \left(1 - \frac{1}{1 + \dfrac{K'_B}{[B]}}\right) \cdot \frac{a}{1 + \dfrac{K_A}{[A]}}. \qquad (62)$$

With application of the Equations (52) and (54), the dissociation constant $K_{AB'}$ can be further replaced by $K_A/\{1 + (q - 1)\beta'\}$.

For a more detailed discussion of the model of OFFERMEIER and BRANDT the reader may be referred to the original publication (BRANDT, 1973). Here it may suffice to stress that the theoretical concentration-effect curves based on this model may differ essentially from those based on the model of ARIËNS et al. (compare Fig. 11 with Fig. 12). Especially if the difference between K_A and $K_{AB'}$ is larger, it is quite probable that in the experimental situation only the first parts of these curves, i.e. the effect caused by interaction with the unchanged receptors, would be observed, so that a metaffinoid antagonist acting according to the model in question would probably be mistaken for a metactoid antagonist. Actually, as the authors point out, it is possible that the conformational change due to the metaffinoid interaction results in the equilibrium dissociation constant of $R_c A$ becoming virtually infinite. This would mean that the agonistic drug would have no affinity for the changed receptors and thus would not be able to exert an effect via these receptors. It would seem as if, in the presence of increasing concentrations of B, the agonist gradually loses its intrinsic activity: substance B would be acting as a metactoid antagonist. This is reflected by the fact that, if the value of $K_{AB'}$ in Equation (62) is supposed to be infinite, this equation can be reduced to Equation (48), which describes complete metactoid antagonism.

D. A More Generalized Metaffinoid Model

The metaffinoid models developed by ARIËNS and coworkers and by OFFERMEIER and BRANDT should not be taken for rival models. It can easily be shown that they only represent special cases of a more generalized model, based on the following assumptions:

1. The agonistic receptors can occur in two conformational states, R_u (unchanged) and R_c (changed); the dissociation constants of $R_u A$ and $R_c A$ are K_A and $K_{AB'}$, respectively. The metaffinoid receptors likewise can occur in two conformational states, R'_u and R'_c; the dissociation constants of $R'_u B$ and $R'_c B$ are K'_B and K'_{BA}, respectively.

2. The interaction between B and a certain fraction of the metaffinoid receptors leads to a conformational change of the same fraction of the agonistic receptors; the interaction between A and a certain fraction of the agonistic receptors leads to a conformational change of the same fraction of the metaffinoid receptors.

It is not supposed that the agonistic and metaffinoid receptors occur in interdependent couples and no assumptions are made concerning the ratio of the numbers of both kinds of receptors; in this aspect the model presented here differs from that of ARIËNS et al. and is in keeping with that of OFFERMEIER and BRANDT. On the other hand, as in ARIËNS' model, it is assumed that the relation between the agonistic and the metaffinoid system allows for reciprocity; it will be clear that this is a more general assumption than that of a one-way influence (cf. also p. 209).

In the presence of [A] in the biophase of the agonistic receptors and of [B] in that of the metaffinoid receptors the following equations will hold:

$$[r] = [R_u] + [R_u A] + [R_c] + [R_c A] \tag{63}$$

and

$$[r'] = [R'_u] + [R'_u B] + [R'_c] + [R'_c B]. \tag{64}$$

For convenience the following indications will be used:

$$\frac{[R_u]}{[r]} = a, \quad \frac{[R_u A]}{[r]} = b, \quad \frac{[R_c]}{[r]} = c, \quad \frac{[R_c A]}{[r]} = d,$$

$$\frac{[R'_u]}{[r']} = e, \quad \frac{[R'_u B]}{[r']} = f, \quad \frac{[R'_c]}{[r']} = g, \quad \frac{[R'_c B]}{[r']} = h,$$

so that the Equations (63) and (64) can be written as

$$a + b + c + d = 1 \tag{65}$$

and

$$e + f + g + h = 1. \tag{66}$$

For the unchanged agonistic receptors the following holds

$$\frac{[R_u A]}{[R_u] + [R_u A]} = \frac{1}{1 + \dfrac{K_A}{[A]}},$$

so that

$$\frac{a}{b} = \frac{K_A}{[A]}. \tag{67}$$

Analogous reasonings for the changed agonistic receptors, the unchanged metaffinoid receptors, and the changed metaffinoid receptors, respectively, show that

$$\frac{c}{d} = \frac{K_{AB'}}{[A]}, \tag{68}$$

$$\frac{e}{f} = \frac{K'_B}{[B]}, \tag{69}$$

and

$$\frac{g}{h} = \frac{K'_{BA}}{[B]}. \tag{70}$$

Finally, from the assumption that the fraction of the agonistic receptors which are changed is equal to the fraction of the metaffinoid receptors which are occupied, and that the fraction of the agonistic receptors which are occupied is equal to the fraction of the metaffinoid receptors which are changed, it follows that

$$c + d = f + h \tag{71}$$

and

$$b + d = g + h. \tag{72}$$

In the simplest case, a linear stimulus-effect relation in the agonistic system, the effect $E_{AB'}/E_{max}$ will be equal to $\alpha([R_u A]/[r] + [R_c A]/[r])$, or to $\alpha(b + d)$. By application of Equations (65—72), which are the mathematical expressions of the presuppositions made in the model, $b + d$ can be expressed in K_A, $K_{AB'}$, K'_B, K'_{BA}, [A] and [B].

If the following indications are used

$$\frac{1}{1 + \dfrac{K_A}{[A]}} = \phi, \quad \frac{1}{1 + \dfrac{K_{AB'}}{[A]}} = \chi, \quad \frac{1}{1 + \dfrac{K'_B}{[B]}} = \psi \quad \text{and} \quad \frac{1}{1 + \dfrac{K'_{BA}}{[B]}} = \omega$$

so that

$$\frac{K_A}{[A]} = \frac{1 - \phi}{\phi}, \quad \frac{K_{AB'}}{[A]} = \frac{1 - \chi}{\chi}, \quad \frac{K'_B}{[B]} = \frac{1 - \psi}{\psi} \quad \text{and} \quad \frac{K'_{BA}}{[B]} = \frac{1 - \omega}{\omega},$$

the Equations (67—70) can be changed to

$$a + b = \frac{1}{\phi} b, \tag{73}$$

$$c + d = \frac{1}{\chi} d, \tag{74}$$

$$e + f = \frac{1}{\psi} f, \tag{75}$$

$$g + h = \frac{1}{\omega} h. \tag{76}$$

Combining Equations (73) and (74) with Equation (65) and Equations (75) and (76) with Equation (66) gives

and

$$b = \phi - \frac{\phi}{\chi} d \tag{77}$$

$$f = \psi - \frac{\psi}{\omega} h \tag{78}$$

Combining Equation (74) with Equation (71) and Equation (76) with Equation (72) gives

$$\frac{1}{\chi}d = f + h \tag{79}$$

and

$$b + d = \frac{1}{\omega}h. \tag{80}$$

Combining Equation (77) with Equation (80) gives

$$\phi - \frac{\phi}{\chi}d + d = \frac{1}{\omega}h$$

or

$$\frac{\chi - \phi}{\chi}d = \frac{1}{\omega}h - \phi \tag{81}$$

and in an analogous way combining Equation (78) with Equation (79) gives

$$\frac{1}{\chi}d = \psi + \frac{\omega - \psi}{\omega}h. \tag{82}$$

Combining Equations (81) and (82) leads to

$$\frac{1}{\omega}h - \phi = (\chi - \phi)\psi + \frac{(\chi - \phi)(\omega - \psi)}{\omega}h,$$

$$\frac{1 - (\chi - \phi)(\omega - \psi)}{\omega}h = \phi + (\chi - \phi)\psi,$$

$$\frac{1}{\omega}h = \frac{\phi + (\chi - \phi)\psi}{1 - (\chi - \phi)(\omega - \psi)}.$$

According to Equation (80), $\frac{1}{\omega}h$ equals $b + d$, and so the final equation is obtained:

$$\frac{E_{AB'}}{E_{max}} = \alpha\frac{\phi + (\chi - \varphi)\psi}{1 - (\chi - \phi)(\omega - \psi)}$$

or

$$\frac{E_{AB'}}{E_{max}} = \alpha\frac{(1 - \psi)\phi + \psi\chi}{1 - (\chi - \phi)(\omega - \psi)}. \tag{83}$$

Now return to the two metaffinoid models discussed in the preceding sections of this chapter. In the model developed by Offermeier and Brandt the interaction between R and A was not assumed to result in a change of K'_B. In the terms of the more generalized model this means that $\omega = \psi$. If this is the case, Equation (83) changes to

$$\frac{E_{AB'}}{E_{max}} = \alpha\{(1-\psi)\phi + \psi\chi\}$$

which is identical with the final equation derived by Offermeier and Brandt [Eq. (62)].

As for the first model, here the special assumption was that $K_A/K_{AB'} = K'_B/K'_{BA}$, or, in the terms of the generalized model:

$$\frac{1-\phi}{\phi} \cdot \frac{\chi}{1-\chi} = \frac{1-\psi}{\psi} \cdot \frac{\omega}{1-\omega}.$$

From this it follows that

$$\omega = \frac{(1-\phi)\chi\psi}{\phi - \phi\chi - \phi\psi + \chi\psi}. \tag{84}$$

Equation (83) can be rearranged:

$$\frac{E_{AB'}}{E_{max}} = \alpha \frac{\phi - \phi\psi + \chi\psi}{1 - \phi\psi + \chi\psi + (\phi - \chi)\omega}$$

$$= \frac{\alpha}{1 + \dfrac{1 - \phi + (\phi - \chi)\omega}{\phi - \phi\psi + \chi\psi}}. \tag{85}$$

By applying Equation (84), ω is eliminated from the second term of the divisor:

$$\frac{1 - \phi + (\phi - \chi)\omega}{\phi - \phi\psi + \chi\psi} = \frac{1-\phi}{\phi - \phi\psi + \chi\psi} + \frac{(\phi - \chi)(1-\phi)\chi\psi}{(\phi - \phi\psi + \chi\psi)(\phi - \phi\chi - \phi\psi + \chi\psi)}$$

$$= \frac{(1-\phi)(\phi - \phi\chi - \phi\psi + \chi\psi + \phi\chi\psi - \chi^2\psi)}{(\phi - \phi\psi + \chi\psi)(\phi - \phi\chi - \phi\psi + \chi\psi)}$$

$$= \frac{(1-\phi)(1-\chi)(\phi - \phi\psi + \chi\psi)}{(\phi - \phi\psi + \chi\psi)(\phi - \phi\chi - \phi\psi + \chi\psi)}$$

$$= \frac{(1-\phi)(1-\chi)}{\phi - \phi\chi - \phi\psi + \chi\psi}.$$

Equation (85) thus can be transformed to

$$\frac{E_{AB'}}{E_{max}} = \frac{\alpha}{1 + \dfrac{(1-\phi)(1-\chi)}{\phi - \phi\chi - \phi\psi + \chi\psi}} \cdot = \qquad (86)$$

The second term of the divisor is further developed as follows:

$$\frac{(1-\phi)(1-\chi)}{\phi - \phi\chi - \phi\psi + \chi\psi} = \frac{(1-\chi)(1-\psi) + (1-\chi)\psi}{\phi(1-\chi)(1-\psi) + \chi\psi(1-\phi)}(1-\phi)$$

$$= \frac{\dfrac{(1-\chi)(1-\psi)}{\chi\psi} + \dfrac{1-\chi}{\chi}}{\dfrac{(1-\chi)(1-\psi)}{\chi\psi} + \dfrac{1-\phi}{\phi}} \cdot \frac{1-\phi}{\phi}$$

$$= \frac{\dfrac{K_{AB'}K_B'}{[A][B]} + \dfrac{K_{AB'}}{[A]}}{\dfrac{K_{AB'}K_B'}{[A][B]} + \dfrac{K_A}{[A]}} \cdot \frac{K_A}{[A]}$$

$$= \frac{K_{AB'}K_B' + [B]K_{AB'}}{K_{AB'}K_B' + [B]K_A} \cdot \frac{K_A}{[A]}$$

$$= \frac{K_A/[A]}{1 + \dfrac{K_A - K_{AB'}}{K_{AB'}} \cdot \dfrac{[B]}{K_B' + [B]}} \cdot$$

This shows that Equation (86) is identical with Equation (53). It follows that also the model proposed by ARIËNS et al. represents a special case of the generalized model presented in this section.

The discussion of metaffinoid interaction may be concluded with the following three remarks concerning the generalized model. First, Equation (83) as such does not differentiate between drugs belonging to the same metaffinoid family but differing in intrinsic activity, and drugs belonging to different metaffinoid families. As mentioned earlier, this can be remedied by replacing the constant $K_{AB'}$ by $K_A/\{1 + (q-1)\beta'\}$. Since the interaction between the R-system and the R'-system was supposed to be mutual, an analogous reasoning holds for the constant K_{BA}', which can be replaced by $K_B'/\{1 + (q^* - 1)\alpha^*\}$, in which q^* equals the ratio of K_B' and the value which the dissociation constant of BR' can acquire as a result of the maximal *metaffinoid* stimulus created via the R-receptors, and in which α^* is the intrinsic activity of substance A with respect to the formation of this metaffinoid stimulus. The value of α^* is not necessarily equal to that of α, the intrinsic activity of A with respect to the formation of the agonistic stimulus.

Secondly, it will be evident that the sets of theoretical concentration-effect curves predicted by the models of ARIËNS et al. and of OFFERMEIER and BRANDT can also be

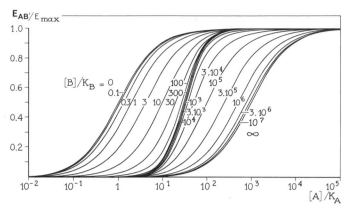

Fig. 13. Metaffinoid antagonism. Theoretical concentration-effect curves of agonist A ($\alpha = 1$) in presence of increasing concentrations of metaffinoid antagonist B. This set of curves is based on Equation (83) with assumption that $K_{AB'} = 1000\,K_A$ and $K'_{BA} = 10^6\,K'_B$ [i.e., $\chi = \varphi/(1000 - 999\,\varphi)$ and $\omega = \psi/(1000000 - 999999\,\psi)$, see text]

obtained on the basis of the generalized model. However, in addition this model predicts other possibilities. An example is given in Figure 13.

Finally, it is worth stressing that the metaffinoid model is remarkably versatile. It was mentioned already that under certain conditions it predicts the same sets of curves as the models of competitive and metactoid antagonism (see p. 212 and p. 216). It should be added that also in many cases of functional interaction, the model to be discussed in the next section, sets of curves are obtained which as such are indistinguishable from certain sets of curves predicted by the metaffinoid model.

VII. Functional Interaction

A. The Model of Functional Interaction

1. The Original Model of Functional Interaction

The concept of functional interaction was introduced by Ariëns et al. (1956c). In a later publication (1964b), the same authors defined functional interaction as follows: "Two drugs, A and B, interact with their own specific receptor system, R_I and R_{II}, respectively, but produce their effect by means of a common effector, E."

The authors continue: "If A and B are agonistic drugs, there is synergism. The effect, $E_{I_A II_B}$, may be represented by

$$\frac{E_{I_A II_B}}{E_{max}} = \frac{E_{I_A}}{E_{max}} + \frac{E_{I_B}}{E_{max}} - \frac{E_{I_A} E_{II_B}}{E_{max^2}} \tag{87}$$

in which E_{I_A} and E_{II_B} are the individual effects of A and B induced on the receptor systems R_I and R_{II}, respectively".

In this model of functional synergism it is implicitly assumed that the maximal effects obtainable with A and B alone are equal to the maximal effect obtainable by their combined action ($E_{A_{max}} = E_{B_{max}} = E_{max}$). E_{max} is defined as "the maximum effect possible with the effector system concerned" (ARIËNS et al., 1956c)[7]. Furthermore the effects caused by A and B, respectively, are supposed to interfere with one another. The interference term $E_{I_A} E_{II_B}/E_{max}^2$ prevents the overall effect $E_{I_A II_B}$ from growing larger than the maximal effect E_{max}.

In the same paper, the authors write: "Another possibility is two drugs which interact with different receptors R_I and R_{II} while they produce their effect by means of a common effector system E in such a way that their contributions to the effect are opposite:

$$\frac{E_{I_A II_B}}{E_{max}} = \frac{E_{I_A}}{E_{max}} - \frac{E_{II_B}}{E_{max}} \text{''} . \tag{88}$$

Here it is implicitly assumed that if the value of $E_{I_A}/E_{max} - E_{II_B}/E_{max}$ is negative, the term $E_{I_A II_B}/E_{max}$ equals zero. Further this model of functional antagonism differs from that of functional synergism expressed in Equation (87) in the absence of an interference term.

2. A New Model of Functional Interaction

Recently a new model of functional interaction was introduced (VAN DEN BRINK, 1973a, b). The reasons why the original model had to be replaced are the following:

First, there is a theoretical reason: the model makes more independent presuppositions than necessary. In the cases of competitive, metactoid, and metaffinoid interactions both synergism and antagonism are described by one and the same equation. The original model of functional interaction, however, uses two essentially different equations, thus assuming different mechanisms for functional synergism and antagonism. This assumption is not justified unless there are compelling reasons to make it. According to the law of parsimony, a single model covering both aspects of functional interaction has to be preferred.

Secondly, there is a practical reason, best illustrated with an example. Figure 14 shows a set of experimental curves of the cholinomimetic drug methacholine in the presence of increasing concentrations of the β-adrenoceptor stimulant l-isoprenaline. This is a clear example of functional antagonism (see ARIËNS et al., 1964b, and OFFERMEIER and VAN DEN BRINK, 1974). The methacholine curves are found to be shifted in a parallel way to higher concentration ranges. However, in the presence of a certain concentration of l-isoprenaline the shift reaches a maximum. Further increase of the isoprenaline concentration is without effect—in other words, the curves become stationary. The magnitude of the maximal effect that can be obtained with methacholine is not influenced.

Figure 15 gives a set of theoretical curves calculated according to Equation (88). It is clear that the overall picture is very different from that in Figure 14. The theoretical curves do not become stationary, whereas the magnitude of the maximal effect of the

---

[7] This is worth mentioning, since in the equations describing simple agonism, E_{max} is defined as "the maximal effect obtainable with a drug of this type", i.e. of the same type as the agonist in question (ARIËNS et al., 1964a). In other words, there E_{max} is the maximal effect obtainable via the *receptor system* concerned.

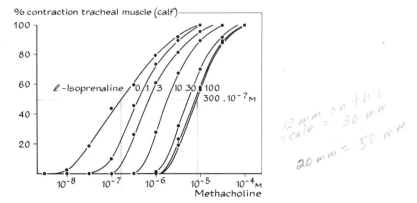

Fig. 14. Experimental concentration-effect curves of methacholine in presence of increasing concentrations of 1-isoprenaline. Note that characteristics of this set of curves agree with these of set of theoretical curves given in Figure 18. Lower concentrations of the functional antagonist cause a parallel shift of methacholine curves, but shift soon reaches a maximum. Magnitude of maximal effect of methacholine not influenced

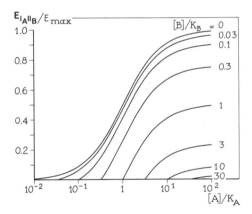

Fig. 15. Theoretical concentration-effect curves of agonist A ($\alpha = 1$) in presence of increasing concentrations of functional antagonist B ($\beta = 1$), calculated according to Equation (88). Effects E_{I_A}/E_{max} and E_{II_B}/E_{max} were calculated according to normal equation for agonistic action [Eq. (18)]. Note that magnitude of maximal effect of agonist decreases as concentration of antagonist increases: curves are not shifted in a parallel manner and do not become stationary. Results differ essentially from set of experimental curves in Figure 14

agonist becomes smaller with increasing concentrations of the antagonist. Obviously here the predictions of the original model disagree with the experimental data. The conclusion that the model had to be revised therefore was inevitable.

Reconsideration of the model of functional antagonism as expressed in Equation (88) led to the supposition that one factor in particular might be responsible for the observed discrepancy with the experimental result (Van den Brink, 1971). To elucidate this it is necessary to touch again on the subject of reserve in the agonistic system.

On p. 205 the concept receptor reserve was introduced. In its definition the overall relation between stimulus and final effect was considered. However, the same concept of a reserve can be applied to parts of the stimulus-effect chain. A reserve may exist in the relation between stimulus and a subeffect (a subeffect is an event occurring in the stimulus-effect chain before the final effect), between two consecutive subeffects or between a subeffect and the final effect. In general it can be said that a relation between a causative and a resultant factor has a reserve when the latter can reach its maximal value at a submaximal value of the former.

Equation (88) shows that the magnitude of the final effect $E_{I_A II_B}$ is supposed to be linearly dependent on the magnitudes of E_{I_A} and E_{II_B}. The maximal value of $E_{I_A II_B}$ can be reached only if the value of E_{I_A} is maximal: the relation between E_{I_A} and $E_{I_A II_B}$ has no reserve. In other words, the model implicitly supposes that reserves—if present at all—occur only in those parts of the stimulus-effect chains which the two receptor-effector systems do not share, so that they have no influence on the functional interaction proper. However, there is no reason to assume that this would be generally the case. The conclusion must be that Equation (88) only gives a description of a special case of functional antagonism.

A schematic representation of the model of functional antagonism published by ARIËNS supports this notion (1969). The scheme in question, adapted to cover both antagonism and synergism, is reproduced in Figure 16a. It should be compared with the more general model of functional interaction given in Figure 16b. In the latter scheme P_{I_A} and P_{II_B} are the last subeffects in the stimulus-effect chains of A and B, respectively, which the two systems do not have in common, whereas $P_{I_A II_B}$ is the first subeffect, the magnitude of which is dependent on both S_{I_A} and S_{II_B} (S_{I_A} being the stimulus created by the interaction of A and receptors of type R_I, S_{II_B} the stimulus caused by the interaction of B and receptors of type R_{II}).

The total stimulus-effect chain can be divided into three parts, which, theoretically, all may or may not have a reserve:

I. The formation of P_{I_A} and P_{II_B} (in the original model: of E_{I_A} and E_{II_B}) as a result of the stimuli S_{I_A} and S_{II_B}, respectively. This part precedes the functional

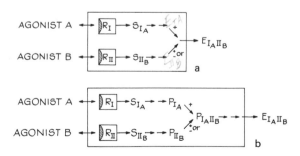

Fig. 16a and b. Schematic representation of two models of functional interactions. Figure 16a (adapted from ARIËNS, 1969) represents old model (top), Figure 16b (bottom) shows adapted version which allows for reserves in second and/or third part of stimulus-effect chain (see text). Note that original model is a special case of relations covered by new model

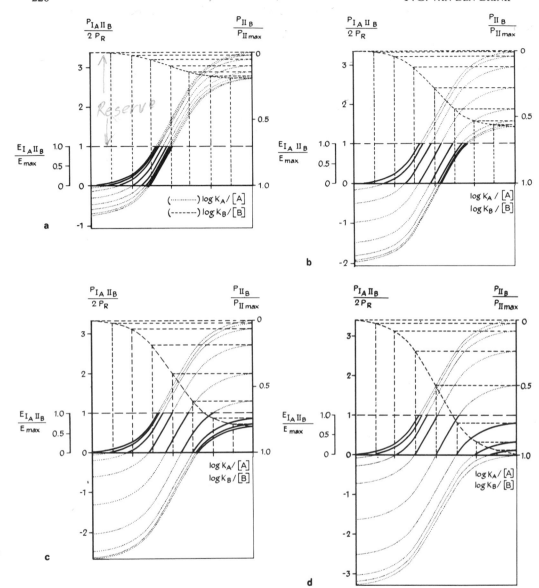

Fig. 17a—h. Diagrams showing theoretical consequences of combinations of functional antagonists with different potencies, according to Equation (92) plus assumptions concerning subeffect-effect relations made in text. Graphs were drawn with supposition that $\alpha = 1$, $p = 3\,^1/_3$, and $q = -3\,^1/_3$. Figures 17a—d give sets of concentration-effect curves of agonist A in presence of increasing concentrations of functional antagonist B; values of β are 0.2, 0.6, 0.8, and 1, respectively. [A] increases continuously from $0.01\,K_A$ to $100\,K_A$ (dotted line: concentration-subeffect curve; continuous line: concentration-effect curve); [B] increases with steps of a factor $10^{\frac{1}{2}}$ from $0.01\,K_B$ to $100\,K_B$ (interrupted lines). Figures 17e—h give sets of concentration-effect curves of functional antagonist B in presence of increasing concentrations of agonist A; values of β again are 0.2, 0.6, 0.8, and 1, respectively. [B] increases continuously from $0.01\,K_B$ to $100\,K_B$ (interrupted line: concentration-subeffect curve; continuous line: concentration-effect curve); [A] increases with steps of a factor $10^{\frac{1}{2}}$ from $0.01\,K_A$ to $100\,K_A$ (dotted lines). For discussion of sets of theoretical curves, see text

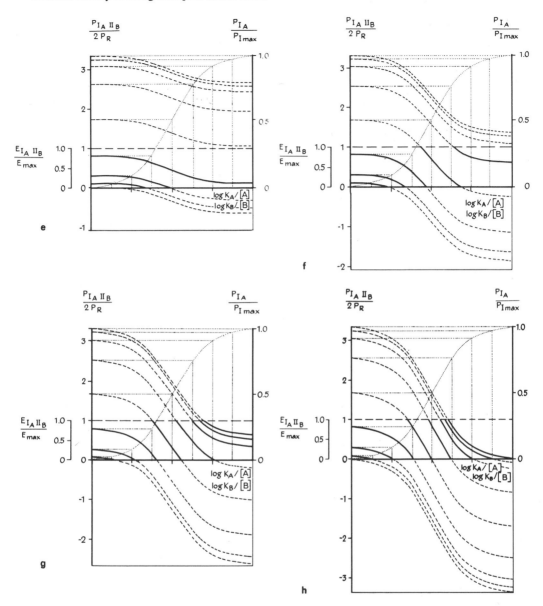

interaction proper. The question whether it has a reserve is immaterial with respect to our problem: although the presence or absence of a reserve may have an influence on the shape of the individual curves, it cannot influence the *character* of the set of curves predicted by the models of functional interaction under consideration.

II. The formation of $P_{I_A II_B}$ as a result of the subeffects P_{I_A} and P_{II_B}. This part is the functional interaction proper.

III. The formation of the final effect $E_{I_A II_B}$ as a result of the subeffect $P_{I_A II_B}$.

In the original model, parts II and III were taken together [see Eqs. (87—88)]. In the case of functional antagonism the relation was supposed to be linear and in that of functional synergism it was nonlinear, but in neither case the relation had a reserve. It was obvious, therefore, that the consequences of the presence of a reserve in this relation had to be examined.

In order to do this, it is necessary to make explicit assumptions concerning the relations in the three parts of the stimulus-effect chain, so that they can be represented by mathematical equations. Theoretically many different nonlinear functions can be assumed for both part II and III, but since we have no information about the true physiological relations, the choice is necessarily arbitrary. It seemed justified, therefore, to test the model with assumptions that would realize the essential difference between the original and the new model, but which would also be as simple as possible.

As mentioned, the presence of a reserve in part I of the stimulus-effect chain has no consequences for the functional model as such. It was assumed, therefore, that part I can be described with the normal equation for agonistic action:

$$\frac{P_{I_A}}{P_{I_{max}}} = \frac{\alpha}{1 + \frac{K_A}{[A]}} \quad \text{and} \quad \frac{P_{II_B}}{P_{II_{max}}} = \frac{\beta}{1 + \frac{K_B}{[B]}}. \tag{89, 90}$$

This implies a linear stimulus-subeffect relation.

The second part, which represents the functional interaction proper, likewise is supposed to be linear:

$$\frac{P_{I_A II_B}}{2P_R} = p\frac{P_{I_A}}{P_{I_{max}}} + q\frac{P_{II_B}}{P_{II_{max}}} \tag{91}$$

in which $p = P_{I_{max}}/2P_R$ and $q = P_{II_{max}}/2P_R$. The value P_R is the reference value of the subeffect $P_{I_A II_B}$, defined as that value of $P_{I_A II_B}$ which corresponds with the final effect $\frac{1}{2}E_{max}$. (An analogous reference value was used in the definition of α^S in the model of agonistic action; see Equation (19), p. 187.) The reason for taking P_R as a reference value instead of P_{max} (the maximal value that $P_{I_A II_B}$ can attain) is that the sum of $p \cdot P_{I_A}/P_{I_{max}}$ and $q \cdot P_{II_B}/P_{II_{max}}$ should be able to attain values larger than 1.

Equation (91) can be combined with Equations (89) and (90) to give

$$\frac{P_{I_A II_B}}{2P_R} = p\frac{\alpha}{1 + \frac{K_A}{[A]}} + q\frac{\beta}{1 + \frac{K_B}{[B]}}. \tag{92}$$

This equation, which covers part I and part II of the stimulus-effect chain, does not yet allow for a reserve. The relation describing part III therefore should do so. In the first instance this was realized by the simple assumption that $E_{I_A II_B}/E_{max} = P_{I_A II_B}/2P_R$ if $0 \leqslant P_{I_A II_B} \leqslant 2P_R$, but that $E_{I_A II_B}/E_{max} = 1$ if $P_{I_A II_B}$ is larger than $2P_R$. In addition it was supposed that $E_{I_A II_B} = 0$ if $P_{I_A II_B} < 0$. The fact that the model allows $P_{I_A II_B}$ to attain negative values may be an anomaly without real meaning, but it is also possible that this has its counterpart in reality, for instance if $P_{I_A II_B}$ has a spontaneous resting value of a certain magnitude and changes would be measured with respect to this resting value.

Figure 17 gives the elaboration of the adapted model [Equation (92) plus the above-mentioned assumptions concerning the subeffect-effect relation] for the case of functional antagonism. In Figures 17a—d, sets of theoretical curves of the agonist A in the presence of various concentrations of the functional antagonist B are presented. In the first two cases, in which the maximal value of P_{II_B} is smaller than the reserve in the agonistic system, the effect curves are shifted over a smaller of larger distance before they become stationary, whereas in the third case, $P_{II_{B_{max}}}$ being larger than the reserve but not large enough to prevent the realization of the subeffect $P_{I_AII_B}$ completely, the curves are shifted and subsequently depressed before they become stationary. In the fourth case, $P_{II_{B_{max}}}$ being large enough to prevent the formation of $P_{I_AII_B}$, the curves are shifted and subsequently depressed until they pass completely below the ordinate base-line. This means that in this case even maximal concentrations of A will be rendered ineffective by a sufficiently high concentration of B.

The Figures 17 e—h give sets of theoretical curves of the functional antagonist B in the presence of various concentrations of the agonist A. In the first case the antagonistic curves are raised and soon pass above the line of maximal effect. This means that with a sufficiently high concentration of A (viz. if the reserve created by A is too large to be completely eliminated by B) the presence of maximal concentrations of B is without visible effect. In the second case the picture is analogous, but the antagonistic curves seem to be shifted towards higher concentration ranges of B before they pass above the line of maximal effect. In the third case, the maximal value of P_{II_B} being larger than the reserve in the agonistic system but smaller than $P_{I_{max}}$, the curves are shifted to the right and raised a certain amount before they become stationary, whereas in the fourth case the curves are shifted and become stationary without being raised.

As may be clear from the discussed figures, the shifting of the curves is a phenomenon that essentially differs from the true shifting observed in competitive and metaffinoid antagonism. In fact the subeffect curve is just moved up and down, but since in each case a different part of this curve is translated into effect, the effect curves may show a pattern of shifting.

Since the theoretical results shown in Figure 17a and b strongly resemble the experimental results in Figure 14, it appeared that the new model was a step in the right direction. A further refinement was realized by making a more realistic assumption about the subeffect-effect relation, viz. that the effect is proportional to the subeffect $P_{I_AII_B}$ up to about 95 percent of E_{max}, and with greater values of $P_{I_AII_B}$ approaches E_{max} asymptotically. Mathematically this assumption was very closely approximated by using the following equation:

$$E = P - \frac{1}{20}\ln(1 + e^{20(P-1)}) \tag{93}$$

in which $E = E_{I_AII_B}/E_{max}$ and $P = P_{I_AII_B}/2P_R$ [8].

---

[8] To avoid misunderstanding, it may be stressed that the Equations (92) and (93) should not be understood as a detailed description of the physiological relations. These are unknown. Equation (93) in itself is arbitrary, but it is acceptable for our limited purpose, which is the calculation of sets of theoretical concentration-effect curves, since the *character* of these sets is not dependent on the exact nature of the subeffect-effect relation but on the presence of a reserve as such. Any relation which implies the possibility of a reserve and which results in a theoretical curve with a shape sufficiently similar to that observed in the experiment, would serve our purpose just as well as the relation chosen.

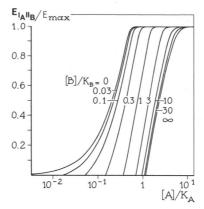

Fig. 18. Theoretical concentration-effect curves of agonist A in presence of increasing concentrations of functional antagonist B, calculated according to Equations (92) and (93) ($p\alpha = 3$, $q\beta = -1.6$). Note that curves are shifted to right in parallel manner and become stationary at higher concentrations of B, whereas magnitude of maximal effect does not change

By means of a computer program based on Equations (92) and (93) the consequences of the new model were explored. Figure 18 gives an example of the results. In this case of functional antagonism the theoretical curves are shifted in a parallel manner and become stationary at higher concentrations of the antagonist; the maximal effect does not change. Comparison with Figure 14 shows a striking agreement between the character of this set of theoretical curves and that of the set of curves obtained experimentally. Next it was checked whether the theoretical curves based on the new model would also correspond with the experimental results in a case of functional synergism. Figure 19 gives such a set of theoretical curves; Figure 20 shows a set of curves obtained in the experiment. Again the agreement between theory and experimental results was quite satisfactory. The fact that the lower parts of the

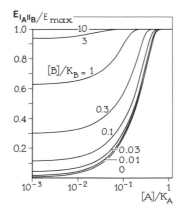

Fig. 19. Theoretical concentration-effect curves of agonist A in presence of increasing concentrations of functional synergist B, calculated according to Equations (92) and (93) ($p\alpha = 3$, $q\beta = 1.25$). Compare with experimental results in Figure 20

compare with curves for competitive synergism, Fig 4, p. 194

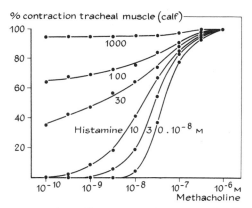

Fig. 20. Experimental concentration-effect curves of methacholine in presence of increasing concentrations of histamine. Compare with set of theoretical curves in Figure 19

experimental curves are shifted slightly to the left before they are raised may be the result of a threshold in the stimulus-effect relation (ARIËNS et al., 1964c). In the case of synergism it appears that a set of theoretical curves based on the adapted model (Fig. 19) does not show characteristic differences from a set of curves based on the original model (cf. Fig. 40 *in* ARIËNS et al., 1964b).

B. Implications of the New Model of Functional Interaction

From the results discussed in the previous section, it appears that the new model of functional interaction meets the requirements:

1. It describes both functional synergism and antagonism with the same equation. If p and q in Equation (92) have the same sign, we are dealing with synergism; if p and q have opposite signs the equation represents functional antagonism.

2. A satisfactory agreement exists between sets of theoretical concentration-effect curves predicted by the model and experimental sets of curves obtained in well-known cases of functional synergism and antagonism. Moreover, these sets of theoretical curves could be obtained with realistic assumptions concerning the affinity and intrinsic activity values.

3. The model predicts the occurrence of some sets of concentration-effect curves with very typical characteristics. Thus it was possible to put it to the test with new, critical experiments.

Since the introduction of the model, the occurrence of sets of curves with characteristics as referred to above has been verified experimentally (VAN DEN BRINK, 1973b; OFFERMEIER and VAN DEN BRINK, 1974). Here a single example has to suffice: in the case of functional antagonism between histamine and 1-isoprenaline on the isolated guinea pig ileum, the histamine curves are shifted and become stationary after being depressed to about 80% of their maximal height (Fig. 21a); repetition of this experiment in reversed form in other guinea pigs produced isoprenaline curves which are raised but become stationary without passing above the line of maximal effect (Fig. 21b). These experimental results should be compared with the theoretical curves

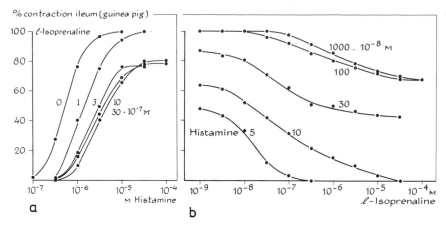

Fig. 21a and b. Functional antagonism between histamine and l-isoprenaline, tested on isolated guinea pig ileum. Figure 21a: experimental concentration-effect curves of histamine in presence of increasing concentrations of l-isoprenaline. Curves are shifted over a relatively small distance and become stationary after being depressed to about 80% of their original height. Figure 21b: experimental concentration-effect curves of l-isoprenaline in presence of increasing concentrations of histamine. Curves clearly show that in this case l-isoprenaline behaves as a partial functional antagonist of histamine. Note similarity of these experimental results to sets of theoretical curves given in Figure 22

in Figure 22. For a number of other experimental results which tally with the predictions of the model, the reader must refer to the original publications.

In the preceding section it was already mentioned that in the case of functional synergism the predictions of the new model do not differ much from those of the original model. It may be added that there is not much difference with sets of curves based on the model of competitive synergism of two full agonists either (compare Fig. 19 with Fig. 4). However, as pointed out by Ariëns et al. (1964b) the predictions of the original functional model and the competitive model are essentially different if it is supposed that a full agonist is combined with a partial agonist. As can be seen by comparing Figure 23 with Figure 5a, this holds also for the new functional model.

A last point to be discussed here concerns the intrinsic activity of functional antagonists. If a just maximal (concentration) of a test organ caused by, e.g., a cholinomimetic drug like methacholine can be antagonized completely by a β-adrenoceptor-agonist, the latter is indicated as a full agonist, and if the maximal antagonism is less than complete, it is called a partial agonist. With respect to β-adrenoceptor-induced relaxation this differentiation was the only distinction based on intrinsic activity that the original model allowed. It is rather improbable, however, that all full agonists would have equal intrinsic activities: if applied at concentrations which cause a maximal degree of interaction with β-adrenoceptors, they may realize reserves of different magnitudes in the relaxation system.

That this indeed is the case can be clearly observed in experiments in which the curve of the spasmogen is shifted in a parallel way by a β-adrenoceptor functional antagonist. According to the new model, the magnitude of the maximal shift is a simple and unequivocal measure of the intrinsic activity of the functional antagonist (the

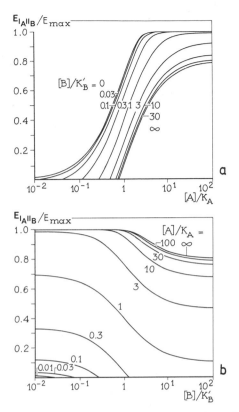

Fig. 22a and b. Theoretical concentration-effect curves of agonist A in presence of increasing concentrations of functional antagonist B (Fig. 22a) and of functional antagonist B in presence of increasing concentrations of agonist A (Fig. 22b), calculated according to equations 92 and 93 ($p\alpha = 1.4$, $q\beta = -0.6$). Note similarity to sets of experimental curves in Figure 21a and b, respectively

maximal shift is comparable to the maximal height of the curve of a normal agonist, cf. Figs. 17a and b).

It follows that here a differentiation between two practical expressions of intrinsic activity is necessary. If B is the functional antagonist under consideration, the expression of intrinsic activity β^E equals $E_{II_{B_{max}}}/E_{II_{max}}$, in which $E_{II_{B_{max}}}$ is the maximal relaxation that can be caused by the interaction of B with its receptors and $E_{II_{max}}$ is the maximal relaxation that can be caused via these receptors (both in presence of that concentration of the agonist A which causes a just-maximal contraction of the organ). The magnitude β^E is completely analogous to the α^E used in the agonistic model. For all full functional antagonists β^E equals 1, so that the presence of a reserve in the antagonistic system does not find expression in this value.

The other expression of intrinsic activity, which may be indicated as β^P, is defined as $P_{II_{B_{max}}}/P_{II_{max}}$. Suppose that two drugs, B and C, which belong to the same family of functional antagonists, cause parallel shifts of the agonistic concentration-effect curve with different maxima. If the assumptions made in the model of functional interaction

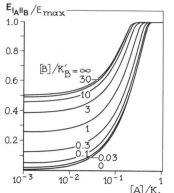

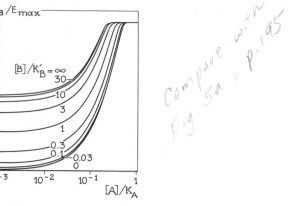

Fig. 23. Theoretical concentration-effect curves of agonist A in presence of increasing concentrations of functional synergist B, calculated according to Equations (92) and (93). B is a partial agonist ($p\alpha = 3$, $q\beta = 0.5$). Note difference with Figure 5a, which shows results of combining a full and a partial agonist in a case of competitive interaction

are correct, it follows that the ratio of these maximal shifts equals the ratio of $P_{II_{B_{max}}}$ and $P_{II_{C_{max}}}$, and, therefore, the ratio of β^P and γ^P. There is no ready way to place these intrinsic activity values on a normalized scale (see p. 185); it is possible, however, to express the β^P's of drugs belonging to one family in relation to one another. For instance, the β^P-values of norfenefrine, l-isoprenaline and l-Cc 25, measured in calf isolated tracheal muscle, are in the ratio of 0.39 to 1 to 1.37 (Van den Brink, 1973b). In β-adrenoceptor structure-activity relation studies such data are highly relevant.

VIII. Plural Affinities

As mentioned before, many drugs have affinity to more than one kind of receptor. In this connection a number of theoretical possibilities, which are borne out in the experiment, have been described (see, e.g., Ariëns et al., 1964b and Van den Brink, 1966). Here a single example may suffice, viz. the case of a drug being a competitive antagonist of a certain agonist and at the same time being able to antagonize the effect of this agonist by means of metactoid antagonism.

If it is supposed that the affinity to the receptors of the metactoid system is higher than to the receptors of the agonist, and if the metactoid system has the possibility of nullifying the effect of the agonist completely (as is usually the case, see p. 204), then the competitive antagonism will stay undetected in the experiment: the effect of the agonist will be reduced to zero before the competition can express itself. If, however, the affinity to the receptors of the agonist is the higher one, a complicated set of concentration-effect curves is obtained, showing mainly a shift with lower concentrations of the antagonist, but a shift plus a depression at the same time with higher ones.

Theoretical curves demonstrating these phenomena (Fig. 24) may be obtained on the basis of an equation which is a simple combination of Equation (24), describing the competitive antagonism, with Equation (44) which represents the noncompetitive

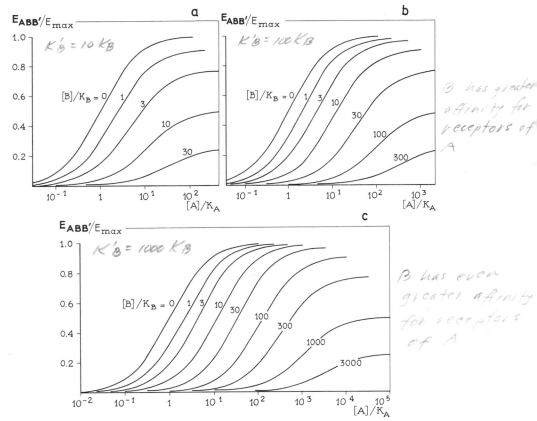

Fig. 24a—c. Plural affinities. Theoretical concentration-effect curves of agonist A ($\alpha=1$) in presence of increasing concentrations of drug B which is a competitive antagonist and a metactoid antagonist, calculated according to Equation (94) ($\beta'=1$, $p=0$). Affinity of B to receptors of agonist is higher than to receptors of noncompetitive system. How far curve is shifted to right before a measurable depression occurs depends on ratio of K_B and K'_B. Figure 24a: $K'_B=10\ K_B$. Figure 24b: $K'_B=100\ K_B$. Figure 24c: $K'_B=1000\ K_B$

interaction:

$$\frac{E_{ABB'}}{E_{max}} = \left\{1+(p-1)\frac{\beta'}{1+\dfrac{K'_B}{[B]}}\right\}\frac{\alpha}{1+\left(1+\dfrac{[B]}{K_B}\right)\dfrac{K_A}{[A]}}. \tag{94}$$

In practice, sets of curves as presented in Figure 24 are often found. More exceptional is the combination of competitive and *incomplete* metactoid antagonism in one drug. Figure 25 gives an example; the incomplete metactoid antagonism expresses itself as a decrease of the maximal height of the agonist curve to about 60 percent of E_{max}, on which the parallel shift caused by competitive antagonism is superimposed (compare with the theoretical concentration-effect curves for incomplete metactoid antagonism in Fig. 8a).

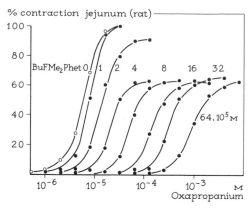

Fig. 25. Plural affinities. Experimental concentration-effect curves of cholinomimetic substance oxapropanium in presence of increasing concentrations of 2-butyl, 4-[N,N-dimethyl, N-(2-phenylethyl) aminomethyl] dioxolane bromide (BuFMe$_2$Phet). Note incomplete metactoid antagonism which expresses itself in a decrease of maximal height of curves to about 60%, on which a competitive antagonism is superimposed as a parallel shift (VAN ROSSUM, 1958)

Theoretically, sets of curves which are nearly identical with those in Figure 24 may also be obtained with a drug which combines metactoid antagonism with a second type of antagonism which is not competitive but results in parallel shifting of the agonist curve, like metaffinoid antagonism or functional antagonism if the agonistic system has a reserve (see above). This would be the case if, in the presence of increasing concentrations of such a drug, the metactoid depression of the agonist curve is complete before the metaffinoid or functional shifting approaches its maximal value.

The interpretation of sets of curves as presented in Figure 24 may not be easy. It is possible to distinguish competitive shifting from metaffinoid or functional shifting, but this may require special experiments (see, e.g., OFFERMEIER and VAN DEN BRINK, 1974). Furthermore, as shown earlier, the action of a purely metactoid antagonist on an agonistic system with a receptor reserve also may result in a shift of the curve—although not an exactly parallel one—before depression occurs. It is true that the sets of theoretical curves representing this situation show certain differences from the curves based on Equation (94) (compare Fig. 24 with Fig. 9, curves d', c', b' a, followed by depression), but the experimental sets of curves may look rather similar.

If the antagonist has very different affinities to the two kinds of receptors, the situation will be clear, for in this case there will be a perfectly parallel shift of the curve over a considerable distance before depression occurs (Fig. 24c). This is a phenomenon that cannot be imitated by a metactoid antagonist in presence of a receptor reserve. If, however, the affinities do not differ very much (Fig. 24a) it may become rather hard to detect the underlying mechanism from the set of experimental concentration-effect curves. Fortunately the mechanism can also be elucidated by other means. The experiments may be repeated with a partial agonist as a reference compound, so that the existence of a receptor reserve in the system is excluded; or else the receptor reserve may be nullified beforehand by incubation of the isolated organ with an irreversible competitive antagonist (FURCHGOTT, 1954, 1955), a technique also known as "non-equilibrium blockade" (NICKERSON, 1956, 1957) or "unsurmountable blockade"

(GADDUM et al., 1955). (See also p. 239.) But even without experiments of this kind a reasonable surmise about the underlying mechanism may be obtained by comparing the sets of curves in question with the curves obtained in the presence of close structural analogs of the antagonist.

IX. Numerical Expressions of Intrinsic Activity and Affinity

It was shown before that the activity of a drug may depend on two properties: its affinity to certain receptors, and the intrinsic activity which determines to what degree the interaction with the receptors results in a stimulus, and thus in an effect. In practice it proves convenient to express these magnitudes as numbers. In the last few sections of this chapter, the derivation of such numerical expressions will be discussed.

On p. 185 a numerical expression of the (relative) intrinsic activity was introduced, viz. the constant α. The affinity on the other hand has been introduced as a concept only, so that first a measure should be chosen in which this characteristic can be expressed. Since the affinity is the tendency of the drug to associate with the receptor, it is inversely proportional with the tendency of dissociation of the pharmacon-receptor complex. In the law of mass action, and in all equations that were derived from it, this tendency is expressed in the dissociation constant, a magnitude with the dimension of a concentration. It is plausible, therefore, to express the affinity as the reciprocal of this dissociation constant, in other words, as $1/K_A$. Since, however, the concentration-effect curves from which K_A may be derived are plotted on a logarithmic concentration scale, it is more practical to use a logarithmic measure of the affinity, viz. $\log 1/K_A$ or $-\log K_A$ (pK_A). Thus the negative logarithm of the molar concentration that corresponds with the dissociation constant of the drug is used as a measure of the affinity.

As may be clear from the discussion of the presuppositions in the agonistic model (cf. pp. 191—192) it is rather improbable that the exact values of α and pK_A (β and pK_B, etc.) can be found from the experimental curves. It is possible, however, to calculate practical affinity and intrinsic activity constants from these curves, constants which approximate the true α and pK_A and which equal these magnitudes if a number of conditions are fulfilled. These constants are α^E (ARIËNS, 1954; VAN ROSSUM, 1958), α^S (VAN ROSSUM, 1966a, b), pD_2 (MILLER et al., 1948; ARIËNS and VAN ROSSUM, 1957) and $pK_A{}^S$ (VAN ROSSUM, 1966a, b) for the agonists,[9] pA_2 (SCHILD, 1947, 1949) for the competitive antagonists, and β'^E and pD_2' (ARIËNS and VAN ROSSUM, 1957; SCHILD, 1957) for the metactoid antagonist. The α^S, $pK_A{}^S$, and pA_2 are better approximations of the true values than the α^E, pD_2, β^E, and pD_2' since the degree of approximation is independent of the stimulus-effect relations in the systems in question (see pp. 187, 240 and 196). Also for metaffinoid drugs an intrinsic activity constant β'^E and an affinity constant pD_2' may be used; their derivations differ from those of the β'^E and the pD_2' of a metactoid drug. Finally, for drugs which act functionally, two measures of intrinsic activity with different applicabilities, β^E and β^P, have been proposed (VAN DEN BRINK, 1973b).

---

[9] α^E was introduced by ARIËNS as α (see footnote on p. 186). The $pK_A{}^S$-value was introduced by VAN ROSSUM as pK_{RA}; this notation has not been accepted since it gives the false impression that this value, as determined experimentally, would simply be the negative logarithm of the dissociation constant.

A. Calculation of α^E and pD_2

The value of α^E is calculated according to Equation (17):

$$\alpha^E = \frac{E_{A_{max}}}{E_{max}}.$$

Under the conditions discussed above, including a linear stimulus-effect relation, pD_2 equals $-\log K_A$. Under the same conditions Equation (11) applies:

$$\frac{E_A}{E_{A_{max}}} = \frac{1}{1 + \dfrac{K_A}{[A]}}.$$

From this it follows that

$$\frac{K_A}{[A]} = \frac{E_{A_{max}}}{E_A} - 1$$

$$\log K_A = \log[A] + \log\left(\frac{E_{A_{max}}}{E_A} - 1\right)$$

$$pD_2 = -\log[A] - \log\left(\frac{E_{A_{max}}}{E_A} - 1\right). \tag{95}$$

Since $[A]$, $E_{A_{max}}$, and E_A are known, the value of the pD_2 can be found from this equation.

It may be noted, that if

$$E_A = \tfrac{1}{2}E_{A_{max}}$$

it follows that

$$\frac{E_{A_{max}}}{E_A} - 1 = 1$$

and

$$\log\left(\frac{E_{A_{max}}}{E_A} - 1\right) = 0.$$

In this case the pD_2 is identical with the negative logarithm of the given concentration of A. The pD_2 may be defined on this basis: it is the negative logarithm of the molar concentration of the agonist which produces 50 percent of the maximal effect of the drug on the receptor-effector system concerned. If, for instance, the concentration corresponding with the effect $\tfrac{1}{2}E_{A_{max}}$ is 10^{-8} molar, the pD_2-value is 8. On this basis the pD_2 can be determined more readily. The 50% point of a concentration-effect curve is projected on the concentration axis; probably the projection will be found somewhere between the points indicating the whole degrees of ten. The distance to the nearest point at the left is measured, and is e.g. 0.4 unit, whereas the distance between two

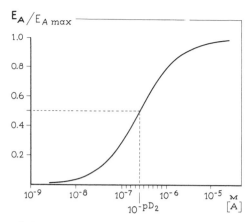

Fig. 26. Determination of the pD_2-value from a (theoretical) concentration-effect curve of agonist A. The pD_2 is identical with negative logarithm of molar concentration corresponding with effect $0.5 E_{A_{max}}$

successive degrees of ten is 1 unit (see before). Since the axis is logarithmic for the concentrations, it is linear for the exponents, so if the nearest point at the left indicates a concentration of 10^{-7} molar, the sought concentration is $10^{-7+0.4}$ or $10^{-6.6}$. The pD_2 is 6.6 (Fig. 26).

B. Calculation of pK_A^S and α^S

As discussed already on p. 187, α^S equals $\frac{1}{2}\phi\alpha$ if certain general suppositions are fulfilled. The stimulus-effect relation should be "drug-independent", but special presuppositions about the character of the stimulus-effect relation have not to be made. Likewise, the pK_A^S-value will equal the pK_A if these conditions are fulfilled (apart from measuring faults).

The calculation of the pK_A^S and α^S of an agonistic drug is possible with the aid of a technique of reducing the concentration of reactive specific receptors in the organ. This may be accomplished by incubating the organ with an irreversible competitive antagonist of the agonist in question during an appropriate period of time (FURCHGOTT, 1954, 1955; GADDUM et al., 1955; NICKERSON, 1956, 1957). First a normal concentration-effect curve is made; the agonist is washed away and the organ is incubated with the irreversible competitive antagonist; then after washing away the molecules of the latter which are not irreversibly bound to the organ, the agonistic curve is made anew. If the stimulus-effect relation of the agonistic system is perfectly linear, the second curve will be less steep and reduced in height but otherwise in the same position on the concentration axis as the original one; if, however, the stimulus-effect relation is nonlinear the slope of the second curve may be less steep with or without a reduction of the maximal height and the curve may be shifted to higher concentrations. Figure 27a gives a theoretical example: in calculating the original curve a it was supposed that the stimulus-effect relation is linear up to an effect of about 85% of E_{max} and that a receptor reserve exists, whereas the interrupted line indicates the further path of the curve for the case where the stimulus-effect relation would have been directly proportional along the whole range; curve *b* is the concentration-effect curve of the same agonist after elimination of 50% of the specific receptors (cf. Figs. 8 and 9). The suppositions made here are arbitrary, the stimulus-effect relation does not play a role in what follows.

If an effect with a given magnitude was caused by the concentration $[A]_1$ before the incubation, a higher concentration, $[A]_{i1}$, will correspond with this effect after that (Fig. 27a). According to Equation (3) the connection of these concentrations with the corresponding relative receptor occupation will be as follows:

$$\frac{[RA]_1}{[r]} = \frac{1}{1 + \dfrac{K_A}{[A]_1}}$$

and

$$\frac{[RA]_{i1}}{[r]_i} = \frac{1}{1 + \dfrac{K_A}{[A]_{i1}}}$$

in which $[r]$ is the total concentration of specific receptors and $[r]_i$ the total concentration of specific receptors which are not occupied by the irreversible competitive antagonist after the incubation. The ratio of these two concentrations ($[r]_i/[r]$) will be called g_i.

Since equal effects in the same organ may be supposed to correspond with equal values for $[RA]$, $[RA]_1$ equals $[RA]_{i1}$ and thus

$$\frac{1}{1 + \dfrac{K_A}{[A]_1}} = g_i \frac{1}{1 + \dfrac{K_A}{[A]_{i1}}}.$$

This equation may be generalized to hold for all pairs of concentrations corresponding with effects of the same magnitude, one concentration before and the other after the incubation:

$$\frac{1}{1 + \dfrac{K_A}{[A]}} = g_i \frac{1}{1 + \dfrac{K_A}{[A]_i}}.$$

The equation is further developed as follows:

$$g_i + g_i \frac{K_A}{[A]} = 1 + \frac{K_A}{[A]_i}$$

$$g_i \frac{K_A}{[A]} - \frac{K_A}{[A]_i} = 1 - g_i.$$

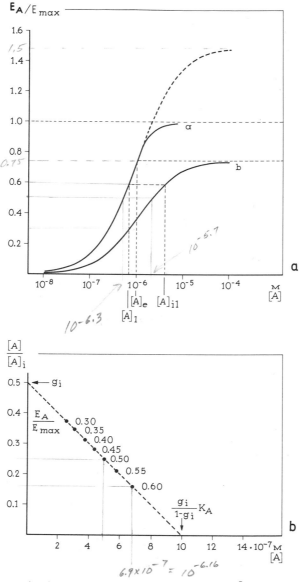

Fig. 27a and b. Determination of magnitudes from which the $pK_A{}^S$-value and α^S-value of agonist A can be calculated. In calculating the theoretical concentration-effect curve a in Figure 27a it was supposed that the stimulus-effect relation is linear up to an effect of about 85% of E_{max} and that a receptor reserve exists, whereas the interrupted line indicates the further path of curve for the case that stimulus-effect relation would have been directly proportional along whole range; curve b is concentration-effect curve of same agonist after elimination of 50% of specific receptors by means of an irreversible competitive antagonist. Figure 27a: determination of concentrations [A] and $[A]_i$ which correspond with effects of same magnitude before and after elimination of a proportion of specific receptors. Figure 27b: determination of g_i, being ratio of total concentration of specific receptors which are not occupied by irreversible competitive antagonist after incubation with this compound and total concentration of specific receptors before this incubation (for further details see text)

All terms are divided by K_A and multiplied with $[A]$:

$$g_i - \frac{[A]}{[A]_i} = [A]\frac{1 - g_i}{K_A}$$

or

$$\frac{[A]}{[A]_i} + \frac{1 - g_i}{K_A}[A] - g_i = 0 . \tag{96}$$

As follows from this equation, the connection between the two variables $[A]/[A]_i$ and $[A]$ can be represented by a straight line (Fig. 27b). The point of intersection of this line with the ordinate represents g_i, the intersection with the abscissa $\frac{g_i}{1 - g_i}K_A$.

Thus in practice the $[A]$ and $[A]_i$ belonging to an effect of a certain magnitude may be determined from a pair of experimental curves and may be used to give one point of the line representing Equation (96); if this procedure is repeated for a number of different effects a number of points will be obtained, a straight line can be drawn through these points and the values of g_i and $\frac{g_i}{1 - g_i}K_A$ can be found by extrapolation. By substitution of the value of g_i in the other term a value of K_A can be determined (a value which can be considered right only under the above mentioned conditions); the negative logarithm of K_A determined in this way is the $pK_A{}^S$ (Van Rossum, 1966a, b).

The value of $\frac{g_i}{1 - g_i}K_A$ can also be found directly from the experimental curves: it is the value of $[A]$ which corresponds with $[A]/[A]_i = 0$ and thus with $[A]_i$ being infinitely large. If before the incubation $[A]_e$ is the concentration which corresponds with the effect that equals the maximal effect after the incubation (Fig. 27a), then

$$K_A = \frac{1 - g_i}{g_i}[A]_e .$$

In the example given in Figure 27, the $g_i = 0.5$ and the $pK_A{}^S = 6.0$, whereas the pD_2 equals 6.30. In practice often much larger differences between $pK_A{}^S$ and pD_2 are found.

The procedure can be simplified by the use of tables connecting the ratio of the concentrations $[A]_i$ and $[A]$ directly to the magnitude of the shift.

The $pK_A{}^S$ being determined, the calculation of a numerical value of the α^S presents little difficulty. According to Equation (19)

$$\alpha^S = \frac{S_{A\text{max}}}{2S_{P\text{max}}} .$$

$S_{P\text{max}}$ is the stimulus which corresponds with the effect $\frac{1}{2}E_{\text{max}}$. The concentration of A needed to create this stimulus and thus the effect $\frac{1}{2}E_{\text{max}}$ may be called $[A]_{50}$.

Application of Equation (7) leads to

$$\frac{S_{P_{max}}}{S_{A_{max}}} = \frac{1}{1 + \dfrac{K_A}{[A]_{50}}}$$

and thus

$$2\alpha^S = 1 + \frac{K_A}{[A]_{50}} \qquad (97)$$

According to the foregoing the negative logarithm of the K_A in this formula is the $pK_A{}^S$; the negative logarithm of $[A]_{50}$ may be called the $pK_A{}^E$.

$$\log(2\alpha^S - 1) = pK_A{}^E - pK_A{}^S$$
$$\alpha^S = \tfrac{1}{2}(1 + 10^{(pK_A^E - pK_A^S)}). \qquad (98)$$

The $pK_A{}^E$ can be defined as the negative logarithm of the molar concentration of the agonist which produces 50 % of the maximal effect that can be caused by any member of the family in question. For full agonists this constant is equal to the pD_2, for partial agonists, however, it will have a different value.

By application of Equation (98) to the example given in Figure 27 an α^S which equals 1.5 is found.

C. Calculation of pA_2-values

For the calculation of the affinity constant of a competitive antagonist Equation (25) serves as starting-point:

$$\frac{[A]_2}{[A]_1} = 1 + \frac{[B]}{K_B} .$$

It follows that

$$K_B = \frac{[B]}{\dfrac{[A]_2}{[A]_1} - 1}$$

$$\log K_B = \log[B] - \log\left(\frac{[A]_2}{[A]_1} - 1\right)$$

$$pA_2 = -\log[B] + \log\left(\frac{[A]_2}{[A]_1} - 1\right). \qquad (99)$$

If logarithmic concentration-effect curves are used, the value of $\dfrac{[A]_2}{[A]_1}$ may be found directly from the shift. On p. 196 it was demonstrated that the shift, measured in

244 F.G. van den Brink

the correct unit, is equal to $\log \dfrac{[A]_2}{[A]_1}$ (Fig. 7). The correct unit is the distance which represents a difference in concentration of a factor 10. If the shift, measured in this way, is called s, from the equation

$$s = \log \frac{[A]_2}{[A]_1}$$

it follows that $\dfrac{[A]_2}{[A]_1} = 10^s$.

A table directly correlating the distance of the standardized curves with the corresponding value of $\log \left(\dfrac{[A]_2}{[A]_1} - 1 \right)$ is a useful help. In the table published by Van Rossum (1963) the distances are given in mm, one unit being 30 mm, whereas $\dfrac{[A]_2}{[A]_1}$ is indicated as x.

As can be seen from the equation derived above, the pA_2 is equal to the negative logarithm of the given concentration of the antagonist if $\log \left(\dfrac{[A]_2}{[A]_1} - 1 \right)$ equals zero. This is the case if $[A]_2 = 2[A]_1$. This datum offers the possibility of a practical definition of the pA_2: it is the negative logarithm of the molar antagonist concentration, in the presence of which twice the original agonist concentration is needed for the original effect.

It is inevitable that a certain experimental error is made when the shift of the concentration-effect curves is measured. For this reason it is desirable to use no shifts of less than a certain magnitude as starting-point for the calculation, otherwise the influence of this error may be too large. In practice, shifts of less than a factor three $\left(\dfrac{[A]_2}{[A]_1} < 3 \right)$ should not be used and, if possible, a shift of a factor ten or more is advisable.

D. Calculation of β'^E and pD_2'

The intrinsic activity constant of a metactoid sensitizer or antagonist is calculated according to Equation (46):

$$\beta'^E = \frac{E_{AB'_{max}} - E_A}{E_{AS'_{max}} - E_A}$$

whereas the intrinsic activity constant of a metaffinoid drug which acts according to Equation (55) may be obtained according to Equation (60):

$$\beta'^E = \frac{[A]_1/[A]_2 - 1}{[A]_1/[A]_3 - 1}.$$

For the calculation of the pD_2' of a metactoid compound, Equation (42) is a suited starting-point:

$$\frac{E_{AB'} - E_A}{E_{AS'_{max}} - E_A} = \frac{\beta'}{1 + \dfrac{K_B'}{[B]}} \cdot \qquad \beta'^E = \frac{E_{AB'max} - E_A}{E_{AS'max} - E_A}$$

In the derivation of this equation it was supposed that the metactoid "effect" is directly proportional to the magnitude of the metactoid stimulus and thus β'^E can be substituted in Equation (42):

$$\frac{E_{AB'} - E_A}{E_{AB'_{max}} - E_A} = \frac{1}{1 + \dfrac{K_B'}{[B]}}$$

$$\frac{K_B'}{[B]} = \frac{E_{AB'_{max}} - E_A}{E_{AB'} - E_A} - 1$$

$$\log K_B' = \log[B] + \log\left(\frac{E_{AB'_{max}} - E_A}{E_{AB'} - E_A} - 1\right)$$

$$pD_2' = -\log[B] - \log\left(\frac{E_{AB'_{max}} - E_A}{E_{AB'} - E_A} - 1\right). \qquad (100)$$

As was to be expected, this equation is quite analogous to the one derived for the pD_2. The pD_2' is equal to the negative logarithm of the given concentration of the metactoid drug, if the caused change in the effect of the agonist equals the half of the maximal change in this effect that can be caused with the metactoid drug in question. (If $(E_{AB'_{max}} - E_A)/(E_{AB'} - E_A) = 2$, the last term of Equation (100) equals zero.)

It should be appreciated that the value of $(E_{AB'_{max}} - E_A)/(E_{AB'} - E_A)$ is independent of the actual value of E_A. It has practical advantages to compare the maximal values of E_A, therefore to use Equation (100) in this form:

$$pD_2' = -\log[B] - \log\left(\frac{E_{A_{max}B'_{max}} - E_{A_{max}}}{E_{A_{max}B'} - E_{A_{max}}} - 1\right) \qquad (101)$$

This is especially true if the compound used is an antagonist with a dualism in action (see below).

If the metactoid compound is a complete metactoid antagonist, $E_{AB'_{max}}$ equals zero and Equation (100) may be written as

$$pD_2' = -\log[B] - \log\left(\frac{E_A}{E_A - E_{AB'}} - 1\right). \qquad (102)$$

Further remodeling leads to the original equation presented by Ariëns and Van Rossum (1957):

$$-\log\left(\frac{E_A}{E_A - E_{AB'}} - 1\right) = -\log\frac{E_{AB'}}{E_A - E_{AB'}} = \log\frac{E_A - E_{AB'}}{E_{AB'}} = \log\left(\frac{E_A}{E_{AB'}} - 1\right)$$

so that $pD_2' = -\log[B] + \log\left(\frac{E_A}{E_{AB'}} - 1\right)$.

Since the form of this equation suggests that the pD_2' corresponds more with the pA_2 than with the pD_2 it may obscure the fact that the noncompetitive compound can be formally seen as an agonist with regard to its own system. Therefore Equation (100) is thought to be preferable.

As for the affinity value of a metaffinoid compound which acts according to Equation (55), it should be stressed that the pD_2' does *not* equal the negative logarithm of the concentration of B which causes 50% of the maximal shift of the agonist curve that can be obtained with this drug. If $[A]_1$ is the agonist concentration which causes a certain (submaximal) effect in the absence of the metaffinoid drug B, whereas $[A]_2$ causes the same effect in the presence of $[B]$ and $[A]_3$ in the presence of $[B]_{max}$, so that $E_{A_1} = E_{A_2B} = E_{A_3B_{max}}$, it follows from Equation (18) and Equation (55) that

$$\frac{K_A}{[A]_1} = \frac{1}{1 + \dfrac{(q-1)\beta'}{1 + \dfrac{K_B'}{[B]}}} \cdot \frac{K_A}{[A]_2} = \frac{1}{1 + (q-1)\beta'} \cdot \frac{K_A}{[A]_3}$$

so that

$$\frac{(q-1)\beta'}{1 + \dfrac{K_B'}{[B]}} = \frac{[A]_1}{[A]_2} - 1$$

and

$$(q-1)\beta' = \frac{[A]_1}{[A]_3} - 1.$$

Combining these equations gives

$$\frac{1}{1 + \dfrac{K_B'}{[B]}} = \frac{[A]_1/[A]_2 - 1}{[A]_1/[A]_3 - 1}$$

$$\frac{K_B'}{[B]} = \frac{[A]_1/[A]_3 - 1}{[A]_1/[A]_2 - 1} - 1$$

$$\log K_B' = \log[B] + \log\left(\frac{[A]_1/[A]_3 - 1}{[A]_1/[A]_2 - 1} - 1\right)$$

$$pD_2' = -\log[B] - \log\left(\frac{[A]_1/[A]_3 - 1}{[A]_1/[A]_2 - 1} - 1\right). \tag{103}$$

It should be noted that $[A]_2$ and $[A]_3$ in this equation do not have the same meaning as in Equation (60) from which the metaffinoid β'^E-value was calculated.

E. Affinity and Intrinsic Activity Values for Functional Antagonists

A drug which acts as a functional synergist of some agonist is a normal agonist itself, and its affinity and intrinsic activity with respect to its receptor-effector system can be expressed as a pD_2- or $pK_A{}^S$-value and an α^E- or α^S-value (see pp. 238—243). If, however, the drug is a functional antagonist which, e.g., causes relaxation of an isolated smooth muscle pretreated with a spasmogenic agonist, it can also be considered an agonist, but the situation is more complicated. The necessity for two different expressions of intrinsic activity, β^E and β^P, for full functional antagonists of this type was discussed on p. 233. The β^P's of drugs belonging to one family can be expressed in relation to one another, but there is no ready way to place them on a normalized scale. This would be possible if $P_{II\text{max}}$ were known, meaning that the maximally potent drug in the family of B (i.e. the drug M for which $P_{II\text{Mmax}} = P_{II\text{max}}$) should be identified, and if realization of $P_{II\text{max}}$ would not depress the agonist curve (or, at least, would not depress this curve so far that the magnitude of the parallel shift is not definable anymore).

To this may be added that, just as β^E may give a wrong indication of the intrinsic activity of the full functional antagonist B, the pD_2-value, calculated from the concentration of B which causes a 50 percent relaxation of an organ that was just maximally contracted by the agonist A, may give a false impression of the affinity between B and its receptors. If the relaxation curve of B can be shifted to the right by application of A in higher concentrations, it is clear that the pD_2-value calculated as described above will be larger than the pK_B. This would not be too disturbing if the error was equally large for all members of the family of drug B, so that the pD_2-values could be used to determine the ratio of the affinities of these drugs with respect to their common receptors. In reality this is not the case: the error will be greater as the intrinsic activity of the full functional antagonist is higher, so that the affinity of a highly potent drug will be overestimated more than that of a less potent member of the family.

F. pA_2 and pD_2' of a Dual (Competitive and Metactoid) Antagonist

A final word may be devoted to the calculation of pA_2 and pD_2' from the curves obtained with a substance which combines the properties of a competitive and a metactoid antagonist. Since either kind of antagonism results from interaction with a different kind of receptor, each one expresses itself as if the other component did not exist: the shift of the curve is as large as would correspond with the competitive antagonism alone, the depression is the same as would be caused by the metactoid antagonism in absence of a competitive one. The pA_2 therefore can be found from the shift and the pD_2' from the depression, as discussed for the competitive and the metactoid drugs, respectively.

In case of a mere competitive antagonism the shift is an unequivocal concept: the curves are parallel, so that the distance between the points indicating equal effects is independent of the actual magnitude of the effect. As may be seen from Figure 28, this does not apply for a dual antagonism. This difficulty is overcome by defining the shift as the distance of the points indicating *relatively* equal effects,—so that the metactoid influence is eliminated.

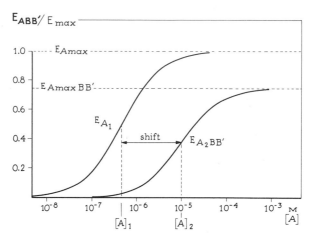

Fig. 28. Determination of magnitude from which the pA_2-value and the pD_2'-value of an antagonist with a dual action (competitive and metactoid) can be calculated. The pA_2 can be found from shift, in this case distance between points indicating *relatively* equal effects (cf. also Fig. 7), by application of Equation (99); the pD_2' can be found from depression of curve ($E_{A_{max}} - E_{A_{max}BB'}$) by application of equation (104), premised that drug B is a complete metactoid antagonist so that $E_{A_{max}BB'_{max}}$ equals 0

Suppose that in absence of B the concentration $[A]_1$ of the agonist causes an effect E_{A_1}, and in its presence the concentration $[A]_2$ causes a different effect $E_{A_2 BB'}$, for which holds that

$$\frac{E_{A_2 BB'}}{E_{A_{max}BB'}} = \frac{E_{A_1}}{E_{A_{max}}}.$$

Application of the Equations (11) and (94) leads to

$$\frac{1}{1+\dfrac{K_A}{[A]_1}} = \frac{\left\{1+(p-1)\dfrac{\beta'}{1+\dfrac{K'_B}{[B]}}\right\}\dfrac{\alpha}{1+\left(1+\dfrac{[B]}{K_B}\right)\dfrac{K_A}{[A]_2}}\cdot E_{max}}{\left\{1+(p-1)\dfrac{\beta'}{1+\dfrac{K'_B}{[B]}}\right\}\dfrac{\alpha}{1+\left(1+\dfrac{[B]}{K_B}\right)\dfrac{K_A}{[A]_{max}}}\cdot E_{max}}.$$

Theoretically $[A]_{max}$ is infinitely large, and thus $\left(1+\dfrac{[B]}{K_B}\right)\dfrac{K_A}{[A]_{max}}$ is infinitely small and may be neglected. It follows that

$$\frac{1}{1+\dfrac{K_A}{[A]_1}} = \frac{1}{1+\left(1+\dfrac{[B]}{K_B}\right)\dfrac{K_A}{[A]_2}}$$

$$1+\frac{[B]}{K_B} = \frac{[A]_2}{[A]_1}.$$

Since this is the same relation as found in case of a single competitive antagonism, for the dual antagonist therefore likewise applies:

$$pA_2 = -\log[B] + \log\left(\frac{[A]_2}{[A]_1} - 1\right).$$

Here the pA_2 may be defined as the negative logarithm of the antagonist concentration (in molars) in the presence of which twice the original agonist concentration is needed to cause an effect that is *relatively* equal to the original effect. It may be remarked that contrary to the situation with a purely competitive antagonist where the possible existence of a nonlinear relation between stimulus and effect of the agonist does not disqualify the definition given on p. 243, the definition of the pA_2 of a dual antagonist as given above is not valid if the concentration-effect relation of the agonist includes a threshold or a receptor reserve. The possible existence of these two phenomena may be detected with other techniques (ARIËNS et al., 1964c), which, however, fall outside the scope of this chapter.

The calculation of the pD_2' does not present special problems, since the depression of the curve can be measured in the same way as if no shift had taken place. Equation (102) may be applied in this form:

$$pD_2' = -\log[B] - \log\left(\frac{E_{A_{max}}}{E_{A_{max}} - E_{A_{max}BB'}} - 1\right). \tag{104}$$

G. Conclusion

In conclusion of this chapter it may be stressed that the numerical expressions of affinity and intrinsic activity, obtained by means of the techniques discussed in the preceding sections, may be important data but should not be overrated. It was pointed out before that if the stimulus-effect relation in the agonistic receptor-effector system departs from linearity, the values of the affinity constant and the intrinsic activity constant of the agonist, calculated on the basis of the presented equations, may differ from the true values. The same applies for metaffinoid, metactoid, and functional antagonists, which formally are agonists with respect to their own systems.

It is true that the $pK_A{}^S$ and α^S of an agonist and the pA_2 of a competitive antagonist are better approximations of the true values, since the stimulus-effect relation has no influence on the calculated constants. As will be clear from the discussion of the models in question, however, this does not mean that these constants would always be perfect expressions of the true affinity or intrinsic activity. The main significance of the calculated constants lies in the fact that they form a basis for comparing closely related compounds within one family, whereas the general characteristics of the sets of experimental curves are the basis for differentiations between various families. In general the meaning of isolated values will be very limited.

References

Åberg, B.: On the effects of weak auxins and antiauxins upon root growth. Physiol. Plantarum 5, 305—319 (1952).

Ahlquist, R.P.: A study of the adrenotropic receptors. Amer. J. Physiol. 153, 586—600 (1948).

Ariëns, E.J.: Affinity and intrinsic activity in the theory of competitive inhibition. Part I. Problems and theory. Arch. int. Pharmacodyn. 99, 32—49 (1954).

Ariëns, E.J.: Receptor theory and structure-action relationships. In: Harper, N.J., Simmonds, A.B. (Eds.) Advances in Drug Research, Vol. 3, pp. 235—285. London-New York: Academic Press 1966.

Ariëns, E.J.: Reduction of drug action by drug combination. J. mond. Pharm. (La Haye) 12, 263—279 (1969).

Ariëns, E.J., de Groot, W.M.: Affinity and intrinsic activity in the theory of competitive inhibition. Part III. Homologous decamethonium-derivatives and succinyl-choline-esters. Arch. int. Pharmacodyn. 99, 193—205 (1954).

Ariëns, E.J., Simonis, A.M.: Affinity and intrinsic activity in the theory of competitive inhibition. Part II. Experiments with para-amino-benzoic acid derivatives. Arch. int. Pharmacodyn. 99, 175—187 (1954).

Ariëns, E.J., Simonis, A.M.: Autonomic drugs and their receptors. Arch. int. Pharmacodyn. 127, 479—496 (1960).

Ariëns, E.J., Simonis, A.M.: A molecular basis for drug action. J. Pharm. Pharmacol. 16, 137—157 (1964).

Ariëns, E.J., Simonis, A.M., de Groot, W.M.: Affinity and intrinsic activity in the theory of competitive and non-competitive inhibition and an analysis of some forms of dualism in action. Arch. int. Pharmacodyn. 100, 298—322 (1955).

Ariëns, E.J., Simonis, A.M., van Rossum, J.M.: Drug receptor interaction: Interaction of one or more drugs with one receptor system. In: Ariëns, E.J. (Ed.): Molecular Pharmacology, Vol. I, pp. 119—286. New York-London: Academic Press 1964a.

Ariëns, E.J., Simonis, A.M., van Rossum, J.M.: Drug receptor interaction: Interaction of one or more drugs with different receptor systems. In: Ariëns, E.J. (Ed.): Molecular Pharmacology, Vol. I, pp. 287—393. New York-London: Academic Press 1964b.

Ariëns, E.J., Simonis, A.M., van Rossum, J.M.: The relation between stimulus and effect. In: Ariëns, E.J. (Ed.): Molecular Pharmacology, Vol. I, pp. 394—466. New York-London: Academic Press 1964c.

Ariëns, E.J., van Rossum, J.M.: pD_x, pA_x and pD_x' values in the analysis of pharmacodynamics. Arch. int. Pharmacodyn. 110, 275—299 (1957).

Ariëns, E.J., van Rossum, J.M., Koopman, P.C.: Receptor reserve and threshold phenomena. I. Theory and experiments with autonomic drugs tested on isolated organs. Arch. int. Pharmacodyn. 127, 459—478 (1960).

Ariëns, E.J., van Rossum, J.M., Simonis, A.M.: A theoretical basis of molecular pharmacology. Part I. Interaction of one or two compounds with one receptor system. Arzneimittel-Forsch. 6, 282—293 (1956a).

Ariëns, E.J., van Rossum, J.M., Simonis, A.M.: A theoretical basis of molecular pharmacology. Part II. Interactions of one or two compounds with two interdependent receptor systems. Arzneimittel-Forsch. 6, 611—621 (1956b).

Ariëns, E.J., van Rossum, J.M., Simonis, A.M.: A theoretical basis of molecular pharmacology. Part III. Interactions of one or two compounds with two independent receptor systems. Arzneimittel-Forsch. 6, 737—746 (1956c).

Ariëns, E.J., van Rossum, J.M., Simonis, A.M.: Affinity, intrinsic activity and drug interactions. Pharmacol. Rev. 9, 218—236 (1957).

Beidler, L.M.: Taste receptor stimulation. In: Progress in Biophysics and Biophysical Chemistry, Eds. Butler, J.A.V., Huxley, H.E., Zirkle, R.E., Vol. 12, pp. 107—151. New York: Pergamon Press 1962.

Belleau, B.: A molecular theory of drug action based on induced conformational perturbations of receptors. J. med. Chem. 7, 776—784 (1964).

Belleau, B.: Conformational perturbation in relation to the regulation of enzyme and receptor behaviour. In: Harper, N.J., Simmonds, A.B., (Eds.): Advances in Drug Research, Vol. 2, pp. 89—126. London-New York: Academic Press 1965.

Belleau, B.: Steric effects in catecholamine interactions with enzymes and receptors. Pharmacol. Rev. 18, 131—140 (1966).

Belleau, B., Lavoie, J.L.: A biophysical basis of ligand-induced activation of excitable membranes and associated enzymes. A thermodynamic study using acetylcholinesterase as a model receptor. Canad. J. Biochem. 46, 1397—1409 (1968).

Bloom,B.M., Goldman,I.M.: The nature of catecholamine-adenine mononucleotide interactions in adrenergic mechanisms. In: Harper,N.J., Simmonds,A.B., (Eds.): Advances in Drug Research, Vol. 3, pp. 121—169. London-New York: Academic Press 1966.

Bovet,D., Bovet-Nitti,F., Bettschart,A., Scognamiglio,W.: Mécanisme de la potentialisation par le chlorhydrate de diéthylamino-éthyldiphénylpropylacétate des effects de quelques agents curarisants. Helv. physiol. pharmacol. Acta **14**, 430—440 (1956).

Brandt,H.D.: The mechanisms by which Beta-Adrenergic Drugs antagonize Different Spasmogens, pp. 1—174. D. Sc. Thesis, University of Potchefstroom, 1971.

Canepa,F.G.: Mechanism of ganglion blocking activity by methonium chains. Nature (Lond.) **195**, 573—575 (1962).

Cavallito,C.J.: Some interrelationships of chemical structure, physical properties and curarimimetic action. In: Bovet,D., Bovet-Nitti,F., Martini-Bettòlo,G.B., (Eds.): Curare and Curare-like Agents, pp. 288—303. Amsterdam-London-New York-Princeton: Elsevier Publ. Co. 1959.

Chagas,C.: The fate of curare during curarization. In: de Reuck,A.V.S., (Ed.): Curare and Curare-like Agents, pp. 2—10. London: J. and A. Churchill Ltd. 1962.

Changeux,J.P., Podleski,T.R.: On the excitability and cooperativity of the electroplax membrane. Proc. nat. Acad. Sci. (Wash.) **59**, 944—950 (1968).

Changeux,J.P., Thiéry,J., Tung,Y., Kittel,C.: On the cooperativity of biological membranes. Proc. nat. Acad. Sci. (Wash.) **57**, 335—341 (1967).

Chargaff,E., Olson,K.B.: Studies on the chemistry of blood coagulation. VI. Studies on the action of heparin and other anticoagulants. The influence of protamine on the anticoagulant effect in vivo. J. biol. Chem. **122**, 153—167 (1937).

Clark,A.J.: The reaction between acetyl choline and muscle cells. J. Physiol. (Lond.) **61**, 530—546 (1926a).

Clark,A.J.: The antagonism of acetyl choline by atropine. J. Physiol. (Lond.) **61**, 547—556 (1926b).

Clark,A.J.: The Mode of Action of Drugs on Cells, pp. 1—298. London: Edward Arnold and Co. 1933.

Clark,A.J.: General pharmacology. In: Heubner,W., Schüller,J., (Eds.): Heffter's Handbuch der experimentellen Pharmakologie, Vol. 4, pp. 1—228. Berlin: J. Springer 1937.

Clark,A.J., Raventós,J.: The antagonism of acetylcholine and of quaternary ammonium salts. Quart. J. exp. Physiol. **26**, 375—392 (1937).

Croxatto,R., Huidobro,F.: Fundamental basis of specificity of pressor and depressor amines in their vascular effects; theoretical fundaments; drug receptor linkage. Arch. int. Pharmacodyn. **106**, 207—243 (1956).

Dagley,S., Freeman,L.O., Tatton,J.O'G.: The kinetics of growth of Bact. lactis aerogenes in the presence of phenol, alcohols, ketones and acetates. Biochem. J. **43**, IV (1948).

Dale,H.H.: The action of certain esters and ethers of choline, and their relation to muscarine. J. Pharmacol. (Lond.) **6**, 147—190 (1914).

Del Castillo,J., Katz,B.: Interaction at end-plate receptors between different choline derivatives. Proc. roy. Soc. B **146**, 369—381 (1957).

Ehrlich,P.: Address in pathology: on chemiotherapy. Lancet **1913 II**, 445—451 and Brit. med. J. **1913 II**, 353—359.

Fastier,F.N.: Structure-activity relationships of amidine derivatives. Pharmacol. Rev. **14**, 37—90 (1962).

Fastier,F.N., Hawkins,J.: Inhibition of amine oxidase by isothiourea derivatives. Brit. J. Pharmacol. **6**, 256—262 (1951).

Fastier,F.N., Reid,C.S.W.: Circulatory properties of amine derivatives. II. Potentiation of the vasoconstrictor action of adrenaline. Brit. J. Pharmacol. **3**, 205—210 (1948).

Ferguson,J.: The use of chemical potentials as indices of toxicity. Proc. roy. Soc. B **127**, 387—404 (1939).

— Furchgott,R.F.: Dibenamine blockade in strips of rabbit aorta and its use in differentiating receptors. J. Pharmacol. exp. Ther. **111**, 265—284 (1954).

— Furchgott,R.F.: The pharmacology of vascular smooth muscle. Pharmacol. Rev. **7**, 183—265 (1955).

Gaddum,J.H.: The action of adrenalin and ergotamine on the uterus of the rabbit. J. Physiol. (Lond.) **61**, 141—150 (1926).

Gaddum, J. H.: The quantitative effects of antagonistic drugs. J. Physiol. (Lond.) **89**, 7p—9p (1937).

Gaddum, J. H.: Symposium on chemical constitution and pharmacological action. Trans. Faraday Soc. **39**, 323—332 (1943).

Gaddum, J. H., Hameed, K. A., Hathway, D. E., Stephens, F. F.: Quantitative studies of antagonists for 5-hydroxytryptamine. Quart. J. exp. Physiol. **40**, 49—74 (1955).

Ginsborg, B. L., Stephenson, R. P.: On the simultaneous action of two competitive antagonists. Brit. J. Pharmacol. **51**, 287—300 (1974).

Goldstein, A.: The interaction of drugs and plasma proteins. Pharmacol. Rev. **1**, 102—165 (1949).

Hahn, F., Schmutzler, W., Seseke, G., Giertz, H., Bernauer, W.: Histaminasefreisetzung durch Heparin und Protamin beim Meerschweinchen. Biochem. Pharmacol. **15**, 155—160 (1966).

Hamilton, W.: Discussion on Philosophy and Literature, Education and University Reform. New York: Harper and Brothers 1868.

Higman, H. B., Bartels, E.: The competitive nature of the action of acetylcholine and local anesthetics. Biochim. biophys. Acta (Amst.) **54**, 543—554 (1962).

Homer, L. D.: The receptor occupation theory of drug responses. J. theor. Biol. **17**, 399—409 (1967).

Karlin, A.: On the application of "a plausible model" of allosteric proteins to the receptor for acetylcholine. J. theor. Biol. **16**, 306—320 (1967).

Katz, B., Thesleff, S.: A study of the "desensitization" produced by acetylcholine at the motor end-plate. J. Physiol. (Lond.) **138**, 63—80 (1957).

Kimelberg, H., Moran, J. F., Triggle, D. J.: The mechanism of interaction of 2-halogenoethylamines at the noradrenaline receptor. J. theor. Biol. **9**, 502—503 (1965).

Koshland, D. E.: The role of flexibility in enzyme action. Cold Spr. Harb. Symp. quant. Biol. **28**, 473—482 (1963).

Langley, J. N.: On the reaction of cells and of nerve-endings to certain poisons, chiefly as regards the reaction of striated muscle to nicotine and to curari. J. Physiol. (Lond.) **33**, 374—413 (1905).

Lasareff, P.: Untersuchungen über die Ionentheorie der Reizung. III. Ionentheorie der Geschmacksreizung. Pflügers Arch. ges. Physiol. **194**, 293—297 (1922).

Lucretius Carus, T.: In: De Rerum Natura, book IV, verse 615 et sqq.

Mackay, D.: A flux-carrier hypothesis of drug action. Nature (Lond.) **197**, 1171—1173 (1963).

Mackay, D.: The mathematics of drug-receptor interactions. J. Pharm. Pharmacol. **18**, 201—222 (1966).

Miller, L. C., Becker, T. J., Tainter, M. L.: Quantitative evaluation of spasmolytic drugs in vitro. J. Pharmacol. exp. Ther. **92**, 260—268 (1948).

Monod, J., Wyman, J., Changeux, J. P.: On the nature of allosteric transitions: a plausible model. J. molec. Biol. **12**, 88—118 (1965).

Nickerson, M.: Receptor occupancy and tissue response. Nature (Lond.) **178**, 697—698 (1956).

Nickerson, M.: Nonequilibrium drug antagonism. Pharmacol. Rev. **9**, 246—259 (1957).

Offermeier, J., van den Brink, F. G.: The antagonism between cholinomimetic agonists and β-adrenoceptor stimulants. The differentiation between functional and metaffinoid antagonism. Europ. J. Pharmacol. **27**, 206—213 (1974).

Paton, W. D. M.: A theory of drug action based on the rate of drug-receptor combination. Proc. roy. Soc. B **154**, 21—69 (1961).

Paton, W. D. M., Rang, H. P.: A kinetic approach to the mechanism of drug action. In: Harper, N. J., Simmonds, A. B., (Eds.): Advances in Drug Research, Vol. 3, pp. 57—80. London-New York: Academic Press 1966.

Paton, W. D. M., Waud, D. R.: Drug-receptor interactions at the neuromuscular junction. In: de Reuck, A. V. S., (Ed.): Curare and Curare-like Agents, pp. 34—54. London: J. and A. Churchill Ltd. 1962a.

Paton, W. D. M., Waud, D. R.: Neuromuscular blocking agents. Brit. J. Anaesth. **34**, 251—259 (1962b).

Paton, W. D. M., Waud, D. R.: A quantitative investigation of the relationship between rate of access of a drug to receptor and the rate of onset or offset of action. Naunyn-Schmiedebergs Arch. exp. Path. Pharmakol. **248**, 124—143 (1964).

Pauling, L.: A molecular theory of general anesthesia. Science **134**, 15—21 (1961).

Renqvist, Y.: Über den Geschmack. Skand. Arch. Physiol. **38**, 97—201 (1919).

Reuse, J. J.: Comparison of various histamine antagonists. Brit. J. Pharmacol. **3**, 174—180 (1948).

Rocha e Silva, M.: Kinetics of recovery from inhibition by antihistaminics, atropine and antispasmodics. Pharmacol. Rev. **9**, 259—264 (1957).

Rocha e Silva, M.: A thermodynamic approach to problems of drug antagonism. I. The "charnière theory". Europ. J. Pharmacol. **6**, 294—302 (1969).

Rocha e Silva, M.: A thermodynamic approach to problems of drug antagonism. II. A microphysical model of the phenomenon of recovery. Physiol. chem. Phys. **2**, 503—515 (1970).

Schild, H. O.: pA, a new scale for measurement of drug antagonism. Brit. J. Pharmacol. **2**, 189—206 (1947).

Schild, H. O.: pA_x and competitive drug antagonism. Brit. J. Pharmacol. **4**, 277—280 (1949).

Schild, H. O.: Drug antagonism and pA_x. In: Symposium on Drug Antagonism. Pharmacol. Rev. **9**, 242—246 (1957).

Simonis, A. M.: Principi di farmacologia molecolare. Farmaco, Ed. sci. **20**, 52—75 (1965).

Stephenson, R. P.: A modification of receptor theory. Brit. J. Pharmacol. **11**, 379—393 (1956).

Stephenson, R. P., Ginsborg, B. L.: Potentiation by an antagonist. Nature (Lond.) **222**, 790—791 (1969).

Storm van Leeuwen, W.: On sensitiveness to drugs in animals and men. J. Pharmacol. exp. Ther. **24**, 13—19 (1925a).

Storm van Leeuwen, W.: On antagonism of drugs. J. Pharmacol. exp. Ther. **24**, 21—24 (1925b).

Storm van Leeuwen, W.: A possible explanation for certain cases of hypersensitiveness to drugs in men. J. Pharmacol. exp. Ther. **24**, 25—32 (1925c).

Stubbins, J. F., Hudgins, P. M., Andrako, J., Beebe, A. J.: Anticholinergic agents based on Ariens' dual receptor site theory. J. pharm. Sci. **57**, 534—535 (1968).

Taylor, D. B., Steinborn, J., Tzu-Chiau Lu: Ion exchange processes at the neuromuscular junction of voluntary muscle. J. Pharmacol. exp. Ther. **175**, 213—227 (1970).

Thron, C. D.: On the analysis of pharmacological experiments in terms of an allosteric receptor model. Molec. Pharmacol. **9**, 1—9 (1973).

Thron, C. D., Waud, D. R.: The rate of action of atropine. J. Pharmacol. exp. Ther. **160**, 91—105 (1968).

Van den Brink, F. G.: Eine Molekulargrundlage für die Wirkung von Pharmaka. 3. Teil: Substanzen mit mehrfacher Wirkung. Arzneimittel-Forsch. **16**, 1403—1412 (1966).

Van den Brink, F. G.: Different kinds of antagonism. In: Histamine and Antihistamines. Molecular Pharmacology, Structure-Activity Relations, Gastric Acid Secretion, pp. 25—28. Nijmegen: Drukkerij Gebr. Janssen N. V. 1969a.

Van den Brink, F. G.: Discussion of the presuppositions in the agonistic model. In: Histamine and Antihistamines. Molecular Pharmacology, Structure-Activity Relations, Gastric Acid Secretion, pp. 43—45. Nijmegen: Drukkerij Gebr. Janssen N. V. 1969b.

Van den Brink, F. G.: The model of metactoid interaction. In: Histamine and Antihistamines. Molecular Pharmacology, Structure-Activity Relations, Gastric Acid Secretion, pp. 49—56. Nijmegen: Drukkerij Gebr. Janssen N. V. 1969c.

Van den Brink, F. G.: The model of metaffinoid interaction. In: Histamine and Antihistamines. Molecular Pharmacology, Structure-Activity Relations, Gastric Acid Secretion, pp. 56—62. Nijmegen: Drukkerij Gebr. Janssen N. V. 1969d.

Van den Brink, F. G.: The interaction of histaminomimetic compounds and of competitive antagonists of histamine with the histamine receptor; the concept additional receptor area. In: Histamine and Antihistamines. Molecular Pharmacology, Structure-Activity Relations, Gastric Acid Secretion, pp. 107—111. Nijmegen: Drukkerij Gebr. Janssen N. V. 1969e.

Van den Brink, F. G.: A new theoretical model of functional interaction. Naunyn-Schmiedebergs Arch. Pharmak. **269**, 385 (1971).

Van den Brink, F. G.: The model of functional interaction. I. Development and first check of a new model of functional synergism and antagonism. Europ. J. Pharmacol. **22**, 270—278 (1973a).

Van den Brink, F.G.: The model of functional interaction. II. Experimental verification of a new model: The antagonism of β-adrenoceptor stimulants and other agonists. Europ. J. Pharmacol. **22**, 279—286 (1973b).

Van Rossum, J.M.: Pharmacodynamics of Cholinomimetic and Cholinolytic Drugs, pp. 9—160. Bruges: St. Catherine Press Ltd. 1958.

Van Rossum, J.M.: Cumulative dose-response curves. II. Technique for the making of dose-response curves in isolated organs and the evaluation of drug parameters. Arch. int. Pharmacodyn. **143**, 299—330 (1963).

Van Rossum, J.M.: Limitations of molecular pharmacology. In: Harper, N.J., Simmonds, A.B., (Eds.): Advances in Drug Research, Vol. 3, pp. 189—234, London-New York: Academic Press 1966a.

Van Rossum, J.M.: Die Pharmakon-Rezeptor-Theorie als Grundlage der Wirkung von Arzneimitteln. Möglichkeiten und Beschränkungen. Arzneimittel-Forsch. **16**, 1412—1426, 1966b.

Van Rossum, J.M., van den Brink, F.G.: Cumulative dose-response curves. I. Introduction to the technique. Arch. int. Pharmacodyn. **143**, 240—246 (1963).

Veldstra, H.: Synergism and potentiation with special reference to the combination of structural analogues. Pharmacol. Rev. **8**, 339—387, (1956).

Watkins, J.C.: Pharmacological receptors and general permeability phenomena of cell membranes. J. theor. Biol. **9**, 37—50 (1965).

CHAPTER 5

A Critical Survey of Receptor Theories of Drug Action

D. MACKAY

I. Introduction

A drug may be defined as a chemical compound which modifies the properties of living cells. The result of the action of a drug may be observed on single cells, isolated tissues, or whole animals but in each case the basic biological unit which is modified is the cell. A drug which produces an observable response is called an agonist, while an antagonist does not itself produce a response but can antagonise the response produced by an agonist. A receptor may be defined as the site, in or on a cell, with which an agonist interacts when it produces a response. Some drugs may interact with cell structures by virtue of their physical properties, but the term receptor implies a close structural relationship between the drug and its site of action, so that an agonist may produce a response from one type of receptor but not from others. Early ideas concerning the existence of specific pharmacologic receptors, which were based on the apparent specificity of action of some antagonists, have now been given strong support by quantitative studies (SCHILD, 1962).

The first quantitative receptor theory of drug action was developed by CLARK (1933). One of the basic assumptions made in Clark's original theory was that the response of a tissue to a drug is due to occupation of the receptors by the drug molecules. For this reason his original theory and subsequent modifications which involve the same assumption, are classified as "occupation theories." At the other extreme is the "rate" theory of drug action proposed by PATON (1961) in which the drug-receptor is assumed to contribute to the production of a response, only at the moment of formation of the drug-receptor complex. Various other theories will also be discussed some of which lie somewhat between these two extremes. The earliest review on receptor theories of drug action is that of CLARK (1937). Later discussions and reviews have been written by GADDUM (1943, 1957); SCHILD (1957), FURCHGOTT (1955, 1964); ARIENS and SIMONIS (1964a, b); MACKAY (1966b); and WAUD (1968b). Other discussions, pertinent to some of the topics dealt with here, are to be found in the report of a symposium, edited by RANG (1973a), and in a lecture presented by RANG (1973b).

It must be emphasised that the use of the term "receptor" is often a tacit admission of our lack of knowledge. The nondividing living cell may be regarded as being in an approximate steady-state condition. This steady-state depends on balances between

1. influx and efflux of ions across membranes,
2. uptake, production, and utilisation of enzyme substrates,
3. production and utilisation of energy,

so that the properties of the cell change very little with time. The effect of a drug on a cell is to cause a change in at least one of these factors, and so produce a response from the cell. The most likely mechanisms of drug action are therefore on the permeability of cell membranes or on the rates of enzyme reactions. The cell membranes which might be modified by drugs include those within the cell, surrounding such intracellular structures as the mitochondria.

However, if the action of a drug is on an enzyme system then it should be possible to isolate the system and to study the mechanism of action of the drug by appropriate biochemical methods. If, on the other hand, the drug acts by modifying the permeability of a membrane then attempts to isolate the receptor by disintegrating the membrane may modify, or even destroy, the receptor. In fact, even when molecules can be isolated which interact with the appropriate agonists and antagonists it is still very difficult to decide whether or not they really are receptors, unless their properties can be accurately compared with those of the receptors in the living tissue (see, e.g., CHAGAS et al., 1958; EHRENPREIS, 1962; NAMBA and GROB, 1967; FEWTRELL and RANG, 1973; O'BRIEN et al., 1973; DE ROBERTIS, 1973; CHANGEUX et al., 1973). The aims of receptor theories or models, may therefore be summarised as follows:

1. to allow one to deduce some of the properties of receptors even if they have not been isolated,

2. to provide a theoretical framework which enables one to summarise experimental data in a suitable form, even though this may have to be interpreted subsequently in different ways,

3. to allow comparison of the properties of receptors in living tissue with those of molecules believed to be isolated receptors.

Many practical and theoretical difficulties arise when attempts are made to study drug-receptor interactions indirectly by observing the responses of living systems to drugs. As was emphasised by CLARK, the experimental system used in such studies should be kept as simple as possible. The simplest system would consist of a drug acting on a single cell. Even in such an experiment the diffusion of the drug to the receptor, the reaction of the drug with the receptor, and the subsequent production of the response, will each take some finite time. The observed response will therefore vary with time and with the concentration of the drug. Although each of these three processes requires a finite time, the rate of the response will be determined mainly by the slowest process. Even in such an apparently simple system, uptake of drug into the cell or metabolism of the drug may cause further complications. It must be emphasised that the various receptor models discussed here are set out on the assumption that the response observed is a graded response from a single cell. Allowances are not usually made in the basic theoretical equations for the problems mentioned above. Such factors must be kept in mind and either eliminated so far as possible by suitable experimental technique, or allowed for separately.

The quantitative interpretation of experimental results in terms of receptor models becomes increasingly difficult as the thickness of the tissue is increased and as the structure of the tissue becomes more complex. If several types of cell are present in an isolated tissue then the overall response may result from the action of the drug on more than one type of cell, or the final observed response may be produced by the action of the initial response on another type of cell. A typical example would be the response produced from smooth muscle cells by the action of nicotine on ganglia. In whole animals the situation becomes still more complicated, with possible responses from various tissues and glands contributing to an overall response, as well as complications from such factors as rates of absorption, distribution, uptake, metabolism, and excretion.

Since most normal isolated tissues have a limited life in vitro, studies on such tissues are necessarily limited to responses obtained within minutes or hours, rather than days. Fortunately the effects of drugs on membrane permeability would be expected to produce fairly rapid responses so that in vitro methods seem best suited to studies of such drug-receptor interactions at the cellular level. The much slower effects produced by some hormones in vivo are probably due to biochemical changes in the cells and should therefore be amenable to studies using biochemical methods. This does not, of course, deny the possibility that some drugs may produce quite rapid responses in isolated tissues by modifying enzyme reactions in the cells.

II. The Mathematics of Drug-Receptor Interactions

All receptor models of drug action require that the drug should interact with a receptor. There is, therefore, a certain amount of mathematical manipulation which is common to most of these models. The various models, or "theories," differ mainly in the mechanism suggested for the production of the observed response by the drug-receptor interaction.

Because of the internal structure of cells it is unlikely that all of the receptors of any single type will be homogeneously distributed throughout the cell. Therefore only a small volume element of a cell will be considered initially. This volume element is chosen so that it contains a fairly uniform concentration of drug molecules, (D), and a concentration $[R]_T$ of receptors. This latter concentration may be in moles/cm^3 if the receptor is a soluble enzyme or in receptor sites/cm^2 if the receptor is on a surface. Curved brackets are therefore used to denote molar concentrations of the drug but the concentrations of the receptors and drug-receptor complexes are indicated by square brackets because their units of concentration are not known. One of the aims of receptor theory is to obtain useful information without knowledge of the absolute concentration of the receptors.

A. Interaction of One Drug with One Type of Receptor

1. The Drug-Receptor Reaction

If the drug molecule is denoted by the symbol D and the receptor site is assumed to be a definite chemical structure given the symbol R, then the interaction of one receptor with the drug is usually represented as a bimolecular reaction,

$$R + D \underset{k_2}{\overset{k_1}{\rightleftharpoons}} RD \tag{1}$$

where k_1 and k_2 are the forward and backward rate constants.

It has recently been emphasised by TAYLOR et al. (1970) that the interaction of an ionised drug molecule with an ionised receptor should be represented as an ion exchange process. For a univalent cationic drug and a univalent anionic receptor the reaction would be

$$R^-X^+ + D^+ \rightleftharpoons R^-D^+ + X^+$$

where X^+ is likely to be an inorganic cation. It has also been pointed out by WERMAN (1969) that, in some cases at least, more than one drug molecule may interact with one receptor. In such cases the process is likely to occur in steps. The second step would be

$RD + D \rightleftharpoons RD_2$, and so on. Appropriate equations can be derived for such situations but these possible complications will be ignored for the present.

2. Onset of Receptor Occupation

Suppose that the system consists initially of a single cell in a volume of physiologic saline. At zero time an amount of drug D is added to the saline. The drug is mixed rapidly through the saline so that the concentration of the drug near the cell rises rapidly from zero to a value $(D)_{aq.}$. Some time later molecules of the drug D will have diffused across the unstirred film of physiologic saline at the cell surface (see CLARK, 1933) and reached the cell membrane. Penetration of the drug into the cell may then be necessary for the drug to reach the receptors. However, attention will now be focussed on a small volume element of the cell which contains receptors.

Suppose that the concentration of the drug in this small volume at time t is $(D)_t$ and that the local concentration of receptors is then $[R]_t$. The rate of change of concentration of drug-receptor complexes in this region is then $d[RD]_t/dt$, given by the equation

$$d[RD]_t/dt = k_1[R]_t(D)_t - k_2[RD]_t . \tag{2}$$

If receptors are neither produced nor destroyed during the experiment their total concentration in the small volume element has some constant value $[R]_T$ where

$$[R]_T = [R]_t + [RD]_t \tag{3}$$

for all values of the time t. Combining Equations (2) and (3) to eliminate $[R]_t$, gives

$$d[RD]_t/dt = k_1(D)_t[R]_T - [RD]_t\{k_2 + k_1(D)_t\} . \tag{4}$$

If $(D)_t$ is a complicated function of time then an exact mathematical solution of Equation (4) may be difficult, if not impossible. However, if the conditions of the experiment are such that $(D)_t$ is independent of time, then the subscript t can be omitted. (However, (D) will not necessarily be equal to $(D)_{aq.}$.) Equation 4 can then be rearranged to give

$$d[RD]_t/(a - b[RD]_t) = dt \tag{5}$$

where a and b are constants given by the equations

$$a = k_1(D)[R]_T \quad \text{and} \quad b = k_2 + k_1(D).$$

Integration of Equation (5) between time zero and time t leads to the equation

$$\ln\left\{1 - \frac{b}{a}[RD]_t\right\} = -bt.$$

Substituting the appropriate values for a and b, and rearranging, the above equation becomes

$$\frac{[RD]_t}{[R]_T} = \{y_D\}_t = \frac{1 - \exp(-[k_2 + k_1(D)]t)}{1 + k_2/k_1(D)} \tag{6}$$

where $\{y_D\}_t$ is the fraction of the receptors occupied by the drug at time t, in the small volume element considered. At sufficiently large values of time Equation (6) reduces to

$$\{y_D\}_{t \to \infty} = \{y_D\}_{eq.} = 1/[1 + k_2/k_1(D)], \tag{7a}$$
$$= 1/[1 + 1/K_D(D)], \tag{7b}$$

where K_D is the affinity constant of the drug for the receptors and $\{y_D\}_{eq.}$ is the fraction of the receptors occupied by the drug at equilibrium. Equations (6) and (7) can then be combined to give the ratio of the number of receptors occupied at time t to the number of receptors occupied at equilibrium,

$$\{y_D\}_t/\{y_D\}_{eq.} = 1 - \exp(-[k_2 + k_1(D)]t). \tag{8}$$

An alternative form of Equation (8) is

$$\ln[1 - \{y_D\}_t/\{y_D\}_{eq.}] = -[k_2 + k_1(D)]t. \tag{9}$$

It can then be shown that the time at which $\{y_D\}_t/\{y_D\}_{eq.}$ is equal to 0.5 is given by

$$t_{1/2} = 0.693/[k_2 + k_1(D)]. \tag{10}$$

This equation shows clearly that under the experimental conditions outlined above the rate of approach to equilibrium occupation of the receptors depends on k_1, k_2, and (D).

3. Offset of Receptor Occupation

If the fraction of receptors occupied by a drug D has been allowed to reach its equilibrium value $\{y_D\}_{eq.}$ and the drug is washed out of the tissue (zero time) then the offset reaction is

$$RD \xrightarrow{k_2} R + D$$

and the rate of decline of receptor occupation is given by $-d[RD]_t/dt = k_2[RD]$, which, on integration, gives

$$\{y_D\}_t = \{y_D\}_{eq.}\ \exp[-k_2 t]\,. \tag{11}$$

B. Interaction of Two Drugs with the Same Receptors

1. Competitive Interactions

If the two drugs are denoted by the symbols A and B then the interactions (assumed to be bimolecular) are respectively

$$R + A \underset{k_{2A}}{\overset{k_{1A}}{\rightleftarrows}} RA\,, \tag{12a}$$

$$R + B \underset{k_{2B}}{\overset{k_{1B}}{\rightleftarrows}} RB\,. \tag{12b}$$

The corresponding kinetic equations are then

$$d[RA]_t/dt = k_{1A}[R]_t(A)_t - k_{2A}[RA]_t \tag{13a}$$

and

$$d[RB]_t/dt = k_{1B}[R]_t(B)_t - k_{2B}[RB]_t\,. \tag{13b}$$

The total concentration of the receptors in the small volume element being considered is

$$[R]_T = [R]_t + [RA]_t + [RB]_t\,. \tag{14}$$

Such a system of differential equations is most easily solved by use of an analog computer. However, if $[R]_T$, $(A)_t$, and $(B)_t$ are independent of time then for equilibrium conditions Equations (13a) and (13b) reduce to

$$[RA]/[R](A) = k_{1A}/k_{2A} = K_A\,, \tag{15a}$$

$$[RB]/[R](B) = k_{1B}/k_{2B} = K_B\,, \tag{15b}$$

where K_A and K_B are the affinity constants of the respective drugs for the receptors. $[R]$ can be eliminated from these equations by use of Equation (14). The resulting equations can then be solved to obtain

$$y_A' = [RA]'/[R]_T = K_A(A)'/[1 + K_A(A)' + K_B(B)']\,, \tag{16a}$$

$$y_B' = [RB]'/[R]_T = K_B(B)'/[1 + K_A(A)' + K_B(B)']\,. \tag{16b}$$

The dash superscript is used to indicate that a second drug is present and occupies some of the receptors.

2. Pseudo-Irreversible Interactions

If one of the drugs, A, has been equilibrated with the receptors and drug B is then added, the rate of approach of y_B to its equilibrium value will depend on the rate of dissociation of RA complexes, if it is assumed that the drugs react only with free receptors. If the rate of dissociation of A from the receptor is slow, and the rate of formation of RB complexes is rapid, then drug B will rapidly reach a pseudo-equilibrium with the unoccupied receptors before reaching the final equilibrium condition given by Equation (16b). In such a case, drug A acts in a "pseudo-irreversible" manner.

Initially drug A occupies a fraction of the receptors given by

$$y_A = K_A(A)/[1 + K_A(A)],\tag{17}$$

[see Eq. (7b)], so that the effective concentration of free receptors available for reaction with drug B is $[1 - y_A][R]_T$. The fraction of these receptors occupied by drug B under pseudoequilibrium conditions is therefore

$$
\begin{aligned}
y_B &= [1 - y_A] K_B(B)'/[1 + K_B(B)'] \\
&= K_B(B)'/\{(1 + K_B(B)')(1 + K_A(A)')\},
\end{aligned}\tag{18}
$$

which is less than the true equilibrium value of y'_B given by Equation (16b). The fraction of the receptors occupied by drug A under pseudoequilibrium conditions is given by Equation (17), and is greater than the value at true equilibrium [see Eq. (16a)].

3. Facilitated Displacement

Although drugs A and B have been assumed to react only with free receptors [see Eqs. (12a, b)] it would be theoretically possible for one drug to displace another from the receptor as in the reaction,

$$RA + B \rightleftharpoons RB + A.$$

Such catalytic displacements have been shown to occur in chemical systems (see, e.g., CORDES and JENCKS, 1962a, b; MACKAY, 1963a). However, such a catalytic displacement would affect only the kinetics of the approach to equilibrium and not the final position of equilibrium. Equations (16a, b) and would therefore still be valid for equilibrium conditions.

4. Specific Noncompetitive Interaction

Another possibility which must be taken into account is that of a reaction of the type

$$RA + B \rightleftharpoons RAB.$$

The equilibrium constant for this process would be

$$K_{AB} = [RAB]/[RA](B).\tag{19}$$

Equations (19) and (15a, b) can then be combined with a modified version of Equation (14) to estimate the fractions of the receptors in the various forms R, RA, RB, and RAB. The modified version of Equation (14) is

$$[R]_T = [R] + [RA] + [RB] + [RAB] . \tag{20}$$

The fraction of the receptors in the form RA is then

$$y'_A = K_A(A)'/[1 + K_A(A)' + K_B(B)' + K_{AB}(B)' \, K_A(A)'] . \tag{21}$$

C. Application of Equations for Receptor Occupation to Macroscopic Tissues

In deriving the equations which describe drug-receptor interactions, it was considered advisable to confine attention to a small volume element of the tissue which contained a fairly uniform concentration of drugs and receptors. This allowed the equations to be developed according to normal chemical principles. The small volume element is analogous to a small volume of the biophase compartment discussed by FURCHGOTT (1955) or of the receptor compartment considered by VAN ROSSUM (1966). It was also assumed in solving the kinetic equations, that the concentration of the drug in this small volume increased instantaneously from zero to some finite value at zero time and was subsequently maintained constant at this value.

These kinetic equations are therefore likely to be valid only if the rate of access of the drug to the receptors is rapid compared with the rate of the drug-receptor reaction. This may be true if the drug-receptor interaction occurs at the outer membranes of single isolated cells, or on the membranes of cells at the surface of a tissue. It is less likely to be true if drugs act intracellularly or if they are applied to the surface of a tissue and react on or in cells which lie deeper inside the tissue.

On the other hand, the equilibrium equations should be valid for each small volume element of the tissue, at sufficiently large values of t, but it must be kept in mind that even when a steady-state distribution of drug has been achieved throughout the interstitial fluid the local concentration of drug may vary with position in the tissue. Such local variations could be produced in the interstitial fluid or inside the cells, by steady uptake or metabolism of the drug. The local concentration of the drug at the receptors is therefore not necessarily equal to that in the external solution nor even to that in the interstitial fluid. More detailed discussions of these and related problems will be found in the articles by FURCHGOTT (1955) and VAN ROSSUM (1966).

D. Drug-Receptor Interactions and the Response

The equations derived in the previous sections refer to the rate of occupation of receptors by drugs and to the fraction of receptors occupied at equilibrium. Although nuclear magnetic resonance has been used to study the interaction of high concentrations of adrenaline with receptors in liver cells (FISCHER and JOST, 1969), there seems to be no physical technique available at the present time which is sufficiently sensitive to allow the direct estimation of the concentration of drug-receptor complexes under normal pharmacologic conditions. When only the result of the drug-receptor interaction can be measured as a response, any information about the interaction must be extracted from such responses. It seems likely that in some cases the observed response is the result of a *series* of changes which occur inside the cell following the drug-receptor interaction (FURCHGOTT, 1955). In such cases the shapes of the dose-response and time-response curves are likely to be only indirectly related to the agonist-receptor interaction (see also WERMAN, 1969).

III. Occupation Theories of Drug Action

A. The Direct Occupation Theory

Since there are several modifications and developments of the original occupation theory, which are nevertheless still occupation theories, the term "direct" occupation theory will be used here when steady occupation by an agonist of some single entity called the receptor, is assumed to determine the response.

If the response results from occupation of the receptors by an agonist then it might also be expected that the response would continue as long as the receptor remains occupied. Since the fraction of receptors occupied by the agonist is zero before addition of the drug, and rises smoothly to some equilibrium value which depends on concentration of drug at the receptors [see Eq. (7b) and Fig. 5a], the variation of the response with time might be expected to follow a similar time course, at least qualitatively. Experimentally such response versus time curves are not always observed. In particular, the peak response is sometimes not maintained. This might be taken to mean that equilibrium occupation of receptors does not necessarily produce a steady peak response. In fact there is no definite evidence that a peak response, or even a steady response, necessarily means that equilibrium occupation of the receptors has been practically attained.

However, in the absence of knowledge as to why some responses are not maintained, it is the usual practice, in applying occupation theories of drug action, to assume that equilibrium occupation of the receptors has occurred when the response versus time curve reaches its maximum value. Inability of the direct occupation theory to explain why some responses are not maintained is sometimes considered to be a major weakness of the theory. However, inability of a tissue to maintain a steady response may be the result of subsequent changes in the properties of the tissue, not directly associated with the drug-receptor interaction itself. Although this problem arises mainly with agonists it can occur also with antagonists (PATON, 1967a).

Another major problem which arises with all drug-receptor theories is lack of knowledge of the relation between the drug-receptor interaction and the response. The most general statement of direct occupation theory is that the equilibrium (or peak) response r, to an agonist A, is some steadily increasing function of the number of receptors occupied by the agonist at equilibrium. This may be written briefly as

$$r = f([RA]) . \tag{22}$$

1. Clark's Original Theory

In the original occupation theory CLARK assumed that the response is proportional to the fraction of the receptors occupied by an agonist, so that

$$r = k\{y_A\} \tag{23}$$

where k is a proportionality constant which was assumed to be the same for all agonists. At sufficiently high concentrations of agonist the receptors become saturated, y_A tends to 1.0 [see Eq. (7b)], and the maximal response becomes equal to k, so that Equation (23) takes the form

$$r/r_{MAX} = \{y_A\} . \tag{24}$$

Clark's assumptions therefore implied that all receptors have to be occupied by an agonist to produce a maximal response from the tissue and that all agonists should produce the same maximal response. As will be seen from Equation (24), his assumptions also led to the conclusion that the fraction of the receptors occupied by an agonist could be estimated from r/r_{MAX}. When the value of r is equal to 0.5 r_{MAX} then y_A should be equal to 0.5. If the concentration of A which produces this response is $(A)_{50}$ then

$$y_A = 0.5 = 1 \Big/ \left[1 + \frac{1}{K_A(A)_{50}} \right] \quad \text{[see Eq. (7b)]} ,$$

and

$$K_A = 1/(A)_{50} , \tag{25}$$

provided that Clark's assumptions are correct.

GADDUM (1937) extended Clark's theory to account for the quantitative effects of specific antagonists. The equation developed by GADDUM was (in the symbols used here)

$$K_A(A)' = [1 + K_I(I)'] \, y'_A/[1 - y'_A] \tag{26}$$

where A represents the agonist and I the antagonist. It was assumed that the antagonist competes with the agonist for the receptors but that receptor-antagonist complexes do not contribute to the production of the response. Gaddum's equation is readily obtained by rearrangement of Equation (16a).

2. Application of the Null Method to Studies of Drug Antagonism

Although CLARK (1933) clearly realised that the response need not be directly proportional to the fraction of receptors occupied by the agonist, he seems to have made this assumption because there was no evidence to the contrary. The assumption, if it is valid, also allows the affinity constants of agonists for receptors to be calculated. However, the assumption is a basic weakness of the original direct occupation theory.

CLARK and RAVENTOS (1937) suggested two methods for estimating the antagonistic power of a drug. The first method was based on the application of Gaddum's equation, which was assumed to describe the dose-response curve of an agonist in the presence of a competitive antagonist. When y'_A is equal to 0.5 Equation (26) reduces to

$$K_A(A)' = 1 + K_I(I)'.$$

If $K_I(I)'$ is also very much greater than unity then

$$(A)'/(I)' = K_I/K_A$$

where, on the basis of Clark's assumption, $(A)'$ is the concentration of agonist which produces a response which is 50% of maximal, in the presence of a concentration $(I)'$ of the antagonist. $(A)'/(I)'$ has been called the drug ratio, but it is not a good measure of drug antagonism (CLARK and RAVENTOS, 1937; GADDUM et al., 1955).

The second method was "to determine the concentration of B (the antagonist) which alters by a selected proportion (e.g., ten-fold) the concentration of A (the agonist) needed to produce a selected effect." This suggestion contains the basis of the null method, which was subsequently applied by SCHILD (1947, 1949, 1954) and by GADDUM et al., (1955) to studies of drug antagonism. In applying the null method to such studies, estimates are made of the concentrations of drugs required to elicit equal responses from the tissue in the absence and in the presence of the antagonist. According to the direct occupation theory, the equilibrium response is some function of y_A, so that it seems reasonable to assume that equal values of y_A produce equal responses from any given tissue.

If a given value of the response, r, is produced by a concentration (A) of the agonist acting alone on the tissue, then the fraction of the receptors occupied at equilibrium is

$$y_A = 1/[1 + 1/K_A(A)] \quad \text{[see Eq. (7b)]}.$$

When a competitive antagonist, I, is also present then the fraction of the receptors occupied by a concentration $(A)'$ of agonist, acting on the same tissue is

$$y_A = 1/\{1 + [1 + K_I(I)]/K_A(A)'\} \quad \text{[see Eq. (16a)]}.$$

This produces a response r'. Therefore when r is made equal to r', y_A should equal y'_A and it follows that

$$(A)'/(A) = 1 + K_I(I). \qquad \textit{Schild equation} \tag{27}$$
see also Rang p. 171

$(A)'$ in the presence of the concentration (I) of the competitive antagonist, produces the same response as does (A) in the absence of the antagonist. Equation (27) should be valid at all values of the response r.

Experimentally Equation (27) can be used in two ways. If $(A)'/(A)$ is kept constant at some value x, then the value of (I) can be altered until r' and r become equal.

Suppose that the value of (I) which achieves this, is $(I)_x$. Then the equation becomes

$$x = 1 + K_I(I)_x, \quad \text{or} \quad (I)_x = [x - 1]/K_I. \quad K_I = \text{affinity constant}$$

Since SCHILD (1947) has defined the pA_x as $[-\log(I)_x]$ it follows that

$$\log K_I = pA_x + \log[x - 1]. \tag{28}$$

Equation (28) is the basis of various methods for testing whether or not antagonism is competitive, and for estimating the affinity constants of competitive antagonists (SCHILD, 1947, 1957; ARUNLAKSHANA and SCHILD, 1959).

If instead of keeping (A)′/(A) constant, the value of (I) is kept constant, then (A)′ can be adjusted until equal responses are obtained from the action of (A)′ and (A) on the tissue. Then Equation (27) gives

$$K_I = \frac{1}{(I)}\left[\frac{(A)'}{(A)} - 1\right] \tag{29}$$

where (A)′/(A) is now the experimentally determined dose-ratio (GADDUM et al., 1955). Since K_I and (I) are both constant, it follows that (A)′/(A) should be independent of r, for a competitive antagonist, and so the log dose/response curves obtained in the absence and in the presence of the competitive antagonist should be parallel. If the log dose/response curves are not parallel then the antagonist is not strictly competitive but, unfortunately the converse is not necessarily true. However, even if the curves are not parallel the dose-ratio may still be used as an arbitrary measure of antagonist potency, provided that the response level at which the dose-ratio is measured is specified (e.g., at 50% of the maximal response). Similar considerations apply to the use of the pA_x in the case of antagonism which is not competitive (SCHILD, 1957).

3. Intrinsic Activity, Efficacy, and the Pharmacologic Stimulus

According to Clark's original theory, drugs which act on one type of receptor must be either agonists or antagonists, since the value of k in Equation (23) was assumed to be the same for all agonists, and zero for antagonists. However, RAVENTOS (1937) studied the action on various tissues of a series of quaternary nitrogen compounds and found that the maximal responses produced by some of these drugs were less than the maximal responses produced by others. These findings were later confirmed by ARIENS (1954) and by STEPHENSON (1956). Agonists which produce maximal responses equal to the maximal response of which the tissue is capable are called full agonists, while those which produce smaller maximal responses are called partial agonists. In order to account for the existence of partial agonists, ARIENS introduced the concept of intrinsic activity and STEPHENSON the idea of efficacy. These concepts are qualitatively similar but quantitatively different. The basic idea is that not all drug-receptor complexes are equally effective in producing a response, so that there is a gradual transition from agonists to antagonists.

a) Intrinsic Activity

ARIENS (1954) defined the intrinsic activity of a drug as a "substance constant determining the effect per unit of pharmacon-receptor complex." He modified Clark's original equation, allowing the value of k [in Eq. (23)] to vary from one drug to another. If the response to any agonist A is written as r_A then

$$r_A = k_A \{y_A\}.$$

At sufficiently high concentrations of A the receptor sites become saturated with agonist and y_A tends to unity [see Eq. (7b)] so that the response tends to a maximum value which is equal to k_A. The above equation can then be written in the form

$$y_A = r_A / \{r_A\}_{MAX}.$$

ARIENS had therefore retained Clark's assumption that the response to an agonist is proportional to the fraction of the receptors occupied, so that a maximal response is obtained only when all of the receptors are occupied. As in the case of Clark's original theory, provided that these assumptions are valid the affinity constant of an agonist for the receptors can be calculated using Equation (25), with the modification that $(A)_{50}$ is now the concentration of A which produces a response equal to one-half of the maximal response which drug A can elicit from the tissue.

If, for each of two drugs A and B, the response is proportional to the fraction of receptors occupied, then the ratio of their intrinsic activities is given by the equation

$$\alpha_A/\alpha_B = \{r_A\}_{MAX}/\{r_B\}_{MAX}$$

where α_A and α_B are the individual intrinsic activities of the two drugs. If drug B produces the maximal response of which the tissue is capable and if its intrinsic activity is set equal to unity, then the intrinsic activity of drug A becomes

$$\alpha_A = \{r_A\}_{MAX}/\{r\}_{MAX}.$$

It will be seen that on this basis the intrinsic activities of all full agonists would be unity, partial agonists would have intrinsic activities lying between zero and unity, and antagonists would have zero intrinsic activity.

However, as has been pointed out by STEPHENSON (1953, 1956), FURCHGOTT (1955), and NICKERSON (1956), it seems probable that some fully active agonists may produce maximal responses from a tissue without occupying all of the receptors. Yet such agonists would still appear to have the same intrinsic activity. Attempts were later made by VAN ROSSUM and ARIENS (1962) to allow for such effects by using irreversible antagonists. In this way they obtained "corrected" intrinsic activities, which could be greater than unity for full agonists.

b) Efficacy and the Pharmacologic Stimulus

STEPHENSON (1956) discarded Clark's assumption that the response is proportional to the fraction of receptors occupied by an agonist, but assumed instead that the most potent member of the group of agonists, which act on the receptors being studied, is able to elicit a maximal response from the tissue when the fraction of receptors occupied by the agonist is very small. This means that for such a highly effective agonist there would be a large surplus of receptors, or a very large proportion of "spare" receptors. It follows that different (full) agonists may produce maximal responses when they occupy different fractions of the receptors. According to Stephenson's ideas, full agonists may therefore have very different efficacies.

An important concept introduced by STEPHENSON (1956) was that of the pharmacologic stimulus, s, which was defined as

$$s = ey$$

where e is the efficacy of the drug and y is the fraction of receptors occupied. The response was then assumed to be some function of this stimulus, or

$$r = f(s) = f(ey) . \tag{30}$$

Then equal values of the stimulus were assumed to produce equal responses from any single piece of tissue.

The idea of the pharmacologic stimulus will be seen to be a generalisation of the null method previously applied to studies of drug antagonism, with the modification that y_A is replaced by $e_A y_A$. If this idea is considered at the molecular level of drug action, it will be seen to imply that a large number of less effective agonist-receptor complexes can produce the same stimulus as a smaller number of more effective complexes. In fact the stimulus could be considered to be the primary response r_p, in the sequence of events

$$R + D \rightleftharpoons RD \rightarrow r_p \ldots \rightarrow r_{obs.} , \tag{31}$$

where $r_{obs.}$ is the response actually measured. Intuitively one might expect some maximum limit to the stimulus per receptor, so that there is presumably some upper limit to the efficacy or intrinsic activity of a drug at the receptor level. Therefore the essential qualitative difference between the assumptions of STEPHENSON and of ARIENS was that the former assumed that if the pharmacologic stimulus was increased, the ability of the tissue to respond soon became the limiting factor. The latter assumed the converse to be true.

By using the stimulus concept, and by assuming that a full agonist occupies a negligible fraction of the receptors even when it produces a maximal response, STEPHENSON (1956) was able to obtain values for the affinity constants of the "partial-agonist" members of a homologous series of alkyl-trimethyl-ammonium compounds. He then estimated the affinity constants of the "full-agonist" members of the series by extrapolating the curve obtained for the affinity constants of the partial agonists. These extrapolated affinity constants were then used to estimate the efficacies of the full agonists.

It now seems to be generally accepted that for some tissues at least, some full agonists may produce maximal responses without occupying all of the receptors (STEPHENSON, 1953, 1956; FURCHGOTT, 1955; NICKERSON, 1956; VAN ROSSUM and ARIENS, 1962). The difficulty of estimating drug parameters such as affinity constants and intrinsic activities or efficacies, is due to uncertainty about the form of the relationship between the response and the fraction of receptors occupied by an agonist. The problem can be restated by saying that the stimulus-response relationship is not known. ARIENS (1954) had, in effect, assumed that the response is proportional to the stimulus, although attempts were later made to eliminate this assumption (VAN ROSSUM and ARIENS, 1962). STEPHENSON (1956) initially assumed that the stimulus is equal to the product of the efficacy and the fraction of the receptors occupied, but in order to estimate efficacies he later had to assume that, for the most potent agonist of the series, the stimulus is given by the product of its efficacy, its affinity constant, and the concentration of the agonist. This led inevitably to the assumption that the response versus stimulus curve is the same as the response versus concentration curve obtained for the most potent agonist (STEPHENSON, 1956, his Fig. 8). The difference between the stimulus-response relationship assumed by ARIENS and that assumed by STEPHENSON is shown in Figure 1, from which it will be clear that the difference becomes greater as the properties of the drug approach those of a full agonist. The affinity constants of full agonists estimated on the basis of Stephenson's assumptions, differed appreciably from those estimated using Arien's assumptions (see, e.g.,

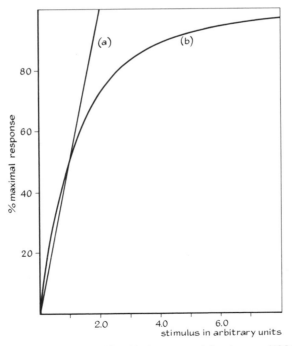

Fig. 1. The stimulus-response relationship. (a) As assumed by ARIENS (1954), (b) as assumed by STEPHENSON (1956)

MACKAY, 1966a). This caused difficulties in the analysis of the structure-activity relationships of agonists.

4. Intrinsic Efficacy

Since the concepts of intrinsic activity and efficacy are similar at the molecular level, and the distinction between them depends on the assumptions made in their evaluation, it seemed advisable to redefine the concept as the primary response or stimulus per drug-receptor complex. The pharmacologic stimulus produced by drug D when it acts on the receptors, is then

$$s_D = f_D[RD], \quad \textit{compare with (12)} \tag{32a}$$
$$= f_D y_D[R]_T \quad \textit{y_D = fraction of receptors} \tag{32b}$$
$$\textit{occupied by D}$$

where f_D has been called the intrinsic efficacy (FURCHGOTT, 1965) or the stimulus coefficient (MACKAY, 1965). The hybrid term "intrinsic efficacy" will be used here to indicate the parameter f_D, with no implications as to how this quantity is to be estimated experimentally.

However, the usefulness of the stimulus concept depends on the assumption that equal responses result from equal stimuli. As has already been mentioned, the stimulus may be regarded as the primary response r_p [see Eq. (31)]. VAN ROSSUM (1966) has pointed out that when the null method is used to compare equal responses, it is implicitly assumed that this primary response is proportional to the product of an intensity factor (the intrinsic efficacy) and the concentration of RD complexes. This implies that any distortion of the proportionality between the response and the concentration of agonist-receptor complexes occurs between r_p and $r_{obs.}$. The magnitude of the distortion will depend on the properties of the tissue and on the nature of the response observed.

However, the relation between the primary response and the concentration of RD complexes may be more complicated than that assumed in Equations (32a) and (32b). A more general relation would be

$$r_p = f\{i_D, [RD]\},$$

where i_D is an intensity factor characteristic of the RD complex. The observed response depends on the primary response, so that

$$r_{obs.} = F\{r_p\},$$

where the function $F\{r_p\}$ is a property of the tissue. As has been emphasised by VAN ROSSUM, the null method cannot be successfully applied if the primary response is not proportional to s_D and if the relation between r_p and [RD] is not known. However, the null method can be applied to more complicated situations if the form of the relation between r_p and [RD] is known or can be predicted. Such situations may require redefinition of the pharmacologic stimulus. The relevance of these comments will become evident later, when the possibility of enzyme-activation by drugs is considered.

5. General Application of the Null Method to the Analysis of Dose-Response Curves

Instead of applying the null method to one or two selected responses the principle can be applied in a general way so as to extract information from dose-response curves obtained on a single tissue. This technique has been used to derive general null equations for drug antagonism and for comparison of the properties of agonists (MACKAY, 1966a).

If reproducible dose-response curves have been obtained for two agonists, A and B, which act on the same receptors in the same tissue, then concentrations $(A)_r$ and $(B)_r$ which produce the same response r, can be read from the dose-response curves. The stimulus produced by drug A is $f_A\{y_A\}_r[R]_T$, while that produced by drug B is $f_B\{y_B\}_r[R]_T$. Equating these two stimuli and substituting for $\{y_A\}_r$ and $\{y_B\}_r$, by use of Equation (7b), the general equation obtained is

$$[1/(A)_r] = [1/(B)_r] [K_A\beta_{AB}/K_B] + K_A(\beta_{AB} - 1) . \tag{33}$$

In this equation, which applies for all values of r, β_{AB} is the ratio of the intrinsic efficacy of drug A to that of drug B. A plot of $1/(A)_r$ against $1/(B)_r$ for a series of values of r should therefore give a straight line of slope ψ_{AB} and intercept I_{AB} where

$$\psi_{AB} = K_A\beta_{AB}/K_B \tag{34a}$$

and

$$I_{AB} = K_A(\beta_{AB} - 1) . \tag{34b}$$

Obviously use of the null method gives two equations which contain the experimental quantities ψ_{AB} and I_{AB}, but which also contain three unknown parameters K_A, K_B, and β_{AB}. These results indicate that it is not possible to estimate the parameters from simple dose-response curves alone. Any value can be arbitrarily chosen for one of these parameters and the other two will take values to fit Equations (34a) and (34b). Each such set of values of K_A, K_B, and β_{AB} represents a possible solution, and each set corresponds to a different stimulus-response relation which can be estimated. Therefore any estimates of these parameters based on an assumption about the form of the stimulus-response relation, could be very much in error.

However, one assumption which is often made and which may sometimes be justified is that for a full agonist A and a partial agonist B, β_{AB} is very much greater than unity, or the intrinsic efficacy of the full agonist is very much greater than that of the partial agonist. If this is true then,

$$I_{AB}/\psi_{AB} = K_B . \tag{35}$$

The above assumption is essentially the same as that introduced by STEPHENSON (1956).

General null equations were similarly derived for antagonism. If $(A)_r$ is the concentration of agonist which produces a response r in the absence of the antagonist, and $(A)'_r$ produces response r in the presence of the antagonist then the corresponding values of the fractions of receptors occupied by A are $\{y_A\}_r$

and $\{y_A\}'_r$. The respective stimuli are $f_A\{y_A\}_r [R]_T$ and $f_A\{y_A\}'_r [R]_T$ so that for equal responses

$$\{y_A\}_r = \{y_A\}'_r .$$

The value of $\{y_A\}_r$ is then given by Equation (7b) while the value of $\{y_A\}'_r$ is obtained from Equation (16a) for competitive inhibition and from Equation (21) for specific noncompetitive inhibition. The resulting null equations are

$$1/(A)_r = [1 + K_I(I)]/(A)'_r \tag{36}$$

for competitive inhibition, and

$$1/(A)_r = [1/(A)'_r] [1 + K_I(I)] + K_A K_{AI}(I) \tag{37}$$

for specific noncompetitive inhibition.

6. Estimation of Affinity Constants and Intrinsic Efficacies of Agonists

A potentially useful method for the estimation of these parameters is the use of specific irreversible antagonists, as suggested by STEPHENSEN (1965, 1966). This method is based on the comparison of dose-response curves obtained for an agonist A acting on the same tissue, before and after treatment of the tissue with a specific irreversible antagonist. The derivation and use of the appropriate equations have been discussed by MACKAY (1966b, c), VAN ROSSUM (1966), FURCHGOTT (1966), FURCHGOTT and BURSZTYN (1968), and WAUD (1968a, b). The irreversible antagonist is assumed to reduce the receptor concentration from an initial value $[R]_T$, to a lower value $[R]_T [1 - y_I]$ where y_I is the fraction of the receptors irreversibly blocked by the antagonist. The general null equation for comparison of the two dose-response curves (see Fig. 2a), is then

$$f_A\{y_A\}_r [R]_T = f_A\{y_A\}'_r [R]_T [1 - y_I] . \tag{38}$$

Substituting the appropriate values for $\{y_A\}_r$ and $\{y_A\}'_r$ by use of Equation 7b, and rearranging, the null equation becomes

$$1/(A)_r = 1/\{(A)'_r [1 - y_I]\} + K_A y_I/[1 - y_I] . \tag{39}$$

A plot of $1/(A)_r$ versus $1/(A)'_r$ should therefore give a straight line of slope $1/[1 - y_I]$ and intercept $K_A y_I/[1 - y_I]$, as shown in Figure 2b. For such a plot of $1/(A)_r$ versus $1/(A)'_r$, the experimental quantity ϱ_A may be defined as

$$\varrho_A = \frac{\text{Intercept}}{\text{Slope} - 1} \tag{40a}$$

and on the basis of the above model,

$$\varrho_A = K_A . \tag{40b}$$

affinity constant

slope $= \frac{1}{1-y_1}$, $1-y_1 = \frac{1}{slope}$, $y_1 = 1 - \frac{1}{slope}$

intercept $= \frac{K_A y_1}{1-y_1} = \frac{K_A(1-\frac{1}{slope})}{\frac{1}{slope}} = slope \cdot K_A - K_A = K_A(slope-1)$

so, $K_A = \frac{intercept}{slope-1}$

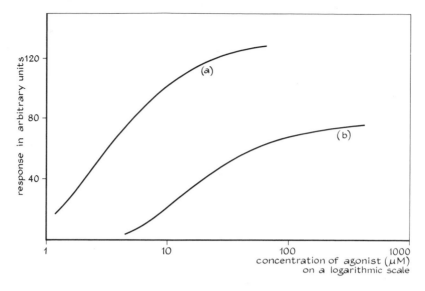

Fig. 2a. Log dose-response curves for action of agonist on tissue. (*a*) before and (*b*) after treatment of tissue with specific irreversible antagonist. Values of $(A)_r$ and $(A)'_r$ can be read from curves (*a*) and (*b*) respectively for any chosen value of response r

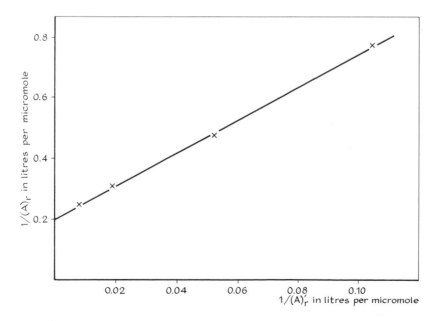

Fig. 2b. Plot of $1/(A)_r$ against $1/(A)'_r$ from results shown in Figure 2a

This last equation should also be valid for pseudoirreversible antagonists, and for specific noncompetitive antagonists if K_{AI} is equal to K_I [see Eq. (37)]. When estimates of the value of the affinity constants K_A and K_B of two agonists have been obtained from Equations (40a) and (40b), their relative intrinsic efficacies can be estimated from the concentration of each required to produce some chosen submaximal response, so that:

$$\beta_{AB} = \{y_B\}_r/\{y_A\}_r$$

$$= \left[1 + \frac{1}{K_A(A)_r}\right] \Big/ \left[1 + \frac{1}{K_B(B)_r}\right].$$

However, a more general approach is to estimate β_{AB} from ψ_{AB}, since from Equations (34a) and (40b),

$$\beta_{AB} = \psi_{AB} K_B/K_A = \psi_{AB}\varrho_B/\varrho_A. \tag{41}$$

Alternatively, from Equations (34b) and (40b),

$$\beta_{AB} = 1 + [I_{AB}/K_A] = 1 + [I_{AB}/\varrho_A]. \tag{42}$$

The fact that β_{AB} can be estimated in two different ways if ψ_{AB}, I_{AB}, ϱ_A, and ϱ_B have all been measured is a consequence of the fact that there are four independent experimental quantities and only three unknown K_A, K_B, and β_{AB} (on the basis of the model).

Combination of Equations (41) and (42) gives

$$\psi_{AB}\varrho_B/\varrho_A = 1 + [I_{AB}/\varrho_A]. \tag{43}$$

Equation (43) contains only experimental quantities, and may therefore be used to test the ability of the model to fit the experimental results.

7. A Discussion of the Direct Occupation Theory of Drug Action

In any discussion of the direct occupation theory it seems advisable to make a clear-cut distinction between the qualitative and quantitative aspects of the theory. The basic assumption of direct occupation theory is that a drug may react with specific receptors to produce a response, and that the magnitude of the response will depend on the number of receptors occupied by the drug. Qualitatively this idea seems reasonable. The qualitative concepts of affinity and intrinsic efficacy also seem logical.

Because of the limited amount of information available from dose-response curves, attempts to obtain quantitative measures of affinity and intrinsic efficacy, necessarily involve some assumptions. Use of the null method has largely eliminated the need for any assumption about the exact form of the relation between the response and the concentration of receptor-agonist complexes, but several other assumptions are still required. In applying the null method to estimate the affinity constant of an antagonist for its receptors, the following assumptions are usually made.

1. The receptor has a definite chemical structure and the interaction between the drug and the receptor is bimolecular.

2. The response measured corresponds to equilibrium or pseudoequilibrium occupation of the receptors by the agonist. When the response is measured in the presence of an antagonist then there is also equilibrium occupation of the receptors by the antagonist.

3. Either a graded response is obtained from each individual cell or the tissue behaves as a syncytium.

4. The observed response results from a primary response or stimulus, this stimulus being proportional to the concentration of receptor-agonist complexes.

5. For any given piece of isolated tissue, the stimulus-response relation is independent of time and constant for all drugs which act on the receptors being studied. The stimulus-response relation is therefore characteristic of the particular piece of tissue and these receptors.

6. The concentration of unbound drug near the receptors can either be estimated, measured, or assumed to be equal to the concentration of unbound drug originally present in the external solution. This latter assumption usually implies that a negligible amount of drug is taken up by the tissue and receptors.

Of the various null methods for the estimation of affinity constants of antagonists for receptors, discussed in Sections III.A.2 and III.A.5, the measurement of pA_x has been used most extensively to characterise both antagonists and their receptors (SCHILD, 1947, 1949, 1957; ARUNLAKSHANA and SCHILD, 1959; ARIENS and VAN ROSSUM, 1957; VAN ROSSUM and ARIENS, 1959; MARSHALL, 1955). The measurement of pA_x is a useful practical method with a sound theoretical basis but it may give low estimates for K_I if insufficient time is allowed for equilibrium occupation of the receptors by the antagonist. The limitations of pA_x have been discussed by SCHILD (1957). The dose-ratio method has been used by Paton and his co-workers (PATON, 1961; PATON and RANG, 1965) and by BARLOW et al. (1963, 1967), as well as by GADDUM et al. (1955).

Extension of the null method to estimate the affinity constant of an agonist for its receptors involves a further assumption.

7. Suitable specific irreversible, pseudoirreversible, or noncompetitive antagonists can inactivate some of the receptors without modifying the stimulus-response relation.

The likely validity of the assumptions listed above must be carefully considered for each drug-receptor system in each tissue. In principle the number of molecules of drug which interact with each receptor can be checked by testing the fit of the experimental results to the appropriate null equations. Ideally responses should be obtained from single cells or from small groups of cells. In the latter case the observed response may be some form of integrated response (MACKAY, 1966a). However, if a tissue behaves as a syncytium, as happens with smooth muscle (see BULBRING et al., 1970) then the observed response may be almost equivalent to the response from a single cell although it may arise from the initial action of the agonist on only a small region of the tissue. Such a situation can cause complications in the interpretation of the *kinetics* of action of agonists and antagonists (WAUD, 1968). As was pointed out by FURCHGOTT (1955), the assumption that the concentration of drug at the receptors is the same as in the external fluid may lead to errors in the estimation of affinity constants. The various errors which can arise have also been discussed by VAN ROSSUM (1966).

The results of TRIGGLE (1965) indicate that even "specific" irreversible alkylating agents react with many tissue sites so that their actions may be more widespread than would be suspected on the basis of pharmacologic tests. On the other hand, this does not necessarily mean that they alter the stimulus-response relation. It may be possible to design more specific irreversible antagonists (see, e.g., GILL and RANG, 1966; RANG and RITTER, 1969; YOUNG et al., 1972).

The assumption that irreversible antagonists do not alter the stimulus-response relation can be tested in several ways. One method is to compare estimates of the affinity constant of an agonist for its receptors, obtained by using different irreversible or pseudoirreversible antagonists. Another is to measure the affinity constant of a partial agonist for its receptors by use of an irreversible antagonist, and subsequently to modify the tissue so as to be able to estimate the affinity constant of the same drug acting as an antagonist (FURCHGOTT and BURSZTYN, 1968). A third method is to use experimental values of ψ_{AB} and I_{AB} as well as the experimental quantities ϱ_A and ϱ_B [see Eq. (40a)] obtained by the use of irreversible or pseudoirreversible antagonists, so as to test the validity of Equation (43) (MACKAY, 1966c).

However, the most serious assumption made in applying direct occupation theory to experimental results is the assumption that the peak responses produced by an agonist correspond to equilibrium or pseudoequilibrium occupation of the receptors. This assumption is not easily defended. The conditions under which it is likely to be valid are discussed in the next section.

8. The Equilibrium Assumption

Generally, a specific antagonist can be left in contact with a tissue for long periods of time without producing any drastic change in the ability of the tissue to respond to agonists which stimulate receptors other than those with which the antagonist interacts. On the other hand, prolonged action of an agonist on a tissue often leads to nonspecific desensitisation. It is therefore usually advisable to reduce the contact time between agonist and tissue to the minimum time necessary to obtain peak or steady responses.

The fractional attainment of equilibrium occupation of receptors by a drug, is given by Equation (8). It will also be seen, from the exponential form of this equation, that absolute equilibrium is reached only after an infinitely long time. Equation (8) may be written in the form

$$\{y_D\}_t = \{y_D\}_{eq.} \left\{ 1 - \exp[-k_2(1 + K_D(D)) t] \right\},$$

where (D) is the concentration of the drug and K_D is its affinity constant for the receptors

Then $\{y_D\}_t$ becomes approximately equal to $\{y_D\}_{eq.}$ only if the exponential term is very much less than unity. This means that the contact time should be very much greater than $t_{1/2}$ [see Eq. (10)]. For example, slightly more than 99% of the equilibrium value of y_A will have been reached after a contact time equal to seven times $t_{1/2}$.

If the above condition is not strictly valid then the equations for equilibrium occupation of receptors by drugs should be replaced by the corresponding non-equilibrium equations when using the null method to compare dose-response curves. For example, if a concentration $(A)_r$ of the agonist A produces a response r, then the stimulus which produces this response at time t is

$$\{s_A\}_t = f_A\{y_A\}_t [R]_T$$
$$= f_A\{y_A\}_{eq.} [R]_T \{1 - \exp[-k_2(1 + K_A(A)_r) t]\},$$

where $[R]_T$ is the total concentration of receptors. If the total concentration of receptors is then reduced to $[R]_T [1 - y_I]$ by use of an irreversible antagonist the general equation for the stimulus becomes

$$\{s_A\}_t' = f_A\{y_A\}_t' [R]_T [1 - y_I]$$
$$= f_A\{y_A\}_{eq.}' [R]_T \{1 - \exp[-k_2(1 + K_A(A)_r') t]\} [1 - y_I].$$

The null equation, for equal responses after a constant time t, is then

$$\{y_A\}_{eq.} \{1 - \exp[-k_2(1 + K_A(A)_r) t]\}$$
$$= \{y_A\}_{eq.}' \{1 - \exp[-k_2(1 + K_A(A)_r') t]\} [1 - y_I],$$

which reduces to Equation (39) if $K_A(A)_r$ and $K_A(A)_r'$ are both very much less than unity, or if the exponential terms are very much less than unity. The former condition is valid under nonequilibrium experimental conditions provided that the agonist would occupy negligible fractions of the receptors even if time were allowed for practical attainment of equilibrium. The latter condition implies that the contact time t should be sufficiently large to allow receptor occupation to reach about 90% of its equilibrium value.

Similar considerations apply to the null equations derived for pseudoirreversible antagonism and for specific noncompetitive antagonism, and also to the null equation for the estimation of the values of ψ_{AB} and I_{AB} [see Eqs. (33), (37), and (39)]. The problem cannot be set out so precisely in the case of reversible competitive antagonism because of the possibility that agonist may displace antagonist from the receptor. However, similar conclusions are likely to be qualitatively valid. The fact that good linear plots are generally obtained by use of the "equilibrium" null equations suggests that one or other of the two conditions discussed above is valid or that there is some other cancellation of error.

9. Variation of the Response with Time

This subject has been discussed by many authors, from various points of view (STRAUB, 1907; GADDUM, 1926; CLARK, 1933; BARSOUM and GADDUM, 1935; CANTONI and EASTMAN, 1946; FURCHGOTT, 1955; PATON, 1961; ARIENS et al., 1964; ELMQVIST and THESLEFF, 1962; TAYLOR and NEDERGAARD, 1965; MACKAY,

1966b; WAUD, 1968; RANG and RITTER, 1970). It includes such fascinating problems as sensitisation, specific and nonspecific desensitisation, and the fade phenomenon. However, in this section attention will be focussed on the time effects only insofar as they may affect the interpretation of response curves in terms of the direct occupation theory of drug action.

Since receptor theory is most likely to be useful when receptors are present in or on membranes, it is interesting to consider the likely consequences of an agonist-induced-change in membrane permeability. If an agonist interacts with receptors so as to cause an increase in the permeability of a cell membrane to some ion X, then the change in permeability would be expected to reach a constant value when the agonist-receptor interaction has resulted in equilibrium occupation of the receptors. If no further changes occur either in the cell or in the receptor sites, then the increased flux of the ion X would be expected to continue until the electrochemical potential of the ion inside the cell is the same as that outside the cell. A new steady-state concentration of X inside the cell should then be reached only when

$$\ln\left[(X)_0/(X)_i\right] = -zF(\varphi_0 - \varphi_i)/RT .$$

where $(X)_0$ and $(X)_i$ are the concentrations of the free ion, and φ_0 and φ_i are the electrical potentials, outside and inside the cell respectively. R in the above equation is the gas constant, T is the absolute temperature, and z is the charge on the ion X. If the tissue is completely depolarised then the new steady-state will occur only when $(X)_i$ is equal to $(X)_0$. If, under these latter conditions, the agonist-receptor interaction goes rapidly to equilibrium then the rate of change of $(X)_i$ with time would be expected to be given by an equation of the form

$$d(X)_i/dt = \lambda\left[(X)_0 - (X)_i\right] ,$$

where λ is proportional to the "equilibrium" permeability change produced by the agonist. By integrating the above equation the ratio of concentration of the ion inside the cell to that outside the cell, at any time t after the addition of the agonist, is found to be

$$(X)_i'/(X)_0 = 1 - \{1 - (X)_i/(X)_0\}\exp\left[-\lambda t\right] ,$$

where $(X)_i$ is the initial concentration of the ion inside the cell and $(X)_i'$ is the concentration at time t. The rate of rise of $(X)_i'$ to its maximum value $(X)_0$ will be seen to depend on the value of λ. However, λ does not affect the final equilibrium state and so the magnitude of the change in permeability produced by the agonist would control only the rate of approach to equilibrium.

If the response depends on the concentration of the ion X inside the cell then it will be apparent that the approach to a steady response would be expected to be slow for depolarised tissues, and the final steady response would be expected to be independent of the concentration of the agonist. However, the results of EDMAN and SCHILD (1962), SCHILD (1964), DURBIN and JENKINSON (1961a, b, and JENKINSON and NICHOLLS (1961) indicate that such slow approaches to a "dose-independent" steady response are not usually observed.

This suggests that other changes do in fact occur, either in the receptors or in the properties of the cell. These changes probably tend to annul the effects of the initial change in membrane permeability, and may explain some forms of desensitisation, tachyphylaxis, and fade.

The type of desensitisation observed with isolated tissues may be divided into two main classes which are

1. specific desensitisation, first reported by BARSOUM and GADDUM (1935), and

2. nonspecific desensitisation, first investigated by CANTONI and EASTMAN (1946).

In order to explain the desensitisation effects which they observed at the neuromuscular junction of frog muscle, DEL CASTILLO and KATZ (1957) postulated a series of time-dependent changes in the acetylcholine-receptor complexes. However, since the specificity of desensitisation can only be tested if a tissue has more than one type of receptor, it is possible that the desensitisation observed in these experiments was of the nonspecific type. Other interesting desensitisation effects have also been interpreted as being due to changes in the properties of receptors (KATZ and THESLEFF, 1957). More recent support for the idea that desensitisation involves the conversion of an active agonist-receptor complex to an inactive form has come from the work of KARLIN (1967) and of RANG and RITTER (1970). PATON (1961) suggested that nonspecific desensitisation might depend "on the rate of loss of potassium under drug action and recovery on the rate at which the cell pumps it back." PATON and ROTHSCHILD (1965) measured the changes in concentration of sodium, potassium, and calcium ions in the longitudinal muscle of guinea pig ileum and concluded that desensitisation might be produced by gain of sodium ions and a resultant stimulation of an electrogenic sodium extrusion mechanism. WAUD (1968) has also put forward the idea that changes in the ionic concentration gradients across the cell membranes (and in unstirred films at the membrane surfaces) may contribute toward desensitisation. MACKAY (1966b) suggested that many pharmacologic phenomena, such as desensitisation and fade, which cannot be explained on the basis of the direct occupation theory itself, might be explained by combining this theory with a negative-feedback mechanism. It was suggested that the feedback might be provided by the sodium pump, which would be expected to be stimulated by an increase in the intracellular concentration of sodium ions. The latter would result from the change in membrane permeability produced by an agonist.

Other explanations of desensitisation and fade have also been suggested and some of these will be discussed later. One obvious possibility is a decrease in the availability of some substance which is essential for the response. This substance might be an enzyme substrate or some essential cofactor such as calcium ions. Specific desensitisation and fade may also be interpreted in terms of the rate theory (see Sect. IV), or as being due to intracellular uptake of drug (see Sect. III.C).

On the other hand, even desensitisation may not be strictly a receptor phenomenan although it may be localised in the area around the agonist-receptor complex. If a tissue consisted of a population of different types of cell, each cell type having only one kind of receptor, then a large dose of an agonist would be expected to produce a maximal response from the appropriate cells, followed by (nonspecific) desensitisation. The other cells of the tissue could still respond to their own appropriate agonists. It may be possible to extrapolate this model down to the submicroscopic scale. Each cell has a complex intracellular structure and there is no evidence as to whether the various types of receptor are uniformly distributed over or within the cell. Each cell might then be regarded as a multi-compartment system, and it may be possible to (nonspecifically) desensitise some compartments withoug seriously affecting others. It is of interest, in this respect, that even the specific desensitisation reported by BARSOUM and GADDUM (1935) had a component of nonspecific desensitisation.

10. A Negative Feedback Model

For the reasons discussed in the previous section it seems likely that when the permeability of the cell membrane is increased by interaction of an agonist with its receptors, changes occur which tend to annul the initial permeability change. Since the presence of feedback mechanisms is one of the characteristic properties of living systems at the physiological and biochemical levels, it seems reasonable to consider the possible consequences of negative feedback on drug action (see also BULBRING, 1964).

Before treatment of the cell with a drug D, the cell is assumed to be in an approximately steady state. The influxes of the various ions balance the effluxes, whether the fluxes are active or passive. Initially the concentration of some ion X inside the cell may be maintained by a pump and leak mechanism. The leak influx, J_L, will be given by an equation of the form

$$J_L = \eta\{(X)_0 - (X)_i\}$$

where η is the initial membrane permeability, and $(X)_0$ and $(X)_i$ are respectively the initial concentrations of the free ion outside and inside the cell. The pump efflux, J_P, would be expected to depend on $(X)_i$, so that its activity may be assumed to be given by an equation of the form

$$J_P = \frac{\zeta(X)_i}{1 + \gamma\zeta(X)_i}, \tag{44}$$

where ζ and γ are constants. For sufficiently small values of $(X)_i$,

$$J_P \simeq \zeta(X)_i, \tag{45}$$

while for sufficiently large values of $(X)_i$, J_P would tend to a maximum value of $1/\gamma$. The effect of the membrane potential and ion charge on the ion fluxes, will be ignored for the time being.

At time zero the drug D begins to react with the receptors and produces a change in the membrane permeability which results in an increase in J_L, from J_L to $J_L + \Delta J_L$. The value of ΔJ_L at time t is

$$\{\Delta J_L\}_t = \{(X)_0 - (X)_i\} f_D\{y_D\}_t [R]_T$$

where $(X)_i'$ is now the concentration of X inside the cell at time t and $\{y_D\}_t$ is given by Equation (8). At sufficiently large values of t,

$$\{\varDelta J_L\} = \{(X)_0 - (X)_i'\}\, f_D\{y_D\}_{eq.}\, [R]_T\,.$$

The increased leakage flux will produce increasing values of $(X)_i'$, which might be expected to stimulate the pump efflux, but it seems unlikely that the response of the pump would be instantaneous. In order to simplify the equations it will also be assumed that the value of $(X)_i'$ is sufficiently low for Equation (45) to be valid. Then the pump efflux might be expected to change from J_P to $J_P + \varDelta J_P$, where

$$\{\varDelta J_P\}_t = \zeta\,[(X)_i' - (X)_i]\,[1 - \exp(-kt)]\,.$$

k is a constant which determines the rate of response of the pump to any change in $(X)_i'$. Obviously this rate might also be some function of $[(X)_i' - (X)_i]$. The net influx of the ion X at time t is, $\{\varDelta J_L\}_t - \{\varDelta J_P\}_t$, and the rate of change of concentration of X inside the cell is therefore given by an equation of the form

$$d(X)_i'/dt = M f_D\{y_D\}_{eq.}\,\{1 - \exp[-(k_2 + k_1(D))\,t]\}\,[(X_0 - (X)_i']$$
$$- N\{1 - \exp(-kt)\}\,[(X)_i' - (X)_i] \tag{46}$$

where M is a constant proportional to the total concentration of receptors $[R]_T$, and N is a constant proportional to the pump constant ζ.

If $d(X)_i'/dt$ is to become equal to zero, corresponding to a new steady-state concentration of the ion X inside the cell then

$$M f_D\{y_D\}_t\,[(X)_0 - (X)_i'] = N\{1 - \exp(-kt)\}\,[(X)_i' - (X)_i]\,. \tag{47}$$

If the pump is inactive, so that N is zero, then a steady state is reached only when $(X)_i'$ is equal to $(X)_0$. This is the case discussed in the previous section. If N has a finite value then a new steady state will be reached, at sufficiently large values of t, when

$$\frac{(X)_i'}{(X)_i} = \frac{M f_D\{y_D\}_{eq.}\,(X)_0/(X)_i + N}{M f_D\{y_D\}_{eq.} + N}\,. \tag{48}$$

Obviously the steady state value of $(X)_i'$ must lie between $(X)_i$ and $(X)_0$. Some examples of the effect of negative feedback have been estimated by numerical integration of Equation (46), and are given in Figure 3.

An interesting point about such a feedback mechanism is the importance of the rate constants k, k_1, and k_2. If k is very much greater than $[k_2 + k_1(D)]$ then the effect of the change in membrane permeability on $(X)_i'$ can be rapidly neutralised by the ion pump, especially for moderate values of f_D. If $(X)_i'$ determines the response then it follows that the rate of the drug-receptor interaction could at least partly determine whether a drug behaves as an agonist, partial agonist, or antagonist. Antagonists could then be of two types,

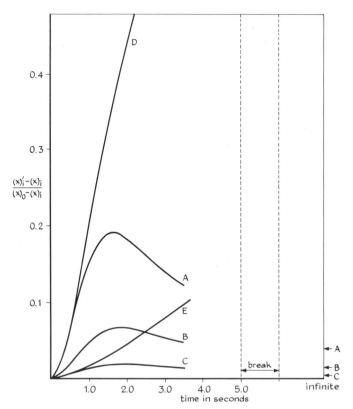

Fig. 3. Effects of negative feedback on changes in intracellular concentration, $(X)_i'$, of some ion X, resulting from drug-induced change in membrane permeability. The quantities $(X)_0$ and $(X)_i$ are extracellular and initial intracellular concentrations of the ion, respectively. The quantity $\{(X)_i' - (X)_i\}/\{(X)_0 - (X)_i\}$ is proportional to change in intracellular concentration of ion X, for given values of $(X)_0$ and $(X)_i$. The curves have been calculated by numerical integration of a modified form of Equation (46), with $M = 1.0$, $f_D = 1.0$, $k_1 = 10^5$ l/mole.s, $k_2 = 1.0\,\mathrm{s}^{-1}$. $k = 0.10\,\mathrm{s}^{-1}$. Curves: A. Agonist concentration, 6.4 μM; $N = 10.0$. B. Agonist concentration, 1.6 μM; $N = 10.0$. C. Agonist concentration, 0.4 μM; $N = 10.0$. D Agonist concentration, 6.4 μM: $N = 0.0$. E. Agonist concentration 0.4 μM; $N = 0.0$. The *arrows* at extreme right of figure indicate final steady-state values of $\{(X)_i' - (X)_i\}/\{(X)_0 - (X)_i\}$ for curves A, B, and C. Final steady-state value for curves D and E is 1.0

1. those which have very low intrinsic efficacies, so that they produce a negligible change in membrane permeability, and

2. those which have somewhat higher intrinsic efficacies but which interact with the receptor at such a slow rate that their effects are neutralised by negative feedback. The increased feedback could cause desensitisation of the tissue to the actions of agonists by effectively changing the stimulus-response relation. The phase II neuromuscular block produced by decamethonium might be of this type.

According to the feedback model, it would be possible for a drug to act as an antagonist on one tissue and as an agonist on another if the feedback system was less effective in the latter tissue or if the overall permeability change in the latter tissue was considerably greater (due for example to a greater receptor density).

Such effects might explain why drugs such as d-tubocurarine and gallamine can produce weak transient depolarisation of chronically denervated muscle (BOWMAN et al., 1968). A less effective feedback mechanism in such muscle and/or increased receptor density may play some part in its increased sensitivity to depolarising agents, and in its spontaneous activity.

Another point of interest is that $(X)'_i$ can pass through a maximum value if k is very much less than $[k_2 + k_1(D)]$, so that peak responses could be obtained. A delay in the onset of increased pump activity would produce even sharper peaks in the graphs of $(X)'_i$ versus time. An initial displacement by an agonist of the ion X from the cell membrane or other structures might also contribute to the production of an initial peak response.

If an agonist is left in contact with the tissue until a steady response is obtained and the agonist is then washed out at zero time, the leakage influx will decrease as the agonist dissociates from the receptors. The pump efflux will then exceed the leakage influx and $(X)'_i$ should decrease toward $(X)_i$. If $(X)'_i$ determines the response then the latter should return slowly to its base level. Just as there is probably some delay in the onset of increased pump activity so there may be a delay in its offset. This would result in overshoot, so that the value of $(X)'_i$ might be reduced below $(X)_i$ before returning again to $(X)_i$. A decrease of $(X)'_i$ below $(X)_i$ would not necessarily show in the response measurement if the response required some critical threshold value of $(X)'_i$. Such an effect might explain desensitisation since the pump could still be hyperactive when a second dose of agonist is applied.

So far consideration has been limited mainly to the effects of drugs which increase the leakage flux J_L. However, some drugs may reduce this leakage flux, in which case removal of the drug could either produce a response or lead to temporary sensitisation. Such effects might explain the "washout phenomenon." Such sensitisation effects are somewhat similar to the withdrawal symptoms produced by drug addiction which may also be the result of negative feedback mechanisms. The possible importance of biochemical feedback systems in drug tolerance and addiction was pointed out by GOLDSTEIN and GOLDSTEIN (1961). When a new steady state has been attained in the presence of a drug its continued presence may be necessary to maintain the steady state.

Other drugs may modify the activity of ion pumps. A drug which stimulates the activity of ion pumps would be expected to stabilise the cell and reduce its sensitivity to the actions of agonists. Relaxation of the isolated rat uterus by isoprenaline could be explained by such effects (SCHILD, 1967). Conversely, drugs which inhibit ion pumps would be expected to slow down the rate of approach to a steady state and to cause increased sensitivity to agonist.

Since the calcium ion seems to be involved in the process of muscle contraction (see, e.g., NIEDERGERKE, 1956, 1963; HODGKIN and HOROWICZ, 1960; ROBERTSON, 1960; DURBIN and JENKINSON, 1961; WINEGRAD and SHANES, 1962; EDMAN and SCHILD, 1962; BULBRING, 1964.), and in the process of secretion (DOUGLAS, 1968) it is tempting to suggest that the ion X is calcium. If this is so then there may be more than one pump mechanism in the cells. One of these pumps may be the calcium accumulating vesicles which seem to be involved in muscle relaxation, while the other may be situated in the cell membrane (GILBERT and FENN, 1957).

It is not clear whether the increased intracellular concentration of free calcium ions, which is assumed to trigger contraction, is the direct result of the penetration of calcium ions through the membrane or release of membranebound or intracellularly bound calcium by an influx of sodium ions or of drug molecules. Interesting discussions of these problems have been presented by SCHATZMAN (1964) and by SCHILD (1964).

It seems likely that the above feedback scheme greatly oversimplifies the problem, but it does seem to offer a possible explanation of pharmacologic phenomena, which cannot be explained by the direct occupation theory alone. If more than one feedback system is present and there are time-dependent interactions between the systems then oscillatory responses could be explained.

11. The Null Method and the Negative Feedback Model

On the basis of the feedback model, it was shown that for steady-state conditions, $(X)_i'/(X)_i$ is given by Equation (48). For any given tissue in a given biochemical state, N, $(X)_0$, and $(X)_i$ may be considered to be constants. Since M is proportional to $[R]_T$ (see previous Section) it follows that the term $M f_D \{y_D\}_{eq.}$ [in Eq. (48)] is proportional to the pharmacologic stimulus $\{s_D\}_{eq.}$ as defined by Equation (32b). Then Equation (48) can be rearranged to give

$$\{(X)_i\}_{ss} = \frac{a\{s_D\}_{eq.} + b}{c\{s_D\}_{eq.} + d}$$

where a, b, c, and d are constants for the tissue and $\{(X)_i\}_{ss}$ is the steady-state concentration of X inside the cell. If the concentration of X determines the response then equal values of the steady-state response may be assumed to correspond to equal values of $\{(X)_i\}_{ss}$.

If the equilibrium pharmacologic stimulus applied to the tissue is modified (either by the use of specific competitive, noncompetitive, or irreversible antagonists or by the use of another agonist), from some value $\{s_1\}_{eq.}$ to another value $\{s_2\}_{eq.}$ then the condition for equal steady-state responses, on the basis of the feedback model, is

$$\frac{a\{s_1\}_{eq.} + b}{c\{s_1\}_{eq.} + d} = \frac{a\{s_2\}_{eq.} + b}{c\{s_2\}_{eq.} + d}.$$

This equation can be cross multiplied and rearranged to give $[bc][\{s_1\}_{eq.} - \{s_2\}_{eq.}] = [ad][\{s_1\}_{eq.} - \{s_2\}_{eq.}]$, which is valid if $[bc]$ is equal to $[ad]$, or if $\{s_1\}_{eq.}$ is equal to $\{s_2\}_{eq.}$. The former condition is valid only for the case when $(X)_i$ is equal to $(X)_0$ and may therefore be ignored. It follows that the general condition for equal steady-state responses, on the basis of the negative feedback model, is that the pharmacologic stimuli [as defined by Eq. (32b)] should be equal.

In fact, provided that peak responses are obtained after some constant time t, Equation (47) can be used to show that the condition for equal peak responses is that

$$\{s_1\}_t = \{s_2\}_t .$$

This is the same condition as that discussed and used in Section III.A.8. The null equations previously derived on the basis of direct occupation theory alone, should therefore also be valid for such peak responses or for final steady-state responses, provided that the feedback model is correct. Such use of the null equations is subject to the conditions already discussed in Section III.A.7 and III.A.8, with the added proviso that the drugs do not affect the feedback mechanism.

B. Agonists as Activators of Enzyme Systems

1. The Conformational Perturbation Theory of Drug Action

This theory, proposed by BELLEAU (1964, 1965), is based on the idea that when a drug interacts with a receptor, the latter undergoes a change in conformation. BELLEAU suggests that a receptor may be a latent enzyme and that the conformational change produced by interaction with an agonist converts the receptor into an active enzyme molecule. These ideas are based on evidence concerning the specific regulatory effects of small molecules on enzyme activity (see review by GRISOLIA, 1964). If the conformational change, and hence the enzyme activation, persists as long as the agonist is present, then the conformational perturbation theory may be considered to be an extension of occupation theory. The symbol * is used to denote a specific conformational change which leads to enzyme activation, while the symbol $\neq$ indicates a nonspecific conformational change which does not lead to activation of the enzyme.

The resting state of the receptor protein is given the symbol P. When a small activator molecule M_a forms a complex with the regulatory site on the receptor then the protein is assumed to be converted to a new active state, P*.

$$P + M_a \rightleftharpoons P^* M_a .$$

The modified receptor is supposed to be effective in catalysing the conversion of the substrate, S, to products, leading to a response.

$$P^* M_a + S \rightleftharpoons P^* M_a S \rightarrow P^* M_a + \text{products} .$$

If another molecule M_i interacts with the regulatory site so as to produce an ineffective complex then this may be written as

$$P + M_i \rightleftharpoons P^{\neq} M_i .$$

The molecules M_a and M_i therefore correspond to agonists and antagonists respectively. In order to take into account the existence of partial agonists, BELLEAU suggested that such a molecule, M_{ai}, may give rise to an equilibrium mixture of P* and P$^+$ complexes, so that

$$P^+ M_{ai} \rightleftharpoons P + M_{ai} \rightleftharpoons P^* M_{ai} \,,$$

where the actual differences in free energy between P$^+$M$_{ai}$ and P*M$_{ai}$ are small. This allows ready interconversion of the two complexes, and an equilibrium mixture which is not entirely composed of either form. According to Belleau's ideas, enzyme activation requires an ordering of the receptor protein molecule toward some optimum structure. Agonists are able to produce such an ordering effect but antagonists produce a relatively disordered conformation. It should therefore be possible to correlate agonist and antagonist activity with the entropy change of the drug-receptor interaction.

Unfortunately these ideas have not yet been tested on actual drug-receptor systems in living tissues, but there is good evidence that these ideas are valid for some isolated enzyme systems. BELLEAU and co-workers (BELLEAU and LACASSE, 1964; BELLEAU et al., 1965) have studied the interaction of members of a homologous series of alkyl-trimethylammonium (alkyl-TMA) compounds with acetylcholinesterase of bovine red blood cells. The alkyl-TMA compounds were first shown to be competitive inhibitors of the enzyme. Measurement of the affinity constant K_I of each compound for the enzyme, allowed the estimation of the corresponding standard free energy change ΔF_0, from the thermodynamic equation

$$- \Delta F_0 = R T \ln K_I \,.$$

The corresponding enthalpy change ΔH_0 was then estimated from measurements of the variation of K_I with temperature since

$$d \ln K_I / d T = \Delta H_0 / R T^2 \,,$$

where T is the absolute temperature and R is the gas constant. The entropy change was then obtained from the equation

$$\Delta S_0 = (\Delta H_0 - \Delta F_0)/ T \,.$$

Some of the results obtained by BELLEAU and his co-workers are shown in Table 1. It will be seen that the entropy change produced by the interaction of an alkyl-TMA compound with bovine acetylcholinesterase is initially negative but increases to positive values as the size of the alkyl group is increased. The observed change in entropy also seems to be related to the agonist or antagonist potency of the compound on muscarinic receptors. BELLEAU has therefore suggested that the cholinergic receptor may be similar in structure to acetylcholinesterase, but that the activated receptor may catalyse the transfer of phosphoryl groups rather than the hydrolysis of acetylcholine.

Belleau's emphasis of the importance of conformational changes, points the way to what may be useful extensions of occupation theory. Besides pointing out the importance of such changes and the possibility of enzyme activation by drug molecules, BELLEAU (1964, 1965, 1967) has discussed the importance of "hydrophobic

Table 1. Thermodynamic quantities for binding of alkyl-trimethylammonium ions to bovine acetylcholinesterase (BELLEAU, 1966)

n^a	$-\Delta F_0$ (K. cal.)	$-\Delta H_0$ (K. cal.)	ΔS_0 (entropy units)	Effect on muscarinic receptors
0	3.61	6.64	—10.2	Agonist
2	3.92	5.95	— 5.95	Agonist
4	3.77	5.51	— 6.1	Agonist
6	4.09	4.37	— 1.0	Partial agonist
8	4.52	4.35	+ 0.6	Partial agonist
11	5.85	2.84	+ 10.1	Antagonist

[a] The general formula of these compounds is $CH_3(CH_2)_n\overset{\frown}{-}\overset{\scriptscriptstyle +}{N}(Me)_3$.

bonding" and entropy changes in drug-receptor interactions. If receptors are latent enzymes then it should be possible to study their biochemical properties in vitro (see, e.g., ROBINSON et al., 1967). Even if the receptors are not latent enzymes, but specialised regions which can modify the permeability of cell membranes, then any marked changes in conformation of the receptors might lead to measurable changes in entropy.

2. The Dynamic-Receptor Hypothesis

BLOOM and GOLDMAN (1966) offered this hypothesis to explain the actions of drugs on adrenergic receptors, but they have also suggested that the hypothesis may be extended to other types of receptors. As far as the adrenergic receptors are concerned the hypothesis is a modification and extension of ideas presented earlier by BELLEAU (1960). The catecholamine agonists are assumed to activate enzymes which are involved in the transfer of phosphoryl groups. BLOOM and GOLDMAN suggest that the α-adrenergic receptor is a complex between adenosine-tri-phosphate (ATP) and a magnesium-activated-ATPase, and that the β-receptor is a complex of ATP with adenylclase. The latter assumption seems to be based on the results of SUTHERLAND and RALL, 1960.

The dynamic receptor hypothesis is similar to Belleau's conformational perturbation theory insofar as the receptor is postulated to be a latent enzyme which can be activated by interaction with an agonist. But whereas BELLEAU left open the detailed mechanism of activation, BLOOM and GOLDMAN suggest that the activation occurs by interaction of agonist with preformed enzyme-substrate complex, so that the reaction is

$$\text{enzyme-substrate complex} \xrightarrow{\text{agonist}} \text{enzyme} + \text{products}$$

The receptor for the agonist is therefore assumed to be the enzyme-substrate complex. Since this is broken down during the reaction, the concentration of receptors depends on the availability of substrate, which is required for their regeneration, hence the term "dynamic-receptor." The postulated reaction mechanism is such as to cause doubts as to whether the hypothesis can really be described as an occupation theory, but the hypothesis is so closely related to Belleau's theory that it seems appropriate to include it here.

The hypothesis is based on the following sequence of reactions.

$$E + S \underset{k_2}{\overset{k_1}{\rightleftharpoons}} ES$$

$$ES + A \underset{k_{4A}}{\overset{k_{3A}}{\rightleftharpoons}} ESA \xrightarrow{k_{5A}} E + A + \text{products}.$$

E is the free latent enzyme, S is the substrate, and A is an agonist. The steady-state solution for the above reaction scheme (SEGAL et al., 1952) can be written in the form

$$v_A = k_{5A} E_T \Big/ \left[1 + \frac{1}{a_{1A}(A)} + \frac{1}{a_{2A}(S)(A)} + \frac{1}{a_{3A}(S)} \right] \tag{49}$$

where v_A is the rate of formation of products, catalysed by the agonist A, E_T is the total concentration of enzyme, and

$$a_{1A} = k_{3A}/[k_{4A} + k_{5A}] = \theta_A, \tag{50a}$$

$$a_{2A} = k_1 k_{3A}/[k_{4A} + k_{5A}] k_2$$

$$= K_S \theta_A \tag{50b}$$

and

$$a_{3A} = k_1/k_{5A}. \tag{50c}$$

$k_{5A} E_T$ is the maximum rate of formation of products when all of the enzyme is in the form of EAS complexes. K_S is the affinity constant of the substrate for the latent enzyme and θ_A is the steady-state constant for the reaction of the agonist with the dynamic receptors. Equation (49) is valid only for essential activation of the enzyme and for steady-state conditions (SEGAL et al., 1952).

It has been pointed out by BLOOM and GOLDMAN that if substrate availability is not a significant rate-determining factor then Equations (49) and (50) reduce to equations which are similar to those obtained on the basis of the direct occupation theory. This condition corresponds to the case when k_1 is very much greater than k_{5A}, so that $1/a_{3A}$ becomes negligibly small. Equation (49) then reduces to

$$v_A = k_{5A} E_T \Big/ \left[1 + \frac{1}{\{a_{1A} + a_{2A}(S)\}(A)} \right]$$

$$= k_{5A} E_T \Big/ \left[1 + \frac{1}{K_1(A)} \right],$$

where K_1 is a constant if (S) remains constant. Then from Equations (50a) and (50b),

$$K_1 = \theta_A[1 + K_S(S)].$$

Also, if $K_S(S)$ is very much less than unity, so that only a small fraction of the enzyme is in the form of ES complexes, and if k_{5A} is very much less than k_{4A}, then the constant K_1 approximates to the affinity constant K_A of the agonist for the dynamic receptor.

Since the magnitude of v_A depends on the concentration of the substrate, it follows that prolonged exposure of the tissue to an agonist could result in depletion of the substrate and so to a fall in the responses. Such effects could therefore explain the occurence of maxima in response versus time curves, and could also explain desensitisation to subsequent doses of agonist.

It has also been pointed out by BLOOM and GOLDMAN that if Equations (49) and (50) are used to estimate v_A as a function of (A) for a series of values of (S), then the resulting curves are very similar in shape and position to those obtained for the action of irreversible antagonists on isolated tissues (see Fig. 2a). These authors have therefore suggested that the so-called irreversible blocking agents may in-activate substrate, rather than receptors in the usual sense.

Although BLOOM and GOLDMAN have discussed a number of experimental results which are explicable on the basis of their assumptions concerning the nature of the adrenergic receptors, none of these results seems to provide conclusive evidence for or against the dynamic-receptor hypothesis itself.

Any attempt to apply the dynamic-receptor hypothesis, or indeed any other receptor hypothesis, to complex resultant responses obtained from living cells, faces the same problem as direct occupation theory, namely lack of knowledge about the relation between the stimulus or primary response and the observed response. It is therefore logical to apply the null method also to such modifications of receptor theory.

3. Application of the Null Method to the Dynamic-Receptor Hypothesis

In order to apply the null method to such an enzyme system it is necessary to modify the definition of the pharmacologic stimulus, which is re-defined as the change in the reaction velocity of the activated enzyme system. The pharmacologic stimulus is therefore proportional to the concentration of EAS complexes (see Sect. III.A.4). Then equal steady-state values of the reaction velocity should produce equal steady-state responses from a single cell. If the dose-response curves of two agonists, A and B, are measured on the same cell or tissue then concentration $(A)_r$ and $(B)_r$ of the agonists, which produce the same response r, can be read from the curves. Then from Equation (49) the rate of the reaction catalysed by agonist A, is

$$v_A = k_{5A} E_T \bigg/ \left[1 + \frac{1}{a_{1A}(A)_r} + \frac{1}{a_{2A}(S)(A)_r} + \frac{1}{a_{3A}(S)} \right].$$

An analogous equation can be set out for the reaction rate, v_B, catalysed by agonist B. Equating v_A with v_B, the condition for equal responses is

$$k_{5A} E_T \bigg/ \left[1 + \frac{1}{a_{1A}(A)_r} + \frac{1}{a_{2A}(S)(A)_r} + \frac{1}{a_{3A}(S)} \right]$$

$$= k_{5B} E_T \bigg/ \left[1 + \frac{1}{a_{1B}(B)_r} + \frac{1}{a_{2B}(S)(B)_r} + \frac{1}{a_{3B}(S)} \right]$$

if it is assumed that E_T and (S) remain constant. The above equation can then be rearranged to obtain a linear equation between $1/(A)_r$ and $1/(B)_r$. The equation obtained, after eliminating a_{1A}, a_{2A}, a_{3A}, a_{1B}, a_{2B}, and a_{3B} by means of Equations (50a), (50b), and (50c), is Equation (T3.1) given in Table 3. It will be seen that Equation (T3.1) is very similar in form to Equation (T.2.1) (see Table 2), which was derived on the basis of the direct occupation theory. However, Equation (T3.1) gives a straight line relationship between $1/(A)_r$ and $1/(B)_r$ only if (S) is a constant. This implies that either the utilisation of substrate is small compared with the store available, or that the rate of production of substrate is automatically increased to keep pace with increased utilisation.

According to the dynamic-receptor hypothesis, the receptor is the enzyme-substrate complex, so that competitive inhibition may be represented as

$$ES + I \underset{k_b}{\overset{k_a}{\rightleftharpoons}} ESI .$$

The affinity constant of the competitive inhibitor for the dynamic receptor is then

$$K_I = k_a/k_b .$$

For a system in which such a competitive antagonist inhibits the activation of dynamic receptors by an agonist A, the steady-state solution is

$$v'_A = k_{5A} E_T \Big/ \left[1 + \frac{1}{a_{1A}(A)} + \frac{1}{a_{2A}(S)(A)} + \frac{1}{a_{3A}(S)} + \frac{(I)}{a_{4A}(A)} \right] .$$

The constants a_{1A}, a_{2A}, and a_{3A} are given by Equations (50a), (50b), and (50c) respectively, and

$$a_{4A} = k_b k_{3A}/[k_a(k_{4A} + k_{5A})]$$
$$= \theta_A/K_I .$$

By applying 'the null method to equal responses obtained in the absence and in the presence of the competitive antagonist, [assuming E_T, (I) and (S) to be constant], the appropriate theoretical equation for equal responses can be derived [Eq. (T3.2), Table 3]. It will be seen from the equation that a plot of $1/(A)_r$ versus $1/(A)'_r$ again gives a straight line from the slope of which $K_I/[1 + 1/K_S(S)]$ can be estimated if (I) is known. According to the dynamic receptor hypothesis, such a plot therefore gives K_I only if $K_S(S)$ is very much greater than unity. Otherwise the quantity obtained is only proportional to K_I.

When the null method is applied to the dynamic receptor hypothesis in order to compare dose-response curves obtained before and after treatment of the cell or tissue with an irreversible antagonist, then two extreme situations must be considered. In the first case the irreversible antagonists may inactivate only the enzyme, reducing its concentration from E_T to a new value E'_T. In the second case the irreversible antagonist may inactivate only substrate, reducing its concentration from (S) to a new steady-state value (S)'.

The appropriate theoretical equations for these two extreme cases are Equations (T3.3) and (T3.4), as given in Table 3. In both cases straight lines should be obtained when $1/(A)_r$ is plotted against $1/(A)'_r$ provided that (S) can be regarded as being practically independent of the response for any given state of the tissue.

If the experimental quantity ϱ_A is estimated from the slope and intercept of such a plot, from the equation

$$\varrho_{A_A} = \frac{\text{Intercept}}{\text{Slope} - 1},$$

then for the case when only enzyme is inactivated,

$$\varrho_A = \frac{\{1 + k_{5A}/k_1(S)\}}{\{1 + 1/K_S(S)\}} \theta_A.$$

When the irreversible blocking agent inactivates only substrate,

$$\varrho_A = k_{5A}\theta_A/k_2.$$

Obviously these values of ϱ_A approximate to K_A under certain circumstances but further discussion of the interpretation of these experimental quantities will be deferred until after the next section.

4. Nondynamic Receptors

The reaction scheme suggested by BLOOM and GOLDMAN is only one of several possible schemes for enzyme activation. Another simple system which might describe enzyme-activation by agonists is shown below

$$E + A \underset{k_{8A}}{\overset{k_{7A}}{\rightleftharpoons}} EA$$

$$EA + S \underset{k_{10A}}{\overset{k_{9A}}{\rightleftharpoons}} EAS \xrightarrow{k_{5A}} EA + \text{products}.$$

Since the agonist is assumed to interact directly with the latent enzyme the receptors are "nondynamic", although the formation of the products still requires the availability of substrate. Therefore lack of substrate could again cause responses to be poorly maintained, and could explain desensitisation. The above scheme could represent the type of activation suggested by BELLEAU (1964). A competitive inhibitor, I, would interact directly with latent enzyme.

$$E + I \underset{k_b}{\overset{k_a}{\rightleftharpoons}} EI$$

and the affinity constant of the inhibitor for the receptor would be

$$K_I = k_a/k_b.$$

The steady-state solutions for the rate of formation of products in the absence and in the presence of such a competitive inhibitor are respectively,

$$v_A = k_{5A} E_T \bigg/ \left[1 + \frac{1}{b_{2A}(S)\,(A)} + \frac{1}{b_{3A}(S)} \right],$$

and

$$v'_A = k_{5A} E_T \bigg/ \left[1 + \frac{(1 + K_I(I))}{b_{2A}(S)\,(A)} + \frac{1}{b_{3A}(S)} \right]$$

where

$$b_{2A} = k_{7A} k_{9A} / k_{8A} [k_{10A} + k_{5A}]$$
$$= K_A \theta_{SA}$$

and

$$b_{3A} = k_{9A} / [k_{10A} + k_{5A}] = \theta_{SA}.$$

These steady-state equations can then be used to derive the appropriate theoretical equations for equal responses, in the same way as in the preceding section. The resulting theoretical equations, obtained by applying the null method to the nondynamic receptor system, are given in Table 4. It will be seen that this reaction scheme also leads to linear plots of $1/(A)_r$ versus $1/(B)_r$ [see Eq. (T4.1)], and of $1/(A)_r$ versus $1/(A)'_r$ [see Eq. (T4.2), (T4.3), and (T4.4)], provided that the steady-state concentration of substrate can be regarded as being independent of the response for any given state of the tissue. Again, the interpretation of the various of the various slopes and intercepts are usually more complex than for the equations derived on the basis of the direct occupation theory (see Table 2).

5. Comparison of Direct Occupation Theory and Latent-Enzyme Activation Hypotheses

The steady-state solutions for various experimental conditions have been set out in Tables 2, 3, and 4, for the direct occupation theory, the dynamic receptor hypothesis, and the nondynamic receptor hypothesis respectively.

The quantities which can be measured experimentally are usually the slopes and intercepts of the various plots. The concentrations of drugs at the receptors are not really known but may be assumed to be equal to their concentrations in the external solution if the tissue is sufficiently thin and if the receptors are all at the cell surface.

According to the direct occupation theory, interaction of a drug with a receptor can be described in terms of two parameters which are the affinity constant and the intrinsic efficacy. It will be seen from Tables 2, 3, and 4, that for a competitive antagonist the three alternative approaches discussed in this section allow the estimation of K_I, or of a quantity proportional to K_I, from the appropriate plots of $1/(A)_r$ against $1/(A)'_r$.

It was shown in Section III.A.6 that according to direct occupation theory, the affinity constant of an agonist for its receptors can be estimated by using a specific irreversible antagonist to reduce the concentration of available receptors,

Table 2. Theoretical equations for equal equilibrium responses, derived on the basis of direct occupation theory of drug action

Second set of conditions[a]		Theoretical equations for equal responses	Equation number
Drugs present	Receptor concentration		
B	$[R]_T$	$[1/(A)_r] = [1/(B)_r] \{f_A K_A/f_B K_B\} + \{f_A/f_B - 1\} K_A$	(T2.1)
A and I	$[R]_T$	$[1/(A)_r] = [1/(A)_r'] \{1 + K_I(I)\}$	(T2.2)
A	$[R]_T'$	$[1/(A)_r] = [1/(A)_r'] \{[R]_T/[R]_T'\} + \{[R]_T/[R]_T' - 1\} K_A$	(T2.3)

[a] Equations apply to equal responses obtained from cell or tissue under two different sets of experimental conditions. Under first set of conditions response is produced by agonist A acting alone on cell or tissue, the concentration of receptors being $[R]_T$. Under second set of conditions another drug (agonist B or antagonist I) may be present, or concentration of receptors may have been changed from $[R]_T$ to $[R]_T'$. These altered conditions are given in table. Methods for obtaining useful information from such null equations are discussed in Section III.A.6 and in Section VI.

Table 3. Theoretical equations for equal steady-state responses, derived on the basis of dynamic-receptor hypothesis

Second set of conditions[a]			Theoretical equations for equal responses	Equation number
Drugs present	Enzyme concentration	Substrate concentration		
B	E_T	(S)	$[1/(A)_r] = [1/(B)_r] \{k_{5A}\theta_A/k_{5B}\theta_B\}$ $+ \{k_{5A}/k_{5B} - 1\} \theta_A/\{1 + 1/K_S(S)\}$	(T3.1)
A and I	E_T	(S)	$[1/(A)_r] = [1/(A)_r'] \{1 + K_I(I)/[1 + 1/K_S(S)]\}$	(T3.2)
A	E_T'	(S)	$[1/(A)_r] = [1/(A)_r'] \{E_T/E_T'\}$ $+ \{E_T/E_T' - 1\} \{1 + k_{5A}/k_1(S)\} \theta_A/\{1 + 1/K_S(S)\}$	(T3.3)
A	E_T	(S)'	$[1/(A)_r] = [1/(A)_r'] \{1 + 1/K_S(S)'\}/\{1 + 1/K_S(S)\}$ $+ k_{5A}\theta_A\{1/(S)' - 1/(S)\}/k_1\{1 + 1/K_S(S)\}$	(T3.4)

[a] Equations apply to equal responses obtained from cell or tissue under two different sets of experimental conditions. Under first set of conditions response is produced by agonist A acting alone on cell or tissue, the total enzyme concentration being E_T and substrate concentration being (S). Under second set of conditions another drug (agonist or antagonist) may be present, or total enzyme concentration or substrate concentration may have been changed. These altered conditions are given in table. Methods for obtaining useful information from such null equations are discussed in Section III.B.3 and in Section VI.

and calculating the experimental quantity ϱ_A [see Eqs. (40a) and (40b)]. The relative intrinsic efficacy, β_{AB}, of two agonists could then be estimated either from Equation (41) or from Equation (42). It was also shown that the internal consistency of the direct occupation model could be checked by testing the validity of Equation (43) which contains only experimental quantities.

However, it can readily be shown that if a specific irreversible antagonist inactivates only receptors and not substrate, then Equation (43) is also theoretically

Table 4. Theoretical equations for equal steady-state responses, derived on the basis of non-dynamic receptor hypothesis

Second set of conditions[a]			Theoretical equations for equal responses	Equation number
Drugs present	Enzyme concentration	Substrate concentration		
B	E_T	(S)	$[1/(A)_r] = [1/(B)_r]\{k_{5A}K_A\theta_{SA}/k_{5B}K_B\theta_{SB}\}$ $+ K_A\theta_{SA}(S)\{[k_{5A}/k_{5B} - 1]$ $+ [k_{5A}/k_{5B}\theta_{SB}(S)] - 1/\theta_{SA}(S)\}$	(T4.1)
A and I	E_T	(S)	$[1/(A)_r] = [1/(A)'_r]\{1 + K_I(I)\}$	(T4.2)
A	E'_T	(S)	$[1/(A)_r] + [1/(A)'_r]\{E_T/E'_T\} + \{E_T/E'_T - 1\}\{1 + \theta_{SA}(S)\}\,K_A$	(T4.3)
A	E_T	(S)'	$[1/(A)_r] = [1/(A)'_r]\{(S)/(S)'\} + \{(S)/(S)' - 1\}\,K_A$	(T4.4)

[a] As for Table 3.

Table 5. Interpretation of derived quantities of β_{AB} and ϱ_A, on the basis of various receptor models, assuming that irreversible antagonists do not inactivate an enzyme substrate

Model	β_{AB}	ϱ_A
Direct occupation theory	f_A/f_B	K_A
Dynamic receptor hypothesis	$k_{5A}\{1 + k_{5B}/k_1(S)\}/k_{5B}\{1 + k_{5A}/k_1(S)\}$	$\theta_A\{1 + k_{5A}/k_1(S)\}/\{1 + 1/K_S(S)\}$
Nondynamic receptor hypothesis	$k_{5A}\{1 + 1/\theta_{SB}(S)\}/k_{5B}\{1 + 1/\theta_{SA}(S)\}$	$K_A\{1 + \theta_{SA}(S)\}$
Allosteric two-state model	$\{K_{RA}/K_{TA} - 1\}/\{K_{RB}/K_{TB} - 1\}$	$K_{TA} + K_{RA} \cdot K_{RT}$

valid for the dynamic and nondynamic receptor models. These three alternative models are therefore indistinguishable on the basis of experimental values of ψ_{AB}, I_{AB}, ϱ_A, and ϱ_B. However, the meanings of the derived quantities β_{AB}, and ϱ_A, depend on which model is correct, as shown in Table 5.

It can also be shown that if the irreversible antagonist acts on a dynamic or nondynamic receptor system by inactivating only substrate, then Equation (43) will not generally be valid although it may be approximately valid in special circumstances. Since the reaction velocity has been regarded as being equivalent to the pharmacologic stimulus when dealing with enzyme activation, the true relative intrinsic efficacy of two agonists A and B, should be k_{5A}/k_{5B}. Table 5 may then be taken to mean that use of the experimental quantities ψ_{AB}, I_{AB}, ϱ_A, and ϱ_B, permits the estimation of a derived quantity β_{AB} which should perhaps be called the apparent relative intrinsic efficacy since its value may differ by some unknown amount from the true value. ϱ_A and ϱ_B might similarly be called apparent affinity constants.

Because of the limited accuracy with which most pharmacologic responses can be measured, and the limited experimental control over the concentrations of molecules (such as drugs and substrates) which may interact with the receptors of the living cell, it seems unlikely that a clear-cut distinction can be made between direct occupation theory and the enzyme-activation hypothesis, unless the latent enzymes can be isolated and characterised in vitro (see, e.g., ROBISON et al., 1967).

C. The Flux-Carrier Hypothesis and Intracellular Uptake of Drugs

1. The Flux-Carrier Hypothesis

This hypothesis was put forward by MACKAY (1963) in an attempt to combine the potential theory of STRAUB (1907) with the occupation theory of CLARK (1933), so as to explain the stimulant actions of quaternary compounds and the variation of their stimulant actions with time. The suggestion was prompted by the ideas and results of CREESE et al., (1959), TAYLOR (1962), and by the autoradiographic results of WASER and LUTHI (1957).

According to the flux-carrier hypothesis, the response results from the influx of an agonist through the cell membrane. This influx was assumed to be carrier-mediated. It was suggested that other agonists and competitive antagonists can compete for the carriers, and that competitive antagonists do not penetrate the cell membrane but reduce the influx of agonists. The reduced influx of agonist might then produce a smaller response.

If the main driving force for the influx of an agonist is assumed to be its concentration gradient across the cell membrane then the carrier-mediated influx of the agonist is

$$J_A = D_A [C]_T [\{y_A\}_0 - \{y_A\}_i]/\delta, \tag{51}$$

where D_A is the diffusion coefficient of the molecular form in which A penetrates the membrane, δ is the membrane thickness, $[C]_T$ is the concentration of carriers in the membrane, and $\{y_A\}_0$ and $\{y_A\}_i$ are respectively the fractions of the carriers occupied by agonist A at the outer and inner surfaces of the cell membrane. If an equilibrium concentration of carrier-agonist complexes is assumed to be maintained at each surface of the membrane then the values of $\{y_A\}$ are obtained from Equation (7b). If the initial value of $\{y_A\}_i$ is zero then the initial flux will be

$$J_A = D_A [C]_T \{y_A\}_0/\delta \tag{52}$$

but this will decrease with time as $\{y_A\}_i$ increases. The maximal initial flux obtained at very high concentrations of agonist in the extracellular fluid, is

$$\{J_A\}_{MAX} = D_A [C]_T/\delta. \tag{53}$$

Competition between agonists and antagonists for the carriers would be analogous to competition for receptors, so that the fraction of carriers occupied by an agonist A in the presence of another competitive drug B, would be given by Equation (16a). The reduced initial flux would then be obtained from Equation (52) by substituting $\{y_A\}_0'$ for $\{y_A\}_0$.

If, however, an agonist penetrates the cell membrane in some cationic form then the initial influx, before depolarisation, might be very much greater than indicated by Equation (52), because the membrane potential would contribute to the driving force on the penetrating molecular species.

The null method can be applied to the flux-carrier hypothesis if the stimulus is assumed to be proportional to the fraction of carriers occupied by the agonist, and therefore to the influx of agonist. The diffusion constant D_A then becomes proportional to the intrinsic efficacy. The equations obtained for equal initial fluxes, and therefore equal initial responses, are identical to those obtained on the basis of the direct occupation theory (see Table 2), except that K_A and K_I become the affinity constants of the drugs for the carriers instead of for the receptors.

One of the aims of the flux-carrier hypothesis was to explain the variation of responses with time. It was suggested that if insufficient time was allowed for the removal of intracellular agonist, which had accumulated as a result of previous treatment with the agonist, then a subsequent dose would produce a smaller influx which might result in a smaller response. Such an effect might explain specific desensitisation. As an explanation of phase II neuromuscular block, which occurs as a result of the prolonged action of a depolarising agent and has some of the properties of a competitive block, it was suggested that the blocking agent might then be competitively reducing the influx of acetylcholine released by nerve stimulation.

2. Discussion of the Flux-Carrier Model

Taken in its simplest form the flux-carrier model predicts that agonists may penetrate cell membranes by carrier-mediated processes whereas pharmacologic antagonists might then be expected to reduce the rate of uptake of agonists.

There seems to be a fair amount of evidence that some cationic agonists are taken up into cells by carrier mechanisms. CREESE et al. (1959) studied the uptake of ^{131}I-labelled iodocholinium and showed that the uptake of this neuromuscular depolarising agent was blocked by d-tubocurarine. WASER and LUTHI (1957) carried out autoradiographic studies on the uptake of ^{14}C-curarine and ^{14}C-decamethonium (C-10) by mouse diaphragm, and showed that the uptake of the latter compound was greater and more diffuse than that of the former. In both cases the labelled drugs were concentrated around the neuromuscular junctions. The location of the uptake of C-10, and inhibition of the uptake by d-tubocurarine, were later confirmed by the use of ^{3}H-labelled C-10 (TAYLOR et al., 1965). Microautoradiographic studies by CREESE and MACLAGAN (1967) suggest that ^{3}H-labelled C-10 penetrates rapidly into muscle fibres, mainly at the neuromuscular junction.

Other studies have shown that C-10 and carbachol are taken up by slices of rat brain in vitro. The uptakes were inhibited by d-tubocurarine and by strychnine, and showed the characteristics of a carrier-mediated process (CREESE and TAYLOR, 1967).

The results of PATON and RANG (1965) also indicate that the cationic agonist methylfurmethide penetrates into the cells of isolated strips of the longitudinal muscle of guineapig ileum. Uptake of this agonist had not reached an equilibrium value after 18 h of incubation of tissue with drug solution. It was suggested that the penetration might be due to a nonspecific increase in membrane permeability resulting from the action of methylfurmethide on muscarinic receptors. Since the uptake of methylfurmethide was markedly reduced when the tissue was depolarised by incubating it in potassium-rich Krebs' solution, it would seem that the membrane potential was a major driving force for the uptake of this cationic agonist. Although PATON and RANG obtained no evidence that the penetration of methylfurmethide into the cells was carrier-mediated, their results do not exclude such a possibility. They also studied the uptake of ^{3}H-labelled atropine by smooth muscle and showed that the equilibrium uptake of atropine exceeded the non-equilibrium uptake of methylfurmethide over a period of 4 h. Comparison of the uptake of atropine with that of the quaternary methyl-atropine suggested that the atropine uptake was partly extracellular and partly intracellular, and that atropine penetrates the cell membrane in the nonionised form.

PATON and RANG were unable to block the uptake of methylfurmethide with low concentrations of atropine. Since the concentration of atropine used should, from the estimated value of K_I, have blocked most of the receptors they concluded that the receptors were not involved in the penetration of methylfurmethide into the smooth muscle cells. However, the validity of this conclusion depends on the assumption that atropine and furmethide compete for the same receptor site. If atropine and methylfurmethide do not act at the same sites then the pharmacologic response could be blocked without affecting the influx of methylfurmethide. There is good evidence that the pharmacologic action of atropine is not competitive in the reversible sense, but is either pseudoirreversible or non-competitive (MACKAY, 1966c). The problem of the relationship between the site of action of agonists and the site of action of selective antagonists is still very far from settled, as will be evident from the article by ARIENS and SIMONIS (1967).

More recently, studies have been carried out on the uptake of ^{3}H-labelled polymethylene bis-onium compounds by isolated mouse diaphragm (MACKAY and TAYLOR, 1970). The rates of uptakes of the methonium homologues of C-10 were found to parallel their ability to depolarise mouse diaphragm. However, when ethyl groups were progressively substituted in place of the methyl groups of C-10 the depolarising ability of the resulting compounds decreased markedly though their uptakes remained nearly as high as that of C-10. Deca-ethonium was shown to behave as a noncompetitive inhibitor of C-10-induced depolarisation and it was suggested that ethyl substitution might produce membrane stabilising properties. The uptakes of the methonium compounds showed the characteristics expected of a carrier-mediated process and were blocked by tubocurarine. The apparent affinity constant of tubocurarine for the carriers was estimated to be in the range 0.3–0.8 μM^{-1} while its affinity for the C-10 receptor was $2.9 \pm 0.6 \mu M^{-1}$ (SE). These results indicate that the C-10 carrier present in the mouse diaphragm is in many ways similar to the C-10 receptor, though there seem to be quantitative differences, which may be significant. Although the C-10 carrier in the mouse diaphragm seems to have a low affinity for C-10 ($K < 0.005 \mu M^{-1}$), recent studies by TAYLOR et al. (1970) indicate that in the guinea pig diaphragm the affinity of C-10 for the carrier is of the same order as that of tubocurarine.

It therefore seems that cationic agonists can penetrate cell membranes by carrier mechanisms and that, in some cases at least, entry may be blocked by pharmacologic antagonists. If intracellular accumulation of a drug were to cause some intracellular change (such as release of calcium ions or a change in enzyme activity) and this change was opposed by a negative feedback system then the rate of influx of agonist could determine its ability to produce an observable response. However, there is no conclusive evidence that either the rate of influx of an agonist, or its intracellular concentration determines the response.

TAYLOR and NEDERGAARD (1965) have presented evidence that phase II neuromuscular blockade may be due to intracellular accumulation of C-10. It has also been suggested that this type of neuromuscular blockade may be due to a change in the ionic composition of the muscle.

3. The Actions of Drugs on Depolarised Tissues, and Possible Intracellular Effects of Agonists

Although most drugs which act on muscle are generally believed to act on receptors located on the cell membranes, there is evidence that some drugs may also have intracellular effects. In a few cases, such as with caffeine and ryanodine, the main action of a drug may be intracellular. In other cases possible intracellular effects may be seen only under nonphysiologic conditions and the possible importance of such intracellular actions under normal circumstances is debatable.

The results of EVANS and SCHILD (1957) and of SINGH and ACHARYA (1957), have shown that agonists can produce contractions from depolarised smooth muscle and similar results have been obtained by JENKINSON and NICHOLLS (1961) for depolarised denervated skeletal muscle. Since the contractions produced from these depolarised tissues are inhibited by the appropriate selective pharmacologic antagonists, they presumably result from interaction of the agonists with the normal receptors (SCHILD, 1964). However, regular contractions can be elicited from such depolarised tissues only when calcium ions are present in the external physiologic saline (DURBIN and JENKINSON, 1961b; ROBERTSON, 1960; EDMAN and SCHILD, 1962). It has also been shown that carbachol causes a marked increase in the ionic permeability of depolarised denervated rat diaphragm (JENKINSON and NICHOLLS, 1961). The increased tension produced in a depolarised tissue as a result of the application of a suitable concentration of agonist, may therefore be explained as being due to an increase in the intracellular concentration of calcium ions arising from the increased membrane permeability.

However, the effect of acetylcholine on membrane permeability may not be the complete explanation of its' action, since the rat isolated uterus immersed in calcium-free sodium chloride-Ringer's solution responds to acetylcholine long after it has failed to respond to potassium-induced depolarisation. The latter result and other similar observations are most readily explained if it is assumed that acetylcholine can also release calcium from some store or from binding sites (see SCHILD, 1964; EDMAN and SCHILD, 1961). Similar views seem to be held by SCHATZMANN (1964) and by SHANES (1965).

It is tempting to try to combine the observations on the intracellular uptake of drugs with these other observations. It might be supposed that an agonist, while penetrating through a cell membrane, causes calcium ions to be displaced from the membrane structure. According to commonly held views on the stabilising effect of calcium on cell membranes (see, e.g., SCHATZMANN, 1964; BUEDING and

BULBRING, 1964; SHANES, 1965), this would be expected to produce an increase in membrane permeability. If the agonist can cause displacement of calcium ions from the membrane structure, then it may also be able to cause the release of calcium from intracellular sites. The tendency of the membrane permeability to reach a peak value sometime after application of the agonist, and subsequently to decrease even in the presence of the agonist (DURBIN and JENKINSON, 1961a), might be due to antagonism of the initial permeability change by the subsequent increase in the intracellular concentration of free calcium ions. Inability to maintain a peak contractile response might be due to loss of calcium ions into the extracellular fluid or to utilisation of ATP. An alternative possibility, which has also been suggested by TAYLOR (personal communication) and which is closely related to some fascinating ideas presented by WATKINS (1965), is that penetration of an agonist through the cell membrane might cause a conformational change leading to a rearrangement of the membrane structure and an increase in the permeability of the membrane to small ions. This could explain the initial effect of a penetrating agonist on the permeability of the cell membrane, but it would also be necessary to postulate an intracellular action on stores of calcium ions, in order to account for the other results mentioned above.

The finding by DEL CASTILLO and KATZ (1955) that intracellular injections of acetylcholine and carbachol at the neuromuscular junction produced no detectable response seems to be good evidence against an intracellular drug action. However, the response which was looked for was a change in membrane potential. The fact that any penetration of the drug cation from the inside of the cell outward through the membrane would be opposed by the membrane potential might explain the lack of effect on the membrane permeability and membrane potential. Any effect on intracellular membranes or on the intracellular concentration of calcium ions would also be expected to be unobservable in such experiments.

If an agonist does act on intracellular receptors then the initial response is likely to depend on the rate at which the drug penetrates the cell membrane, since this rate will largely determine the intracellular concentration of the drug for short times of contact between drug and tissue. This rate would in turn be expected to depend on such factors as the lipid solubility of the drug or the availability of suitable carrier mechanisms. In the latter case there would be two different sites at which antagonists might act, the first being the carrier and the second the intracellular receptor.

See the Monod-Wyman-Changeux model for cooperativity in "Drug Receptors", p. 160

D. The Allosteric Two-State Model   *see Thron, Mol. Pharmacol., 9, 1-9 (1973)*

1. Basis of the Model   *see Lester, Sci. Amer., 107 (Feb. 1977)*
Perutz, ibid. 239, No. 6, 92 (Dec. 1978)

According to this model, which was offered by KARLIN (1967) and independently by CHANGEUX et al. (1967), a receptor can exist in only one or the other of two states. One of these is an active state R, while the other is an inactive state T. These forms may correspond to open and closed channels, respectively in the cell membrane. These two forms are assumed to be in equilibrium at all times. In the untreated tissue the number of receptors in the active state might be expected to be small. Then the value of the equilibrium constant for the

see Mol. Pharmacol., 20, 498 (1981)

conversion of T to R, $K_{RT} = [R]/[T]$, would be very much less than unity. In the general models presented by KARLIN (1967) and by CHANGEUX et al. (1967) each receptor unit was considered to be able to adsorb n molecules of drug. However, for a discussion of the qualitative basis of the model, n will be set equal to one. When a drug A is added to the system it may therefore interact with either T or R, or both, as shown in Figure 4.

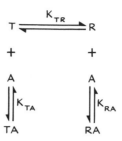

Fig. 4. The diagram represents the simplest form of allosteric two-state model of drug-receptor interaction. A represents a drug, and T and R are respectively the inactive and active forms of receptors

Usually when applying the direct occupation theory the assumption is made that when an agonist interacts with the receptor the latter is changed in some way and this change ultimately produces the response. According to the allosteric two-state model, active and inactive receptors are always present. An agonist interacts with active receptors but does not alter their active state. It merely converts them to RA complexes which are still active. This allows more inactive receptors to change into active receptors. The effect of an agonist is therefore to increase the overall number or concentration, $[\bar{R}]$, of receptors in the active form by a mass action effect, since

$$[\bar{R}] = [R] + [RA].$$

The response of the cell or tissue may then be assumed to be some function of $[\bar{R}]$. Similarly if the drug interacts with inactive receptors to form TA complexes these remain inactive. The distribution of the total number or concentration of available receptors between the active forms, R and RA, and the inactive forms T and TA, is therefore determined by the affinity of drug A for the two forms of the receptor.

If the drug has a much greater affinity for R than for T then it can greatly increase the number of active receptors and will behave as an agonist. If, on the other hand, the affinity constant K_{RA} is only somewhat greater than K_{TA} then the drug may be a partial agonist. If K_{RA} and K_{TA} are exactly equal the drug should act as a competitive antagonist, but if K_{TA} is greater then K_{RA} the net result of the interaction will be a reduction in the number of active receptors below that present in the untreated tissue. Under these circumstances the drug may either behave as an antagonist or as a negative agonist, depending on whether a reduction in the number of active receptors can produce an observable change in the tissue.

If more than one drug molecule can interact with each receptor unit then co-operative interaction may occur, so that the amount of drug bound to the receptors may increase much more rapidly with increasing drug concentration, than would occur in the absence of cooperative binding. According to the allosteric model, the response is not in any case a pure function of the fraction of adsorption sites occupied by an agonist. Nevertheless, from a qualitative point of view, cooperative binding would be expected to lead to a greater rate of increase in the number of active receptors with increasing drug concentration. Such an effect could result in the production of steep log-dose response curves.

2. Application of the Null Method to the Allosteric Two-State Model, and Comparison of the Results with those Obtained on the Basis of the Direct Occupation Theory

As originally presented by KARLIN (1967) and by CHANGEUX et al. (1967), the allosteric two-state model was not combined with the use of the null method. Although the model could explain why most log-dose response curves do not fit accurately, an equation of the same form as the simple Langmuir adsorption isotherm or the Michaelis-Menten equation, there seems to be no valid reason to assume that the response is always directly proportional to the total concentration, $[\bar{R}]$, of receptors in the active form. Instead the response may be assumed to be some function of $[\bar{R}]$.

The appropriate null equations for this model, which have been derived by THRON (1973) and by COLQUHOUN (1973) are presented in Table 6 and are generally applicable for any value of n [except for Equation (T5.3) which takes the form shown only when $n = 1$ and $K_{RA}(A) \gg 1$]. These equations may be compared with those shown in Table 2 which were derived on the basis of the direct occupation theory. It will be seen that the corresponding equations have the same mathematical form. The experimentally determined constants can therefore be derived from suitable data by the methods already discussed in Sections III.A.5 and III.A.6. Alternative methods of estimating the experimental constants from suitable data are also available and are discussed in Section VI.

The main point which becomes clear from a comparison of the null equation derived from the direct occupation theory and from the allosteric two-state model, is that the interpretation of the experimental constants depends on which model is considered to be valid. According to the allosteric model,

$$\psi_{AB} = (K_{RA} - K_{TA})/(K_{RB} - K_{TB});$$

$$I_{AB} = (K_{RA} \cdot K_{TB} - K_{RB} \cdot K_{TA})/(K_{RB} - K_{TB});$$

and

$$\varrho_A \doteqdot (K_{TA} + K_{RA} \cdot K_{RT})$$

If it is assumed that for a full agonist, A, $K_{RA} \gg K_{TA}$, and that for a partial agonist B, $K_{RB} \ll K_{RA}$ and $K_{TB} \gg K_{TA}$ then:

$$I_{AB}/\psi_{AB} \doteqdot K_{TB}.$$

This result may be compared with Equation (35).

Table 6. Theoretical equations for equal equilibrium responses, derived on the basis of allosteric two-state model

Second set of conditions[a]		Theoretical equations for equal responses	Equation number
Drugs present	Total Receptor concentration		
B	$[R]_T$	$[1/(A)_r] = [1/(B)_r]\{f_A K_{TA}/f_B K_{TB}\} + \{f_A/f_B - 1\}K_{TA}$	(T5.1)
A and I	$[R]_T$	$[1/(A)_r] = [1/(A)'_r]\{1 + K_{TI}(I)\}$	(T5.2)
A	$[R]'_T$	$[1/(A)_r] = [1/(A)'_r]\{[R]_T/[R]'_T\} + \{[R]_T/[R]'_T - 1\}\{K_{TA} + K_{RA} \cdot K_{RT}\}$	(T5.3)

[a] Equations apply to equal responses obtained from a cell or tissue under two different sets of experimental conditions. Under first set of conditions response is produced by agonist A acting alone on cell or tissue, the concentration of receptors being $[R]_T$. Under second set of conditions another drug (agonist B or antagonist I) may be present, or concentration of receptors may have been changed from $[R]_T$ to $[R]'_T$. These altered conditions are given in table. Methods for obtaining useful information from such null equations are discussed in Section III.D.2 and in Section VI.

Equations in this table were derived by THRON (1973) and have been modified so that terminology is similar to that used here. According to this model, $f_A = \{K_{RA}/K_{TA} - 1\}$ and $f_B = \{K_{RB}/K_{TB} - 1\}$. Equation (T5.3) is strictly valid only if each receptor unit has one site which interacts with drugs, and if $K_{RA}(A) \gg 1$.

In general the allosteric model interprets the affinity constants of partial agonists and antagonists estimated by means of the null equations of the direct occupation theory, as being affinity constants for the inactive form of the receptor. However, the alternative interpretation of ϱ, estimated by use of irreversible antagonists, is not so clear. On the basis of the direct occupation theory, ϱ_A is equal to the affinity constant K_A of the agonist for its receptor. According to the allosteric model, ϱ_A may be close to the affinity constant for the inactive receptor in the case of a partial agonist, but for a full agonist it probably tends toward $K_{RT} \cdot K_{RA}$.

Values of ϱ for full agonists are usually very much less than the affinity constants of antagonists for their receptors. According to the allosteric model, K_{RT} would be expected to be very much less than unity so that K_{RA} should be considerably greater than ϱ_A, and therefore somewhat nearer in magnitude to the affinity constants of antagonists. However, agonists are generally smaller molecules than antagonists and it is still an open question whether the low, apparent affinity constants of full agonists, estimated on the basis of the direct occupation theory, are physically unreasonable. If K_{RT} and K_{RA} are different then the sites with which A combines when it interacts with the two forms of the receptor must also be different either in location or in detailed structure. Therefore, in a sense, full agonists and antagonists interact with different sites and there is no reason to assume that their affinity constant should be of similar magnitude.

A major attraction of the allosteric two-state model is that it provides a simple physical meaning for intrinsic efficacy since on basis of this model

$$f_A = (K_{RA}/K_{TA} - 1).$$

In other words intrinsic efficacy is determined by the relative affinities of the drug for the two forms of the receptor. Since each receptor unit is either in the active form or in the inactive form, differences in intrinsic efficacy are supposed to be due to differences in the *number* of active receptors, each active receptor being in a *fully* active state. By contrast the direct occupation theory merely postulates the existence of intrinsic efficacy. The derivation of the stimulus concept and subsequent application of the null method to the latter theory might, however, be taken to imply that the stimulus (or primary response) per drug-receptor complex is a graded quantity, as discussed in Section III.A.3.b.

IV. The Rate Theory of Drug Action

This theory was offered by PATON (1960, 1961) as an alternative to occupation theory. He suggested that instead of attributing excitation to the occupation of receptors by drug molecules, it should be attributed to the *process* of occupation, each association between a drug molecule and a receptor providing one quantum of excitation (PATON, 1961). This quantum was initially assumed to be the same for all drugs interacting with one type of receptor. "Instead of thinking of the receptor as, say, a note on an organ, such that as long as it is depressed a note is emitted, we think of it like a piano, one burst of sound and then silence" (PATON, 1960). He pointed out that the onset of action of agonists is generally rapid and that their effects are readily reversed when the agonist is washed out of the tissue. On the other hand, the onset of action of antagonists is usually much slower and their effects are not so rapidly reversed. According to rate theory, these facts can be explained in terms of the individual forward and backward rate constants of the drug-receptor interaction, and the backward rate constant is the factor which determines whether a drug acts as an agonist or as an antagonist. The fading of the response with time, and the phenomenon of specific desensitisation are also interpreted in terms of these rate constants.

A. Agonist Action and the Rate Theory

1. The Kinetics of the Response

According to rate theory, the drug-receptor interaction proceeds in the usual way, as shown in Equation (1). PATON assumes that the response is determined by the forward rate of formation of RD complexes. If this rate, at time t, is written as $\{V_f\}_t$ then

$$\{V_f\}_t = k_1 [R]_t (D),$$ (54)

where (D) is assumed to be independent of time. Since receptors are assumed to be neither produced nor destroyed, Equation (3) is applicable and Equation (54) may be written as

$$\{V_f\}_t = k_1\{[R]_T - [RD]_t\}\,(D)$$
$$= k_1[R]_T\,[1 - \{y_D\}_t]\,(D),$$

where $\{y_D\}_t$ is given by Equation (8). (Of course, the use of these equations involves the various assumptions discussed in Section II.) The forward rate of formation of RD complexes per receptor, at time t, is then

$$Q_t = \{V_f\}_t/[R]_T = k_1[1 - \{y_D\}_t]\,(D) \qquad (55a)$$

This quantity Q is the same as the quantity A used by PATON (1961), but the latter symbol has already been used here to represent an agonist. Initially $\{y_D\}$ is zero, so that

$$Q_0 = k_1(D). \qquad (55b)$$

Then from Equation (55a)

$$Q_t = Q_0[1 - \{y_D\}_t], \qquad (55c)$$

so that Q_t has an initial value Q_0 and decreases with time as $\{y_D\}_t$ increases to its equilibrium value $\{y_D\}_{eq.}$. The equilibrium value of Q is then

$$Q_{eq.} = Q_0[1 - \{y_D\}_{eq.}]. \qquad (55d)$$

In order to obtain estimates of the rate constants of the agonist-receptor interaction from the variation of response with time, PATON assumed that the observed response is directly proportional to the forward rate of formation of RD complexes. Equations (55b), (55c), and (55d) then take the forms

$$r_0 \propto k_1(D), \qquad (56a)$$
$$r_t/r_0 = 1 - \{y_D\}_t, \qquad (56b)$$

and

$$r_{eq.}/r_0 = 1 - \{y_D\}_{eq.} \qquad (56c)$$

For any given values of k_1, k_2, and (D), $\{y_D\}_t$ can be estimated as a function of time by use of Equation (8). The results of such a calculation are given in Figure 5a. According to Clark's theory the response is proportional to y_D, so that the response versus time curve would be expected to have a similar shape. The corresponding values of r_t/r_0, on the basis of rate theory, can be estimated from Equation (56b), and plotted against time, as shown in Figure 5b. Since r_0 is constant for any given values of k_1 and (D), this latter curve represents the corresponding variation of response with time predicted by rate theory. Figure 5a, b therefore illustrates the essential differences between occupation theory and rate theory.

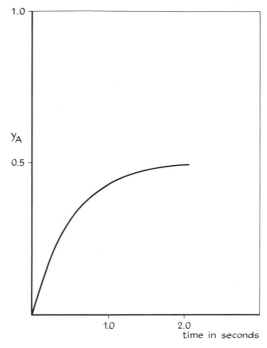

Fig. 5a. A plot of fraction of receptors occupied by drug A, y_A, versus time; y_A has been estimated from Equation (8) with $k_1 = 10^5$ 1/mole·s, $k_2 = 1.0\,\text{s}^{-1}$, $(A) = 10^{-5}$ M. On the basis of direct occupation theory of drug action variation of response with time would be expected to produce similar curve

The most obvious difference between the two theories is the prediction of fade by the rate theory (see Fig. 5b). The extent of fade is best expressed as the fractional fade which is

$$\{r_0 - r_t\}/r_0 = \{1 - r_t/r_0\}$$
$$= \{y_D\}_t, \text{ from Equation (56b)}.$$

At equilibrium the fractional fade becomes

$$\{r_0 - r_{\text{eq.}}\}/r_0 = \{y_D\}_{\text{eq.}}, \qquad \text{from Equation (56c)}.$$

The fractional fade at any time t can therefore be compared with the fractional fade at equilibrium. The ratio of these two quantities is

$$\{r_0 - r_t\}/\{r_0 - r_{\text{eq.}}\} = \{y_D\}_t/\{y_D\}_{\text{eq.}}$$
$$= 1 - \exp\{-[k_2 + k_1(D)]\,t\},$$

from Equation (8). It follows that the time constant for the onset of fade is the same as the time constant for occupation of the receptors. In fact, fade may be considered as being produced by occupation of the receptors.

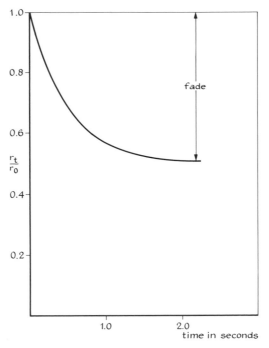

Fig. 5b. A plot of r_t/r_0 versus time, estimated from equation 56b. Variation of y_A with time is shown in Figure 5a; $k_1 = 10^5$ l/mole · s, $k_2 = 1.0$ s^{-1}, (A) $= 10^{-5}$ M. Curve represents variation of response with time, expected on basis of rate theory of drug action

Under equilibrium conditions the net rate of formation of RD complexes is zero, so that the forward and backward rates of reaction are equal. Then the forward rate of formation of RD complexes is

$$k_1[R]_{eq.} (D) = k_2[RD]_{eq.} , \tag{57}$$

and if the response is assumed to be proportional to the forward rate of formation of complexes, it follows that

$$r_{eq.} \propto k_2[RD]_{eq.} \tag{58a}$$

A more general statement of rate theory would be to define the stimulus as the forward rate of formation of RD complexes, the response being some unknown function of this stimulus. Equation (57) would then give the equilibrium stimulus as

$$s = k_2[RD]_{eq.} \tag{58b}$$

If the above equation is compared with Equation (32a), it will be seen that according to rate theory, the intrinsic efficacy of a drug is determined by k_2, the rate constant for dissociation of the RD complex. Rate theory therefore predicts that k_2 should be very much greater for an agonist than for an antagonist. It follows that for any given value of k_1, an antagonist would be expected to have a higher affinity for a receptor than would an agonist for the same receptor.

2. Specific Desensitisation

According to rate theory, specific desensitisation and fade are closely related since both are assumed to be due to increased occupation of the receptors (PATON, 1961; PATON and RANG, 1966). If a drug has been left in contact with a tissue until equilibrium occupation of the receptors has been attained and the drug is then rapidly washed out of the tissue, the drug-receptor complexes should dissociate according to the equation

$$RD \xrightarrow{k_2} R + D .$$

Ideally the forward rate of formation of RD complexes is zero so that on the basis of rate theory the response should also decrease to zero. This prediction of rate theory is in contrast to that of occupation theory, according to which there should be a slower offset of agonist action as receptor occupation decreases with time [see Eq. (11)].

Since rate theory predicts zero response during washout even though receptors are still occupied by the drug, it follows that disappearance of the response would not necessarily indicate removal of the drug from the receptors. If a second dose of the drug is applied before dissociation of the previously formed RD complexes is complete, then the initial peak response obtained from this second dose would be expected to be less than that obtained from the first dose because the initial rate of formation of RD complexes is reduced by the presence of preformed complexes. This desensitisation of the receptors should be observable using either the same agonist D or any other agonist which interacts with the same receptors. In this sense the receptor desensitisation is specific. The rate of offset of specific desensitisation should then depend on k_2, the dissociation rate constant of the drug-receptor complex. For any given agonist, specific desensitisation would be expected to occur only in the case of peak responses, and *not* with equilibrium plateau responses.

B. Antagonists and the Rate Theory

According to rate theory, an essential difference between agonists and antagonists is that the latter dissociate more slowly from the receptors. If the forward rate constant for interaction of an antagonist with its receptors is similar to that of an agonist (see, e.g., BURGEN, 1966) then an initial response might be expected even from an antagonist (PATON, 1961). However, when equilibrium occupation of the receptors by the antagonist has been attained, the equilibrium response is presumably not detectable because of the small value of k_2 [see Eqs. (58a) and (58b)]. Nevertheless the presence of the antagonist still reduces the number of receptors available for interaction with an agonist. If the fraction of the receptors occupied by the antagonist is y_I then the concentration of free receptors is reduced to $[R]_T [1 - y_I]$, and the forward rate of formation of RD complexes, in the presence of the antagonist, is initially

$$Q_0 = k_1(D)' [1 - y_I] .$$

The initial rate of formation of agonist-receptor complexes in the absence of the antagonist, is given by Equation (55b), so that the condition for equal initial peak responses in the presence and absence of antagonist is that

$$(D)' [1 - y_I] = (D) .$$

If y_I corresponds to equilibrium occupation of receptors by the antagonist then it follows that

$$K_I = \{(D)'/(D) - 1\}/(I) \quad [cf., Eq. (29)] .$$

For equilibrium plateau responses, the stimulus, on the basis of rate theory, is given by Equation (58b) which is identical in form to Equation (32a). All of the equilibrium null equations derived on the basis of the direct occupation theory of drug action can therefore also be derived on the basis of rate theory. The only differences are that according to rate theory the responses to be compared are the equilibrium plateau responses rather than the initial peak responses, and the intrinsic efficacy is regarded as being equal to the dissociation rate constant k_2 instead of being a separate parameter of the drug-receptor interaction.

C. Discussion

There are several points which can be made in favour of rate theory. One major point is that it eliminates the need for intrinsic efficacy as a separate parameter of the drug-receptor interaction, since this is then supposed to be equal to the rate constant for dissociation of the drug-receptor complexes. Rate theory also predicts the existence of fade and of specific desensitisation. The more rapid rates of onset and offset of action of agonists, as compared with antagonists, follow logically from the rate theory of drug action, as do the higher affinity constants of antagonists for receptors. These predictions may be considered to provide some good qualitative support for the theory.

PATON (1961) tested the quantitative predictions of his theory by studying the actions of members of a homologous series of alkyl-TMA compounds on the isolated ileum of the guineapig. Using co-axial stimulation of the ileum, he studied the rates of onset and offset of the antagonistic action of the higher members of the series, including some partial agonists. Assuming that these rates were controlled by the rate of the drug-receptor interactions, he was able to obtain estimates of the individual forward and backward rate constants, k_1 and k_2. The values of k_1 for the various drugs were found to be fairly constant but the values of k_2 decreased markedly as the size of the alkyl group was increased. The values of k_1 and k_2, obtained in this way for each compound, gave values of the ratio k_1/k_2 which were in fairly good agreement with the corresponding values of K_I estimated from equilibrium responses using the dose-ratio method.

Attempts to use the fade phenomenon to test the rate theory were not so successful. The fade observed with the partial agonist nonyl-TMA, gave values of k_1 and k_2 which were in fair agreement with the values estimated from its antagonistic action as described above. However, the initial peak responses observed with the higher homologues were smaller than would be expected on the basis of the rate theory.

It will be seen from Equation (56c) that in order to obtain a measurable fractional fade, $\{y_D\}_{eq.}$ must not be too small. The rate of fade depends on the rate constant $[k_2 + k_1(D)]$ and this should not be too large if the rate of fade is to be followed. Both the fractional fade and the rate of fade would therefore be expected to increase with increasing concentrations of the drug. PATON (1961) suggested that the unexpectedly small initial peak responses obtained with homologues higher than nonyl-TMA might be due to a limited rate of response by the tissue, so that when the rate of fade becomes fast compared with the response time of the tissue then the peak response is cut short by fade before the tissue has responded.

The limited rate of response of the tissue was also suggested to be the reason why the observed initial peak responses do not increase indefinitely with increasing doses of agonist, as would otherwise be expected from Equation (56a). Another complicating factor in any study of the kinetics of drug action is the possibility that the rate of formation of drug-receptor complexes may be controlled by the rate of access of the drug to the receptors.

The net result of all these complicating factors is that fade might be expected to be detected only in special circumstances (PATON, 1961; PATON and WAUD, 1964). Nevertheless, since the prediction of fade is a major experimental distinction between rate theory and occupation theory, a better understanding of the fade phenomenon is important. Studies of the kinetics of drug action on tissues other than guineapig ileum have not produced support for the rate theory (see results of HIGMAN et al., 1963; WAUD, 1967; PATON, 1967a).

PATON (1967b) has expressed doubts as to whether the last vestiges of stimulation detected with some antagonists are "large enough to be compatible with a quantum" (of excitation) "which is constant for all drugs".... "One may note that a constant quantum is not an essential ingredient of the kinetic theories. On the other hand, if it is not constant then an ad hoc element of efficacy is reintroduced." Such a modification of rate theory would make an experimental distinction between rate theory and occupation theory even more difficult.

The rate theory has focussed attention on the problems of the kinetics of the drug-receptor interaction and on the kinetics of the resultant response. The studies of PATON and RANG (1965) on the kinetics of action and the kinetics of uptake of atropine and related compounds are therefore of general interest, as are the results of RANG (1966) on the kinetics of action and the kinetics of displacement of acetylcholine antagonists.. The problem of reconciling the rates of uptake and washout of labelled antagonists with the rates of onset and offset of their pharmacologic action, is essentially one of deciding whether or not the rate of access of the antagonists to the receptors controls the rate of formation of drug-receptor complexes and the rate of response (THRON and WAUD, 1968; WAUD, 1968). However, the kinetics of action of antagonists do not allow any distinction to be made between rate theory and occupation theory, and the fact that the rates of interaction of antagonists

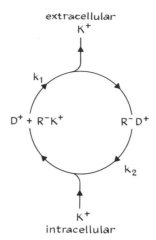

Fig. 6. An ion exchange model for rate theory of drug action (PATON, 1961). Drug D displaces potassium ions from membrane site R^-. These potassium ions are assumed to be able to move only into extracellular fluid. $R^- D^+$ complex is reconverted to $R^- K^+$ by means of intracellular K^+ only. Drug D does not penetrate cell membrane but facilitates removal of K^+ from the cell

with receptors seem to be slower than those of agonists does not by itself provide strong support for the rate theory (see ARIENS and SIMONIS, 1967). Such relative rates of interaction can be explained on the basis of almost any receptor theory of drug action, including the direct occupation theory.

PATON (1961) suggested that his equations might represent an ion exchange mechanism (see Fig. 6). The model was presented only qualitatively and implied some sort of forced extraction of potassium ions from the cells of the tissue, but with no actual exchange of drug for potassium across the cell membrane. It is not clear how this model would operate energetically.

As was mentioned earlier, KATZ and THESLEFF (1957) suggested a cyclic model to explain desensitisation of receptors. As set out originally, this model could be regarded as a modification of occupation theory. The receptor inactivation theory of GOSSELIN (1970) uses such a cyclic model and unifies both the occupation and rate theory. See GOSSELIN (this volume). RANG and RITTER (1970) have also pointed out that the equations derived for this model can also be interpreted in terms of a modified rate theory.

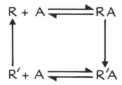

Fig. 7. Cyclic model for receptor desensitisation. Receptor R reacts rapidly with agonist A to produce RA complex which then slowly changes to desensitised complex R'A. The desensitised complex can dissociate rapidly to release desensitised receptor R' which slowly reverts to its initial state

The cyclic model is discussed in detail in the chapter by GOSSELIN (this volume). It will only briefly be discussed in this paragraph. The model is shown in Figure 7. The complex RA is the active form of the agonist-receptor complex which can slowly change to the inactive form R′A. This inactive complex can dissociate rapidly to release desensitised receptors R′, which slowly revert to their initial state R. RANG and RITTER found that for a number of agonists and partial agonists the same amount of desensitisation was produced by those concentrations which produced equal responses. They point out that their results indicate that efficacy is related to the rate constant k_d, and suggest that the stimulus may be a quantal event associated with a transient intermediate conformation between RA and R′A.

The idea of such a transient intermediate conformation raises some interesting possibilities (see GOSSELIN, this volume). When an agonist interacts with the receptor site on a membrane, it is usually assumed that the formation of the complex instantaneously confers new properties on the receptor and hence on the membrane. The cyclic model introduces the idea of two states of the drug-receptor complex each with somewhat different properties. It is tempting to go further and suggest that when the RA complex has been formed various rearrangements will occur in the components which make up the membrane structure, before the system comes to a new equilibrium state. During these changes the local permeability at the receptor site could pass through some maximum value and the stimulus per RA complex would also vary with time. If the agonist equilibrates rapidly with the receptors then the total stimulus might be given by an equation of the form

$$s_A = y_A[R]_T \left\{ F(1 - e^{-k_1 t}) - G(1 - e^{-k_2 t}) \right\}$$

where F, G, k_1, and k_2 are constants which may vary from one drug to another. Similarly, if rapid dissociation of the drug occurred on washout, the modified local membrane permeability at the receptor site might be expected to return slowly to its initial value after a series of time-dependent structural changes.

V. A General Discussion of the Various Receptor Models

In this survey of receptor models of drug action an attempt has been made to present the merits and weaknesses of the various models. The direct occupation theory has the advantage that, superficially at least, it presents a simple picture. However, if the interaction of an agonist with a receptor produces a change in the permeability of the cell membrane, then the direct occupation theory itself fails to take into account subsequent time effects. This point was discussed fully in Section III.A.9. It may be that greater attention should be paid to the possible importance of feedback mechanisms such as that discussed in Sections III.A.10 and III.A.11.

If, on the other hand, receptors are latent enzymes which can be activated by interaction with an agonist (as discussed in Section III.B), then due account must be taken of the availability of substrate and cofactors. Biochemical feedback mechanisms might then also be of importance in determining the variation of response with time. It seems likely that changes in membrane permeability can modify enzyme activity either at the membrane or intracellulary. The converse may also apply. An interesting paper on the effects of various drugs on the Na/K-dependent-ATP-ase system and on the adenyl cyclase system has recently been published by MOZSIK (1969), who also discusses the possibility of interaction between these two systems.

One of the great attractions of the allosteric two-state model is that it provides a simple physical picture of the meaning of intrinsic efficacy. Another attraction is that the switching of the receptor between two states fits in well with modern ideas concerning the generation of membrane action potentials. Although cooperative binding of agonist molecules to the receptor could explain very steep log-dose response curves, there is as yet little evidence that such cooperative binding is of major importance. However, the allosteric two-state model is probably the most attractive alternative to the direct occupation model at the present time.

In its original form, the flux-carrier hypothesis, discussed in Section III.C, side-stepped the problem of how an influx of drug might produce a response. Various possibilities have now been considered. Some of these ideas may have relevance if drugs act either intracellularly or by penetrating cell membranes. It is possible that intracellular uptake of drugs is purely coincidental and is in no way related to their pharmacologic action. Such a suggestion certainly cannot be refuted at the present time.

The original rate theory of drug action, discussed in Section IV, suffers from lack of a clear-cut physicochemical model. It is very difficult to test this theory, especially if the idea of a variable quantum of excitation is introduced. Nevertheless it has been useful in focussing attention on the kinetics of the response. Although there does seem to be a relationship between the rates of onset and offset of action of drugs and their intrinsic efficacies, this may merely reflect the fact that effective antagonists are usually larger molecules than agonists. The latter fact in turn could be explained if agonists have to penetrate into or through membranes, or if agonists must interact *only* with a small region of the receptor. The relationship between intrinsic efficacy and the rate of onset and offset of action of a drug, could also be explained by the access model of THRON and WAUD (1968) or by the existence of negative feedback mechanisms. If such feedback mechanisms exist then both the rate of access of drug to the receptor and the rate constants of the drug-receptor interaction would be important factors in determining whether a response would be observed and, if so, its magnitude.

It therefore seems possible that there may be useful elements in each of the models discussed. At least a large number of possibilities have been suggested and the importance of using the null method for testing the applicability of any model is now fully appreciated. It is obviously too much to expect that any one simple model can be presented as a universal theory of drug action, and it seems likely that each type of receptor will have to be investigated as a separate problem.

VI. A General Discussion of the Possible Uses of Receptor Models

There are now so many models of drug-receptor interaction that it is not unreasonable to ask if they are of any use whatsoever.

The answer to such a question depends, to some extent, on one's point of view. If a pharmacologist merely wants to know if one drug is more potent than another in producing some chosen response from a suitable biological system then usually he has no need of any receptor model. The same conclusion applies if he wishes to estimate the relative potencies of the two drugs, provided that the two log-dose response curves are parallel.

An interesting point that has become clear from the analyses of the various receptor models is that the null equations derived are usually of the same mathematical form. When applying the null equations it is necessary to compare two sets of dose response data obtained from the same piece of isolated tissue. The first set of data is for any agonist A acting alone on the tissue. The second set may be obtained using

(i) a different agonist B, or

(ii) the same agonist A acting in the presence of a reversible antagonist, or

(iii) the same agonist A, after the tissue has been treated with a specific irreversible antagonist.

In each case the general null equation takes the form

$$1/C_{1r} = I_{12} + \psi_{12}(1/C_{2r})$$

where C_{1r} and C_{2r} are the concentrations of agonist required to produce the same response r during the determination of the first and second sets of dose response data respectively. Depending on which of these examples [(i) to (iii)] is being studied, the two sets of dose response data may be obtained using a single agonist or using two different agonists. The quantities I_{12} and ψ_{12} may be regarded as experimental, or phenomenological, constants which summarise the relation between the first and second dose-response curves.

The fact that all of the receptor models lead to null equations of the above form is in one way a disadvantage since it becomes extremely difficult to distinguish between the possible models on the basis of dose response data. However, this situation has one compensatory advantage since, on the basis of any of the models considered, the quantities I_{12} and ψ_{12} should have some basic meaning and would therefore be expected to be reproducible from one sample of tissue to another, and even perhaps from one type of tissue to another. Obviously the reproducibility of such experimental constants ought first to be checked and if the reproducibility is satisfactory then such constants can be used to summarise experimental data with no commitment as to which model may be applicable and regardless of whether the pairs of dose response curves are parallel or not.

The experimental constants I_{12} and ψ_{12} may be regarded as being the intercept and slope respectively of a plot of $1/C_{1r}$ versus $1/C_{2r}$. The equieffective concentrations C_{1r} and C_{2r} have usually been obtained by drawing smooth curves, by eye, through the experimental points plotted as response versus log dose, and reading from these smooth curves the concentrations required to produce equal responses at a number of arbitrarily chosen response levels. However, the fitting of curves by eye is notoriously subjective. Improved methods for estimating various constants from dose-response data have been suggested by PARKER and WAUD (1971) (see also WAUD and PARKER, 1971). These authors used the logit transformation to fit curves to each set of experimental data. Another method, based on a different transformation, has been put forward by MACKAY and WHEELER (1974), MACKAY (1975). The latter method gives estimates of I_{12} and ψ_{12}, as well as approximate values of their standard errors and fiducial limits. From these, the affinity constants of agonists or antagonists (together with estimates of their errors) can be obtained in suitable cases on the basis of the direct occupation theory or other appropriate models.

Affinity constants and relative intrinsic efficacies estimated from the experimental constants should perhaps be prefixed by the word "apparent", unless there is very good evidence that the model being applied is the correct one.

It may seem that the way out of these problems would be to work only with isolated receptors. Unfortunately most tissues contain several macromolecular components capable of interacting with agonists and antagonists. Dependable isolation of receptors therefore requires knowledge of the properties of the receptors in the living tissue. Studies on living tissues, using receptor models, are therefore complementary to any studies on isolated receptors. Where such alleged receptor molecules, or acceptors, have been isolated, detailed studies of the interaction between agonists, antagonists, and acceptors should provide enough information to allow a suitable model to be chosen. Application of the null method to this model and comparison of the quantative results of experiments on the isolated tissue with those on isolated acceptors should then provide good evidence for deciding whether the acceptors are identical with the receptors in situ. In order to make such comparisons it is obviously important to have not only estimates of the various affinity constants of drugs for the receptors and for the acceptors but also estimates of their errors.

Finally, where receptor or acceptor molecules have not been isolated there seems to be no reason why pharmacologic data should not be summarised in terms of experimental constants and tentatively interpreted in terms of the model preferred by the individual research worker. At some later date when more fundamental information becomes available it would then be possible to interpret the experimental constants in other ways, if necessary.

Appendix

Glossary of Symbols

Table of major symbols

A	Drug (usually an agonist)
B	Drug (agonist or antagonist)
C	Carrier
D	Drug (agonist or antagonist)
D_A	Diffusion coefficient of drug A
e_A	Efficacy of drug A
E	Enzyme
ES	Enzyme-substrate complex
ESA	A complex of enzyme with substrate S and drug A
f_A	Intrinsic efficacy of drug A
I	Inhibitor or antagonist
I_{AB}	Intercept obtained by plotting $1/(A)_r$ against $1/(B)_r$, where $(A)_r$ and $(B)_r$ are concentrations of A and B which produce same response r from the tissue

	This quantity may also be estimated by using other suitable transformations, but is essentially an experimental quantity.
J_A	Flux of drug A across the cell membrane
J_L	Leakage flux of some ion X across the cell membrane
J_P	Pump flux of ion X across the cell membrane
k, k_D, etc.	Proportionality constants, as defined in appropriate section of the text
k, k_{1D}, etc.	Rate constants, as defined in appropriate section of the text
K_D, K_A, etc.	Affinity constants of appropriate compounds for receptors, carriers, or enzymes. These are generally expressed in litres/mole. Affinity constant is reciprocal of the dissociation constant
K_{AB}, K_{AI}, etc.	Equilibrium constants as defined in appropriate section of the text
K_{RA}	Affinity constant of drug A for active form of the receptor, where this has to be distinguished from its affinity for an inactive form
K_{TA}	Affinity constant of drug A for an inactive form of the receptor
M	Moles/litre. Also used, in Sections III.A.10 and III.A.11, for a quantity proportional to $[R]_T$
M_a	Activator molecule
M_i	Inhibitor molecule
N	Quantity proportional to ζ
P	Protein molecule
Q	Forward rate of formation of drug-receptor complexes, per receptor
r	Response
R	Receptor. Also used on a few occasions to denote gas constant
RD, RA, RAB, etc.	Receptor-drug complexes
s	Pharmacologic stimulus
S	Substrate
t	Time
T	Absolute temperature
v_D	Velocity of an enzyme reaction activated by drug D
V_f	Forward rate of formation of drug-receptor complexes
x	Dose-ratio
X	Ion
y_D	Fraction of receptors or carriers occupied by drug D. Unless otherwise indicated, y_D refers to equilibrium occupation of receptors or carriers by the drug (see section below on subscripts)
α_D	Intrinsic activity of drug D
β_{AB}	Intrinsic efficacy of drug A relative to that of drug B
γ	Constant, characteristic of pump mechanism
δ	Thickness of cell membrane
Δ	Change in some quantity
ζ	Constant, characteristic of ion pump
η	Initial permeability of cell membrane

θ_A, θ_{SA}, etc.   Steady-state constants, as defined in appropriate section of the text

ϱ_D Ratio {Intercept}/{Slope -1} estimated from plot of $1/(D)_r$ against $1/(D)'_r$, where $(D)_r$ and $(D)'_r$ are concentrations of D which produce same response r, before and after treatment of tissue with a specific irreversible antagonist.

This quantity may also be estimated in other ways but is essentially an experimental constant

ψ_{AB} Slope of plot $1/(A)_r$ against $1/(B)_r$, where $(A)_r$ and $(B)_r$ are concentrations of agonists A and B which produce same response r from tissue.

This quantity may also be estimated in other ways but is essentially an experimental quantity

( )   Molar concentration of compound indicated by symbol enclosed in brackets

[ ]   Concentration of compound indicated by symbol enclosed enclosed in brackets, in arbitrary units

Subscripts:

A, B, etc.   Indicate that quantity applies to compound indicated by subscript

eq.   Indicates that quantity corresponds to equilibrium occupation of receptors by the drug. Where only equilibrium conditions are being considered the subscript eq. may be omitted

i   Indicates that quantity referred to is that *inside* the cell

o   Usually indicates that quantity is that which applies at zero time. In some sections this subscript has been used to indicate that quantity referred to is that *outside* the cell

r   Indicates that quantity is that which corresponds to response r

t   Indicates that quantity is that which applies at time t

T   Indicates *total* concentration of some compound or molecular species

Superscripts:

'   A dash superscript is generally used to indicate that a quantity is that which applies when second drug is also present, or when state of tissue has been altered from some earlier state. This applies to all sections except Sections III.A.9 to III.A.11, where dash superscript is used to indicate that $(X)'_i$ is intracellular concentration of ion X at any time t

References

Ariens, E. J.: Affinity and intrinsic activity in the theory of competitive inhibition. Arch. int. Pharmacodyn. **99**, 32—49 (1954).

Ariens, E. J., Rossum, J. M. Van: pD_x, pA_x and pD_x values in the analysis of pharmacodynamics. Arch. int. Pharmacodyn. **110**, 275—299 (1957).

Ariens, E. J., Simonis, A. M.: A molecular basis for drug action. J. Pharm. (Lond.) **16**, 137—157 (1964a).

Ariens, E. J., Simonis, A. M.: A molecular basis for drug action. J. Pharm. (Lond.) **16**, 289—312 (1964b).

Ariens, E. J., Simonis, A. M., Cholinergic and anticholinergic drugs. Do they act on common receptors? Ann. N.Y. Acad. Sci. **144**, 842—868 (1967).

Ariens, E. J., Simonis, A. M., Rossum, J. M. Van: In: Ariens, E. J. (Ed.): Molecular Pharmacology, Section III.6. New York London: Academic Press 1964.

Arunlakshana, O., Schild, H. O.: Some quantitative uses of drug antagonists. Brit. J. Pharmacol. **14**, 48—58 (1959).

Barlow, R. B., Scott, K. A., Stephenson, R. P.: An attempt to study the effects of chemical structure on the affinity and efficacy of compounds related to acetylcholine. Brit. J. Pharmacol. **21**, 509—522 (1963).

Barlow, R. B., Scott, K. A., Stephenson, R. P.: The affinity and efficacy of onium salts on the frog rectus abdominis. Brit. J. Pharmacol. **31**, 188—196 (1967).

Barsoum, G. S., Gaddum, J. H.: The pharmacological estimation of adenosine and histamine in blood. J. Physiol. (Lond.) **85**, 1—14 (1935).

Belleau, B.: Relationships between agonists, antagonists and receptor sites. In: Vane, J. R., Wolstenholme, G. E. W., O'Connor, M. (Eds.): Ciba foundation symposium on adrenergic mechanisms, p. 223—245. London: J. and A. Churchill (1960).

Belleau, B.: A molecular theory of drug action based on induced conformational perturbations of receptors. J. med. Chem. **7**, 776—784 (1964).

Belleau, B.: Conformational perturbation in relation to the regulation of enzyme and receptor behaviour. In: Harper, N. J., Simmonds, A. B. (Eds.): Adv. in drug research, Vol. **2**. London New York: Academic Press 1965.

Belleau, B.: Water as the determinant of thermodynamic transitions in the interaction of aliphatic chains with acetylcholinesterase and the cholinergic receptors. Ann. N.Y. Acad. Sci. **144**, 705—719 (1967).

Belleau, B., Lacasse, G.: Aspects of the chemical mechanism of complex formation between acetylcholinesterase and acetylcholine-related compounds. J. med. Chem. **7**, 768—775 (1964).

Belleau, B., Tani, H., Lie, F.: A correlation between the biological activity of alkyltrimethyl-ammonium ions and their mode of interaction with acetylcholinesterase. J. Amer. chem. Soc. **87**, 2283—2285 (1965).

Bloom, B. M., Goldman, I. M.: The nature of catecholamineadenine mononucleotide interactions in adrenergic mechanisms. In: Harper, N. J., Simmonds, A. B. (Eds.): Adv. in drug research, Vol. **3**. London and New York: Academic Press 1966.

Bowman, W. C., Rand, M. J., West, G. B.: Textbook of pharmacology, Chapter 26. Oxford-Edinburgh: Blackwell Sci. Publ. 1968.

Bueding, E., Bulbring, E.: The inhibitory action of adrenaline. Biochemical and biophysical observations. In: Bulbring, E. (Ed.): Proceedings of the 2nd international pharmacological congress, at Prague (1963), Vol. **6**. Pharmacology of smooth muscle. Prague: Czechoslovak Medical Press 1964.

Bulbring, E.: In a preface to: Bulbring, E. (Ed.): Proceedings of the 2nd international pharmacological congress, at Prague (1963), Vol. **6**. The pharmacology of smooth muscle. Prague: Czechoslovak Medical Press 1964.

Bulbring, E., Brading, A. F., Jones, A. W., Tomita, T.: Smooth muscle. London: Arnold 1970.

Burgen, A. S. V.: The drug-receptor complex. J. Pharm. (Lond.) **18**, 137—149 (1966).

Cantoni, G. L., Eastman, G.: On the response of the intestine to smooth muscle stimulants. J. Pharmacol. exp. Ther. **87**, 392—399 (1946).

Chagas, C., Penna-Franca, E., Nishie, K., Garcia, E. J.: A study of the specificity of the complex formed by gallamine triethiodide with a macromolecular constituent of the electric organ. Arch. Biochem. **75**, 251—259 (1958).

Changeux, J.-P., Meunier, J.-C., Olsen, R. W., Weber, M., Bourgeois, J.-P., Popot, J. L., Cohen, J. B., Hazelbauer, G. L., Lester, H. A.: Studies on the mode of action of cholinergic agonists at the molecular level. In: Rang, H. P. (Ed.): Drug receptors pp. 273—294. London: Macmillan 1973.

Clark, A. J.: In: Mode of action of drugs on cells. London: Arnold 1933.

Clark, A. J.: General pharmacology. In: Heffter's Handbuch der Experimentellen Pharmakologie, Ergänzungswerk, Vol. **4**, pp. 1—223. Berlin: Springer 1937.

Clark, A. J., Raventos, J.: The antagonism of acetylcholine and of quaternary ammonium salts. Quart. J. exp. Physiol. **26**, 375—391 (1937).

Colquhoun, D.: The relation between classical and cooperative models for drug action. In: Rang, H. P. (Ed.): Drug receptors, pp. 149—182. London: Macmillan 1973.

Cordes, E. H., Jencks, W. P.: Nucleophilic catalysis of semicarbazone formation by anilines. J. Amer. chem. Soc. **84**, 826—831 (1962a).

Cordes, E. H., Jencks, W. P.: Semicarbazone formation from pyridoxal, pyridoxal-phosphate, and their Schiff bases. Biochemistry **1**, 773—778 (1962b).

Creese, R., Maclagan, J.: Autoradiography of decamethonium in rat muscle. Nature (Lond.) **215**, 988—989 (1967).

Creese, R., Taylor, D. B.: Entry of labelled carbachol in brain slices of the rat and the action of d-tubocurarine and strychnine. J. Pharmacol. exp. Ther. **157**, 406—419 (1967).

Creese, R., Taylor, D. B., Tilton, B.: The effect of curare on the uptake and release of a depolarising agent labelled with I^{131}. In: Bovet, D., Bovet-Nitti, F., Marini-Bettolo, G. B. (Eds.): Curare and curare-like agents. Amsterdam: Elsevier 1959.

Del Castillo, J., Katz, B.: On the localisation of acetylcholine receptors. J. Physiol. (Lond.) **128**, 157—181 (1955).

De Robertis, E.: The isolation and molecular properties of receptor proteolipids. In: Rang, H. P. (Ed.): Drug receptors, pp. 257—272. London: Macmillan 1973.

Douglas, W. W.: Stimulus-secretion coupling: the concept and clues from chromaffin and other cells. The first Gaddum memorial lecture. Brit. J. Pharmacol. **34**, 451—474 (1968).

Durbin, R. P., Jenkinson, D. H.: The effect of carbachol on the permeability of depolarised smooth muscle to inorganic ions. J. Physiol. (Lond.) **157**, 74—89 (1961a).

Durbin, R. P., Jenkinson, D. H.: The calcium dependence of tension development in depolarised smooth muscle. J. Physiol. (Lond.) **157**, 90—96 (1961b).

Edman, K. A. P., Schild, H. O.: The need for calcium in the contractile response induced by acetylcholine and potassium in the rat uterus. J. Physiol. (Lond.) **161**, 424—441 (1962).

Ehrenpreis, S.: Electroplax and nerve activity. Science **136**, 175—177 (1962).

Ehrenpreis, S.: Possible nature of the cholinergic receptor. Ann. N.Y. Acad. Sci. **144**, 720—734 (1967).

Elmqvist, D., Thesleff, S.: Ideas regarding receptor "desensitisation" at the motor end-plate. Rev. Canad. Biol. **21**, 229—234 (1962).

Evans, D. H. L., Schild, H. O.: Reactions of the isolated amnion of the chick, suspended in isotonic KCl, to acetylcholine and to electrical stimulation. J. Physiol. (Lond.) **136**, 36P (1957).

Fewtrell, C. M. S., Rang, H. P.: The labelling of cholinergic receptors in smooth muscle. In: Rang, H. P. (Ed.): Drug receptors, 211—224. London: Macmillan 1973.

Fischer, J. J., Jost, M. C.: Nuclear magnetic resonance studies of drug-receptor interactions. The binding of epinephrine to isolated mouse liver cells. Molec. Pharmacol. **5**, 420—424 (1969).

Furchgott, R. F.: The pharmacology of vascular smooth muscle. Pharmacol. Rev. **7**, 138—265 (1955).

Furchgott, R. F.: Receptor mechanisms. Ann. Rev. Pharmacol. **4**, 21—50 (1964).

Furchgott, R. F.: At the symposium on the interactions of drugs with receptors, Chelsea College of Science and Technology, London 1965.

Furchgott, R. F.: The use of β-haloalkylamines in the differentiation of receptors and in the determination of dissociation constants of receptor-agonist complexes. In: Harper, N. J., Simmonds, A. B. (Eds.): Adv. in drug research, Vol. 3. London-New York: Academic Press 1966.

Furchgott, R. F., Bursztyn, P.: Comparison of dissociation constants and of relative efficacies of selected agonists acting on parasympathetic receptors. Ann. N.Y. Acad. Sci. **144**, 882—898 (1967).

Gaddum, J. H.: The action of adrenaline and ergotamine on the uterus of the rabbit. J. Physiol. (Lond.) **61**, 141—150 (1926).

Gaddum, J. H.: The quantitative effects of antagonistic drugs. J. Physiol. (Lond.) **89**, 7—9 p (1937).

Gaddum, J. H.: Introductory address: Symposium on chemical constitution and pharmacological action. Trans. Faraday Soc. **39**, 323—332 (1943).

Gaddum, J. H.: Theories of drug antagonism. Pharmacol. Rev. **9**, 211—218 (1957).

Gaddum, J. H., Hameed, K. A., Hathway, D. E., Stephens, F. F.: Quantitative studies of antagonists for 5-hydroxytryptamine. Quart. J. exp. Physiol. **40**, 49—74 (1955).

Gilbert, D. L., Fenn, W. O.: Calcium equilibrium in muscle. J. gen. Physiol. **40**, 393—408 (1957).

Gill, E. W., Rang, H. P.: An alkylating derivative of benzilylcholine with specific and long-lasting parasympatholytic activity. Molec. Pharmacol. **2**, 284—297 (1966).

Goldstein, D. B., Goldstein, A.: Possible role of enzyme inhibition and repression in drug tolerance and addiction. Biochem. pharmacol. **8**, 48 (1961).

Gosselin, R. E.: Drug receptor inactivation: a new kinetic model. Brit. J. Pharmacol. **39**, 215 (1970).

Grisolia, S.: The catalytic environment and its biological implications. Physiol. Rev. **44**, 657—712 (1964).

Higman, H. B., Podleski, T. R., Bartels, E.: Apparent dissociation constants between carbamyl-choline, *d*-tubocurarine and the receptor. Biochim. biophys. Acta (Amst.) **75**, 187—193 (1963).

Hodgkin, A. L., Horowicz, P.: Potassium contractures in single muscle fibres. J. Physiol. (Lond.) **153**, 386—403 (1960).

Jenkinson, D. H., Nicholls, J. G.: Contractures and permeability changes produced by acetylcholine in depolarised denervated muscle. J. Physiol. (Lond.) **159**, 111—127 (1961).

Karlin, A.: On the application of a "plausible model" of allosteric proteins to the receptor for acetylcholine. J. theor. Biol. **16**, 306—320 (1967).

Katz, B., Thesleff, S.: A study of the "desensitisation" produced by acetylcholine at the motor end plate J. Physiol. (Lond.) **138**, 63—80 (1957).

Mackay, D.: The reaction of thiol amino acids with pyridoxal-5'-phosphate in the absence and in the presence of L-glutamic acid. Biochim. biophys. Acta (Amst.) **73**, 445—453 (1963a).

Mackay, D.: A flux-carrier hypothesis of drug action. Nature (Lond.) **197**, 1171—1173 (1963b).

Mackay, D.: At the symposium on the interactions of drugs with receptors, Chelsea College of Science and Technology, London 1965.

Mackay, D.: A general analysis of the drug-receptor interaction. Brit. J. Pharmacol. **26**, 9—16 (1966a).

Mackay, D.: The mathematics of drug-receptor interactions. J. Pharm. (Lond.) **18**, 201—222 (1966b).

Mackay, D.: A new method for the analysis of drug-receptor interactions. In: Harper, N. J., Simmonds, A. B. (Eds.): Adv. in drug research, **3**. London-New York: Academic Press 1966c.

Mackay, D.: An improvement in the use of the L-transformation. J. Pharm. (Lond.) **27**, 216 (1975).

Mackay, D., Taylor, D. B.: Uptake of ^{3}H-labelled polymethylene bisquaternary ammonium ions by mouse isolated diaphragm. Europ. J. Pharmacol. **9**, 195—206 (1970).

Mackay, D., Wheeler, J.: A useful transformation for comparing dose-response curves. J. Pharm. (Lond.) **26**, 569—581 (1974).

Marshall, P. B.: Some chemical and physical properties associated with histamine antagonism. Brit. J. Pharmacol. **10**, 270—278 (1955).

Mozsik, G.: Some feedback mechanisms by drugs in the interrelationship between the active transport system and adenyl cyclase system localized in the cell membrane. Europ. J. Pharmacol. **7**, 319—327 (1969).

Namba, T., Grob, D.: Cholinergic receptors in skeletal muscle: Isolation and properties of muscle ribonucleoprotein with affinity for *d*-tubocurarine and acetylcholine, and binding activity of the subneural apparatus of motor end plates with divalent metal ions. Ann. N.Y. Acad. Sci. **144**, 772—802 (1967).

Nickerson, M.: Receptor occupancy and tissue response. Nature (Lond.) **178**, 697—698 (1956).

Niedergerke, R.: The potassium chloride contracture of the heart and its modification by calcium. J. Physiol. (Lond.) **134**, 584—599 (1956).

Niedergerke, R.: Movements of calcium in frog heart ventricles at rest and during contractures. J. Physiol. (Lond.) **167**, 515—550 (1963).

O'Brien, R. D., Eldefrawi, M. E., Eldefrawi, A. T.: The isolation of functional acetylcholine receptor. In: Rang, H. P. (Ed.): Drug receptors, pp. 241—256. London: Macmillan 1973.

Parker, R. B., Waud, D. R.: Pharmacological estimation of drug-receptor dissociation constants. Statistical evaluation. I. Agonists. J. Pharmacol. exp. Ther. **177**, 1—12 (1971).

Paton, W. D. M.: The principles of drug action. Proc. roy. Soc. Med. **53**, 815—820 (1960).

Paton, W. D. M.: A theory of drug action based on the rate of drug-receptor combination. Proc. Roy. Soc. B. **154**, 21—69 (1961).

Paton, W. D. M.: Adrenergic receptors viewed in light of general receptor theories. Ann. N.Y. Acad. Sci. **139**, 632—644 (1967a).

Paton, W. D. M.: Kinetic theories of drug action with special reference to the acetylcholine group of agonists and antagonists. Ann. N.Y. Acad. Sci. **139**, 869—881 (1967b).

Paton, W. D. M., Rang, H. P.: The uptake of atropine and related drugs by intestinal smooth muscle of the guinea-pig in relation to acetylcholine receptors. Proc. roy. Soc. B **163**, 1—44 (1965).

Paton, W. D. M., Rang, H. P.: A kinetic approach to the mechanism of drug action. In: Harper, N. J., Simmonds, A. B. (Eds.): Adv. in drug research, **3**. London-New York: Academic Press 1966.

Paton, W. D. M., Rothschild, A. M.: The changes in response and in ionic content of smooth muscle produced by acetylcholine action and by calcium deficiency. Brit. J. Pharmacol. **24**, 437—448 (1965).

Paton, W. D. M., Waud, D. R.: A quantitative investigation of the relationship between rate of access of a drug to receptor and the rate of onset or offset of action. Naunyn-Schmiedebergs Arch. exp. Path. Pharmak. **248**, 124—143 (1964).

Rang, H. P.: The kinetics of action of acetylcholine antagonists in smooth muscle. Proc. roy. Soc., B. **164**, 488—510 (1966).

Rang, H. P.: Drug receptors. Report of a Symposium held at the Middlesex Hospital Medical School, London, 1972. Rang, H. P. (Ed.) London: Macmillan 1973a.

Rang, H. P.: Receptor mechanisms. Fourth Gaddum memorial lecture. Brit. J. Pharmacol. **48**, 475—495 (1973b).

Rang, H. P., Ritter, J. M.: A new kind of drug antagonism: evidence that agonists cause a molecular change in acetylcholine receptors. Molec. Pharmacol. **5**, 391—411 (1969).

Rang, H. P., Ritter, J. M.: On the mechanism of desensitisation at cholinergic receptors. Molec. Pharmacol. **6**, 357—382 (1970).

Raventos, J.: Pharmacological actions of quaternary ammonium salts. Quart. J. exp. Physiol. **26**, 361—374 (1937).

Robertson, P. A.: Calcium and contractility in depolarised smooth muscle. Nature (Lond.) **186**, 316—317 (1960).

Robison, G. A., Butcher, R. W., Sutherland, E. W.: Adenylcyclase as an adrenergic receptor. Ann. N.Y. Acad. Sci. **139**, 703—723 (1967).

Rossum, J. M. Van: Limitation of molecular pharmacology. Some implications of the basic assumptions underlying calculations on drug-receptor interactions and the significance of biological drug parameters. In: Harper, N. J., Simmonds, A. B. (Eds.): Adv. in drug research, **3**, London-New York: Academic Press 1966.

Rossum, J. M. Van, Ariens, E. J.: Pharmacodynamics of drugs affecting skeletal muscle. Structure-action relationships in homologous series of quaternary ammonium salts. Arch. int. Pharmacodyn. **118**, 393—417 (1959).

Rossum, J. M. Van, Ariens, E. J.: Receptor reserve and threshold phenomena. II. Theories on drug-action and a quantitative approach to spare receptors and threshold vaues. Arch. int. Pharmacodyn. **136**, 385—413 (1962).

Schatzmann, H. J.: Excitation, contraction and calcium in smooth muscle. In: Bulbring, E. (Ed.): Proceedings of the 2nd international pharmacological congress, at Prague 1963, Vol. **6**. The pharmacology of smooth muscle. Prague: Czechoslovak Medical Press 1964.

Schild, H. O.: pA, a new scale for the measurement of drug antagonism. Brit. J. Pharmacol. **2**, 189—206 (1947).

Schild, H. O.: pA$_x$ and competitive drug antagonism. Brit. J. Pharmacol. **4**, 277—280 (1949).

Schild, H. O.: Non-competitive drug antagonism. J. Physiol. (Lond.) **124**, 33—34 P (1954).

Schild, H. O.: Drug antagonism and pA$_x$. Pharmacol. Rev. **9**, 242—246 (1957).

Schild, H. O.: Introduction Receptors. In: Mongar, J. L., de Reuck, A. V. S. (Eds.): Enzymes and drug action (Ciba Found. Symposium). 435—439. London: J. and A. Churchill 1962.

Schild, H. O.: Calcium and the effects of drugs on depolarised smooth muscle. In: Bulbring, E. (Ed.): Proceedings of the 2nd international pharmacological congress, at Prague, 1963, Vol. 6. Pharmacology of smooth muscle. Prague: Czechoslovak Medical Press 1964.

Schild, H. O.: Need for calcium in isoprenaline-induced relaxation of the depolarised rat uterus. Nature (Lond.) **215**, 650—651 (1967).

Segal, H. L., Kachmar, J. F., Boyer, P. D.: 1. Further considerations of enzyme inhibition and analysis of enzyme activation. Enzymologia **15**, 187—198 (1952).

Shanes, A. M.: Possible mechanisms of acetylcholine action in muscle. In: Koelle, G. B., Douglas, W. W., Carlsson, A. (Eds.): Proceedings of the 2nd international pharmacological congress, at Prague, 1963. Pharmacology of cholinergic and adrenergic transmission. Prague: Czechoslovak Medical Press 1965.

Singh, I., Acharya, A. K.: Excitation of unstriated muscle without any ionic gradient across the membrane. Indian J. Physiol. Pharmacol. **1**, 265—269 (1957).

Stephenson, R. P.: Acetylcholine receptors and alkyltrimethylammonium salts. Abstr. of commun., 19th international physiological congress, at Montreal, pp. 801—802 (1953).

Stephenson, R. P.: A modification of receptor theory. Brit. J. Pharmacol. **11**, 379—393 (1956).

Stephenson, R. P.: At the symposium on the interactions of drugs with receptors, Chelsea College of Science and Technology, London, 1965.

Stephenson, R. P.: Measurement of affinity constants of partial agonist and agonist drugs. Proceedings of the 3rd international pharmacological congress, at Sao Paulo, p. 1 (1966).

Straub, W.: Zur chemischen Kinetik der Muskarinwirkung und des Antagonismus Muskarin-Atropin. Pflügers Arch. ges. Physiol. **119**, 127—151 (1907).

Sutherland, E. W., Rall, T. W.: The relation of adenosine-3′, 5′-phosphate and phosphorylase to the actions of catecholamines and other hormones. Pharmacol. Rev. **12**, 265—299 (1960).

Taylor, D. B.: Influence of curare on uptake and release of a neuromuscular blocking agent labelled with I^{131}. In: de Reuck, A. V. S. (Ed.): Ciba found. study gp. No. 12. Curare and curare-like agents. London: J. and A. Churchill 1962.

Taylor, D. B., Creese, R., Nedergaard, O. A., Case, R.: Labelled depolarising drugs in normal and denervated muscle. Nature (Lond.) **208**, 901—902 (1965).

Taylor, D. B., Nedergaard, O. A.: Relation between structure and action of quaternary ammonium neuromuscular blocking agents. Physiol. Rev. **45**, 523—554 (1965).

Taylor, D. B., Steinborn, J., Lu, T. C.: Ion exchange process at the neuromuscular junction of voluntary muscle. J. Pharmacol. exp. Ther. **175**, 213—227 (1970).

Thron, C. D.: On the analysis of pharmacological experiments in terms of an allosteric receptor model. Molec. Pharmacol. **9**, 1—9 (1973).

Thron, C. D., Waud, D. R.: The rate of action of atropine. J. Pharmacol. exp. Ther. **160**, 91—105 (1968).

Triggle, D. J.: 2-Halogenoethylamines and receptor analysis. In: Harper, N. J., Simmonds, A. B. (Eds.): Adv. in drug research, Vol. 2. London-New York: Academic Press 1965.

Waser, P. G., Luthi, U.: Autoradiographische lokalisation von C-14-calebassen-curarin I und C-14-decamethonium in der motorischen end platte. Arch. int. Pharmacodyn. **112**, 272—296 (1957).

Watkins, J. C.: Pharmacological receptors and general permeability phenomena of cell membranes. J. theor. Biol. **9**, 37—50 (1965).

Waud, D. R.: The rate of action of competitive neuromuscular blocking agents. J. Pharmacol. exp. Ther. **158**, 99—114 (1967).

Waud, D. R.: On the estimation of receptor occlusion by irreversible competitive pharmacological antagonists. Biochem. Pharmacol. **17**, 649—653 (1968a).

Waud, D. R.: Pharmacological receptors. Pharmacol. Rev. **20**, 49—88 (1968b).

Waud, D. R., Parker, R. B.: Pharmacological estimation of drug-receptor dissociation constants. Statistical evaluation. II. Competitive antagonists. J. Pharmacol. exp. Ther. **177**, 13—24 (1971).

Werman, R.: An electrophysiological approach to drugreceptor mechanisms. Comp. Biochem. Physiol., **30**, 997—1017 (1969).

Winegrad, S., Shanes, A. M.: Calcium flux and contractility in guinea-pig atria. J. gen. Physiol. **45**, 371—394 (1962).

Young, J. M., Hilley, R., Burgen, A. S. V.: Homologues of benzilylcholine mustard. J. Pharm. (Lond.) **24**, 950—954 (1972).

CHAPTER 6

Drug-Receptor Inactivation: A New Kinetic Model

R. E. GOSSELIN

I. Introduction

In this volume MACKAY (1977) has reviewed various drug-receptor theories that have been proposed over the past 30 to 40 years. We offer here a new hypothesis for consideration. As a scheme of drug-receptor kinetics it appears to be at least as successful as earlier models in accounting for a variety of experimental phenomena. The resulting explanations are plausible and attractive but certainly not demonstrably correct. Indeed, like many explanations derived from rival theories, they apparently are not susceptible to rigorous proof by any experimental technique available today. The new proposal, however, does offer an alternative way to interpret experimental data on receptor mechanisms. It also serves to reconcile several rival models by incorporating them into a unifying hypothesis.

Before describing what has been referred to as the "receptor inactivation model" (GOSSELIN, 1968), it is useful to trace its antecedents and thus to establish relationships with alternative schemes. This effort will serve to expose some of the possibilities and impossibilities that are seldom recognized in speculations about receptor mechanisms.

II. Energetics of Receptor Activity

We are aware of no evidence that receptor activation is tightly coupled to effector response. Indeed it seems likely that the interaction between receptor and drug leads not to one but to a sequence of biochemical and biophysical events that are coupled in an orderly array, culminating in the observed macroscopic phenomenon that we call the "pharmacological" effect. In some way the interaction between drug and receptor generates what STEPHENSON (1956) has called a "stimulus" that serves to initiate this complex series of events and to control its intensity from moment to moment.

This stimulus or signal must find a molecular expression at the receptor level, but in spite of several intriguing proposals molecular aspects of stimulus formation have not yet been clarified. Because no satisfactory experimental approaches to this problem are know, speculation has flourished. Many theoretical models of drug-receptor action have been entertained since the original formulations of CLARK (1933, 1937), and each of them contains an implicit or explicit assumption about the nature of stimulus formation.

From the point of view of energetics, two general categories of drug-receptor models can be recognized: (a) those which assume that a continuous expenditure of chemical energy is required for maintaining the stimulus intensity and (b) those which assume an energy expenditure only at the initiation or termination of the stimulus. The former assert that a thermodynamic equilibrium between drug and receptor is incompatible with stimulus formation, while the latter insist that equilibrium is equivalent to a finite and constant stimulus intensity. Whereas other possibilities are conceivable, it appears that any realistic model would have to fit one pattern or the other.

Although the argument can be phrased in rigorous thermodynamic terms (GOSSELIN, unpublished), an analogy is a convenient way to clarify the distinction. All models recognize that large expenditures of metabolic energy are involved in responses of such biological effectors as muscles and glands. The immediate source of this energy is believed to be ATP and other labile metabolites stored in the resting cell. Drug-receptor mechanisms act only to initiate the release of this large store of energy and to control its rate of expenditure. Two fundamentally different types of controlling devices are represented by the trigger of a loaded revolver and the trigger of any automatic weapon such as a "machine gun". In both cases the operator controls the release of enormous amounts of energy by a rather trivial amount of work against the trigger mechanism.

In contrast to the revolver, which requires that work be performed as long as firing is continued and at a rate proportional to the rate of firing, the operator of an automatic weapon is required only to initiate the process, i.e., he expends metabolic energy only to set the trigger to the "on" position (ignoring any "static" work required to hold a spring-loaded trigger). In the "on" position the weapon continues indefinitely to discharge at an "intrinsic" rate without requiring any further trigger energy. Clearly the "stimulus" for the firing is merely the favorable position of the trigger.

The same assertion is implicit in the classic occupation theory of receptor action and its several modern variants (BELLEAU, 1964; BELLEAU and LACASSE, 1964; CHANGEUX et al., 1967; KARLIN, 1967; VAN ROSSUM, 1968). Such models are discussed extensively in this volume (VAN DEN BRINK, 1977) and elsewhere (ARIËNS, 1964; FURCHGOTT, 1964). Whereas considerable evidence can be cited in their support, they are as yet unproved. For this reason it seems premature to discard alternative hypotheses, specifically those based on the revolver analogy. We shall limit our attention to such models because they have been relatively neglected.

III. Models in Which Trigger Energy is Generated

Inspired by the original proposals of RENQVIST (1919), CROXATTO and HUIDOBRO (1956) and PATON (1961), one can formulate a family of receptor models analogous to the revolver. We shall consider only the simplest possibilities. Apparently some of these proposals have not been stated before in an explicit way, and some others have received only superficial treatment. At least the principles are implicit in several earlier speculations about receptor mechanisms (e.g., WAUD, 1968).

PATON and RANG (1966) state: "Thus stimulation is seen, not as an influence emanating from a persisting drug-receptor complex, but as a succession of quantal events each corresponding in the formation of a single drug-receptor complex". This statement was made in a description of the "rate theory" (PATON, 1961). A more general hypothesis might read: stimulation is seen as a succession of quantal events, each corresponding to the progression of one drug molecule through whatever cycle of chemical reactions characterizes its interaction with the receptor. Considerations of energetics require one further stipulation, namely that useful energy can be derived from this molecular cycling.

In the revolver analogy this energy corresponds to the work that must be expended on the trigger. For such energy to be useful in the cell, that step in the drug-receptor interaction which provides the trigger energy must be coupled in such a way that it drives some metabolic reaction that leads ultimately to an effector response. Accordingly the stimulus intensity is equivalent to the number of quanta of trigger energy generated per unit time, corresponding to the rate of molecular cycling. As in the revolver, the size of the quantum is irrelevant as long as it exceeds some threshold value. Within this conceptual framework a variety of models can be entertained.

The simplest possibility is a reversible, 1:1 molar reaction between drug (D) and receptor (R):

$$D + R \underset{k_2}{\overset{k_1}{\rightleftharpoons}} DR. \tag{1}$$

Unlike occupation theories, however, the stimulus is now assumed to depend upon trigger energy generated by the formation of the drug-receptor complex. Accordingly, the stimulus intensity is equal to (or at least proportional to) the net rate of formation of DR. This mechanism has been postulated on several occasions (e.g., RENQVIST, 1919; FEHER and BOKRI, 1961). Because the stimulus depends on a change in the composition of the system, both stimulus and response become zero when reaction (1) attains equilibrium. This scheme has been invoked to explain such related phenomena as fatigue, adaptation, and accommodation to continued chemical stimulation. For some biological chemoreceptor systems the response does appear to cease in the presence of a persisting concentration of the excitatory chemical. Thus an infusion of acetylcholine together with a cholinesterase inhibitor produces excitation of the superior cervical ganglion of the cat. As judged by contraction of the nictitating membrane, however, this excitation ceases in less than 1 min even though the acetylcholine infusion is maintained (FEHER and BOKRI, 1961). At one time the intensity of taste sensation was also thought to be related to the rate of taste receptor occupation, but BEIDLER (1962) has shown that taste adaptation is never complete.

Certainly most drug receptors and other chemoreceptors continue to function during prolonged exposures to agonists and related excitatory chemicals, even though the responses may be distinctly attenuated. For example, in the presence of n-butyl-trimethylammonium bromide the isolated frog rectus muscle maintains a relatively stable level of shortening for almost 24 h (ARIËNS, personal communication). Therefore, as a general basis for generating trigger energy, reaction (1) is highly unlikely. If drug effects require trigger energy from receptor mechanisms, it is apparent that drug and receptor do not generally attain equilibrium or any other truly stationary state, at least not under the usual experimental conditions. The most likely reason for this failure is the existence of one or more irreversible steps in the reaction sequence.

One special kind of stationary state, however, is compatible with the synthesis of trigger energy. Thus it is possible to derive useful work from a chemical cycle in which the final or regenerative phase of the cycle occurs at a different temperature from that of the initial phase, even when the concentrations of all chemical species remain constant in time and space. Conceivably the drug-receptor mechanism is such a heat engine, converting thermal energy into useful trigger energy on the basis of an intracellular temperature gradient generated and maintained by the normal oxidative metabolism of carbohydrates and other foodstuffs. Because cellular respiratory activity is concentrated in mitochondria and not distributed uniformly throughout the cell, stable temperature gradients of microscopic and submicroscopic dimensions must exist. Of course the temperature differences must be quite small, and at least conventional chemical reactions are modified very little by temperature changes of a few degrees. Therefore the rates at which useful energy can be generated by such a heat engine are minute, even if a mechanism exists for shuttling the reactants between temperature zones at a high cycling frequency. The possibility of such a scheme, however, cannot be dimissed completely because there exist no data on which to base an estimate of the trigger energy required for a threshold stimulus. The unique feature of trigger energy is not its magnitude but the special way it is coupled to the effector mechanism. The highly organized structure of cellular organelles may well provide the basis for such specialized coupling.

Admittedly the heat engine is an improbable principle on which to generate a biological stimulus. It seems far more likely that the trigger energy is derived from some irreversible chemical change within the stimulus generator, namely a change in the chemical structure of the drug molecule, of the receptor, or of both.

IV. Models Involving Irreversible Alterations of Agonist or Receptor

First we will consider models in which the agonist drug is altered chemically as a result of its reaction with the receptor. That receptor activation may involve destruction of the agonist has been proposed on several occasions (BECKETT et al., 1956; WILLIAMS, 1962). The simplest possibility of this type can be diagrammed as follows:

$$D + R \xrightarrow{k_1} DR \xrightarrow{k_2} D' + R. \tag{2}$$

The receptor R behaves like an enzyme that metabolizes the drug agonist D to an inactive product D'. Obviously the system cannot achieve equilibrium as long as drug is present. If the amount of D, however, far exceeds that of R, as is probably the usual case, then the reaction consumes drug only slowly and the concentrations of D and DR may stay sensibly constant. Thus the system may achieve and maintain a quasi-steady state. In the above scheme both phases of the reaction are regarded as irreversible. Either phase might generate the trigger energy, i.e., the energy that is coupled to some subsequent metabolic reaction in which DR, R, D, and D' do not participate directly.

Of the two possibilities, the more interesting is the hypothesis that only the association reaction (k_1) generates the trigger energy, so that the stimulus intensity is equal to the rate of receptor occupation. Obviously this model is inspired by the Paton "rate" theory (1961). The fundamental difference is the assertion in the original rate theory that a steady pharmacologic response can be generated and maintained by an equilibrium interaction between agonist and receptor. Because no energy can be derived from a system operating at equilibrium, this assertion is equivalent to denying the need for trigger energy. Unless they share common reactants or products, however, it is impossible for any two chemical systems to be coupled in a kinetic sense without such energy transfer. Accordingly such systems cannot be coupled if either is operating at equilibrium.

The reaction sequence proposed above is in essence a restatement of the rate theory in which the thermodynamic difficulties of the latter are removed. As long as metabolism changes the drug concentration only very slowly, this model is the kinetic equivalent of the original rate theory, and all of the rate equations are identical. One merely substitutes "stationary state" for "equilibrium" and recognizes that k_2/k_1 is not a true dissociation constant and has no thermodynamic significance.

In exploring other models in which drug is consumed, the next order of complexity is represented by the assumption that the occupation reaction is reversible, i.e., possesses a property which in thermodynamics is called "microscopic reversibility":

$$D + R \underset{k_2}{\overset{k_1}{\rightleftharpoons}} DR \xrightarrow{k_3} D' + R. \tag{3}$$

Again no true equilibrium is possible in the presence of drug D, but a quasi-steady state is attainable if the reaction does not consume D too rapidly.

Either of the two forward steps of (3) might be the source of the trigger energy, but the more interesting model is that in which the k_3 reaction is responsible. Accordingly the stimulus intensity by definition is equal to the rate of production of the drug metabolite D'. Because this rate equals $k_3 \cdot [DR]$, the stimulus is also proportional to the concentration (or number) of occupied receptors. Therefore this hypothesis is properly classified as an "occupation" model. Indeed if k_3 is much smaller than k_1 and k_2, its kinetic properties are identical with those of the classic occupation model in both stationary and transient states. One merely substitutes k_3 for the intrinsic activity α, ($k_2 + k_3$) for k_2, and "stationary state" for "equilibrium". That α is at least analogous to the k_3 rate constant in enzymology has been appreciated for some time (ARIËNS et al., 1957).

Of course it is not difficult to devise more complex receptor cycles in which drug is consumed. No convincing evidence can be cited, however, to indicate that agonists are invariably destroyed in their interaction with specific receptors. For a given agonist one might seek for some hopefully unique drug metabolite in amounts that are larger the greater the response of the effector. In a series of related partial agonists tested separately, high concentrations should result in the production of D's with similar if not identical chemical structures in amounts proportional to their respective intrinsic activities. LÜLLMANN and ZIEGLER (1968: also personal communication) failed to find any labelled metabolites of C^{14}-arecaidine ethyl ester in extracts of contracting longitudinal muscle of the guinea pig ileum or of the isolated, beating guinea pig atrium. Similarly JENSEN and JACOBSEN (1962) and JENSEN et al. (1968) found no estrogen metabolites in extracts or homogenates of the isolated rat uterus under circumstances in which the hormone was demonstrably active. Very few careful studies of this type are available, however, and because the detection of a labelled metabolite in trace amounts in the presence of a large quantity of unmodified drug is a technically formidable task, negative evidence is far from conclusive.

Drug-metabolizing models of receptor activation seem far less appropriate for simple agonist molecules lacking reactive groups than for labile compounds like acetylcholine (WILLIAMS, 1962) or for complex substances such as the opium alkaloids (BECKETT et al., 1956). Of course there is no a priori reason to insist that covalent bonds which resist attack by liver microsomal enzymes are necessarily stable in the presence of specialized tissue receptor-enzymes. Nevertheless the existence of such well-defined receptor agonists as the tetramethylammonium ion makes it improbable that drug metabolism is a general mechanism of receptor activation.

The alternative possibility is that the receptor is the entity which is irreversibly altered by its encounter with any effective agonist. The simplest scheme of this type can be depicted as follows:

$$D + R \xrightarrow{k_1} DR \xrightarrow{k_2} R' + D \tag{4}$$

where R' represents an altered receptor which is no longer capable of reacting with drug or of generating a stimulus. With the stipulation that the second of the two reactions is the source of the trigger energy, this scheme has already been proposed and called the "dissociation theory" (PATON and RANG, 1966). Paton regards it as an alternative to his "rate" theory. Indeed, as we will see later, one reinterpretation of the original rate theory identifies it with the above reaction sequence in which the first of the two steps furnishes the trigger energy. In either case it is necessary to postulate some extraneous mechanism for repairing the biochemical lesion, i.e., for reactivating R' or synthesizing new receptor substance. The dissociation theory seems to have been presented only sketchily (PATON and RANG, 1966); no complete theoretical analysis has been offered. It represents, however, only a special case of a more general theory to be considered next.

V. A Receptor Inactivation Theory

The next order of complexity arises when one introduces in the above scheme the simple assumption that the first of the two reactions is reversible:

$$D + R \underset{k_2}{\overset{k_1}{\rightleftharpoons}} DR \xrightarrow{k_3} R'. \tag{5}$$

Again receptor exists in three different forms: free receptor (R), occupied receptor (DR), and inactivated receptor (R'), where the latter is generated from DR by an irreversible reaction. As a chemically modified receptor, R' may or may not incorporate all or part of the agonist molecule, but in any case it cannot react with further drug. The hypothesis says nothing about the fate of the agonist D. Whether it is consumed or conserved is immaterial insofar as the kinetic analysis is concerned, as long as there are many more drug molecules than receptor units.

Whereas either of the two reactions might be the source of the trigger energy, we shall make the important assumption that the k_3 step is responsible. Accordingly the stimulus intensity by definition is equal to the rate of receptor inactivation. Because this rate is always equal to $k_3 \cdot [DR]$, the stimulus is also proportional to the concentration (or number) of occupied receptors. Therefore the new hypothesis is in essence a further modification of the occupation theory. It possesses, however, most of the dynamic (transient state) characteristics of the Paton rate theory. It has been referred to as the "receptor inactivation theory" (GOSSELIN, 1968).

In order to explore the kinetic properties of this model, it is essential to recognize that there must exist some further reaction by which R is regenerated from R' or else synthesized de novo. Otherwise one must accept the implausible argument that the receptor reserve is adequate to last a lifetime. As a possible mechanism of repair, receptor synthesis accords with the observation that various inhibitors of protein synthesis prolong recovery from drug-induced local anesthesia (KNAPP and MEJIA, 1969). The experimental literature, however, offers essentially no clues upon which to base a hypothesis about the kinetics of the reparative process. Consequently we adopt the simplest assumption, namely that reactivation (or resynthesis) is first-order in terms of R':

$$R' \xrightarrow{k_4} R. \tag{6}$$

Perhaps the repair reaction occurs spontaneously and perhaps it requires metabolic energy. In the latter case it is conceivable that the agonist is conserved, whereas in the former case drug must be consumed somewhere in the cycle. For greatest generality we admit the possibility that every agonist generates an R' with a unique chemical structure as evidenced by its own characteristic rate of recovery expressed in terms of k_4.

For convenience the postulated reaction sequence is summarized in Figure 1, and the kinetic properties of the model are described below. For the present it is sufficient to note its behavior under certain limiting circumstances. For example, if $k_3 \ll k_4$, then R' is reconverted to R as fast as it is formed, so that no significant amounts of inactivated receptor can possibly accumulate. Indeed, if $k_2 \gg k_3 \ll k_4$, the receptor inactivation model becomes indistinguishable on kinetic grounds from the classic and modified occupation theories [viz. (3)].

At the other extreme the following possibility is of interest: $k_3 \gg k_1, k_2, k_4$. Under these circumstances no appreciable amounts of DR appear, and in effect receptor exists only in two forms, free R and R'. The conversion of the former to the latter is controlled by k_1, representing the slower of the two consecutive reactions. This degenerate model can be depicted as follows:

$$D + R \underset{k_4}{\overset{k_1}{\rightleftharpoons}} R'. \tag{7}$$

This representation, however, is formally equivalent to the rate theory, and aside from the choice of symbols, all equations describing its kinetic behavior in steady and transient states are identical with those proposed by PATON (1961). It is also equivalent to the modified rate theories depicted in (2) and (4). Thus, judged solely in terms of

RECEPTOR   INACTIVATION   THEORY

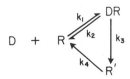

Fig. 1. Chemical reaction sequence postulated by receptor inactivation theory. Fate of drug D is unspecified. It may be conserved or destroyed. In whole or in part it may or may not be incorporated in R'

kinetics, both the classic occupation theory and the original "rate" theory represent special cases of the receptor inactivation model.

Before examining the properties of this inactivation hypothesis we should note that still more complex models of drug-receptor inactivation have been proposed. Based on the observation that acetylcholine and other cholinergic drugs are able to desensitize the motor end-plates so that they resist drug-induced depolarization, DEL CASTILLO and KATZ (1957) and KATZ and THESLEFF (1957) suggested that these drugs produce temporary inactivation of cholinergic receptors. Various kinetic models were entertained in which depolarization (receptor activation) and desensitization (receptor inactivation) were regarded as independent processes occurring either contemporaneously or sequentially. Whatever the merit of these schemes, we note that they differ importantly from the receptor inactivation theory described above in two major respects: they assume that receptor inactivation is incidental to and not an essential part of excitation, and they consider that excitation arises from the existence of DR, not from the rate of any reaction in the cycle. Thus these models are elaborations of the occupation theory.

The "dynamic receptor" hypothesis of BLOOM and GOLDMAN (1966), however, is a receptor inactivation model of the type proposed here. It too asserts that drug-induced excitation of the receptor mechanism leads inevitably to receptor inactivation. The kinetic behavior of their model in transient states has not been described, but in terms of mathematical formalism their scheme is equivalent to the receptor inactivation model, except that the latter postulates a simpler reactivation step, namely an irreversible monomolecular reaction [viz. (6)] in contrast to the reversible bimolecular reaction of BLOOM and GOLDMAN (1966).

VI. Stationary State Behavior with Single Agonists

Table 1 summarizes stationary state equations for the various models proposed here, as well as for the original rate theory (PATON, 1961). The classic occupation theory can be represented by an equation like that in Table 1 for the "modified" occupation theory, except that the intrinsic activity α replaces k_3 and k_2 replaces $(k_2 + k_3)$. All of these equations can be derived simply by applying conventional kinetic postulates to a receptor population that is assumed to be homogeneous before exposure to drug. For the dissociation theory the derivation requires an additional assumption not contained in the original description of this model (PATON and RANG, 1966), namely, that receptor reactivation is first order in terms of the concentration of R' [viz. (6)]. In every case the equation in Table 1 describes the dependency of the stimulus intensity (s) upon the stationary state value (x) of the agonist concentration in the biophase. According to these formulations, s represents the stimulus intensity per receptor. The total stimulus is the product of s and r, where r equals the number or concentration of receptors in the total population under consideration. The latter consists of all receptors that are identical and available to react with the agonist when it is first applied. In the stationary state this includes receptors that are free, occupied, and even inactivated (if the inactivation is not "permanent").

For generality we shall avoid any assumption about the relationship between stimulus intensity (s) and effector response intensity (E), except to suppose, in accord

Table 1. Stationary state equations for single agonists[a]

Reference to equation in text	Postulated source of trigger energy	Stationary state values of		Maximal stimulus/r (when $x\to\infty$)
		$s=$ Stimulus intensity (per receptor r)		
Renqvist theory — 1	k_1-k_2 reaction	0		0
Original rate theory — 1	k_1 reaction	$k_2\left[\dfrac{x}{x+k_2/k_1}\right]$		k_2
Modified rate theory — 2	k_1 reaction	$k_2\cdot\left[\dfrac{x}{x+k_2/k_1}\right]$		k_2
Modified occup. theory — 3	k_3 reaction	$k_3\cdot\left[\dfrac{x}{x+(k_2+k_3)/k_1}\right]$		k_3
Modified dissoc. theory — 4 and 6	k_2 reaction	$\dfrac{k_2k_3}{k_2+k_3}\cdot\left[\dfrac{x}{x+k_2k_3/(k_1(k_2+k_3))}\right]$		$\dfrac{k_2k_3}{k_2+k_3}$
Receptor inactiv. theory — 5 and 6	k_3 reaction	$\dfrac{k_3k_4}{k_3+k_4}\cdot\left[\dfrac{x}{x+k_4(k_2+k_4)/(k_1(k_3+k_4))}\right]$		$\dfrac{k_3k_4}{k_3+k_4}$

[a] $x=$ concentration of agonist in biophase (= receptor compartment).

with the postulates of STEPHENSON (1956), that E is some invariant, real, single-valued, monotonically increasing function of s. Whatever the character of this function in any particular biological preparation, it is obvious that no experimental protocol can hope to distinguish among the models of Table 1 if only stationary state responses are measured. Even if s could be measured independently of E, stationary state data would not lead to any definitive conclusion because in every one of these models s is a hyperbolic function of the dose x. As noted above, the same assumption is implicit in the classical occupation theory and its several modern variants. Thus, experimental values of E measured in stationary states offer no basis for preferring any one of these models over any other one.

The formulas in Table 1 are nevertheless of interest. One notes that, in contrast to almost all other receptor theories, the receptor inactivation model denies the possibility of complete receptor occupancy in stationary states. Thus as the agonist concentration x is raised, the fraction of the receptor population in the form of DR approaches $k_4/(k_3 + k_4)$ as a maximal value. Therefore the largest possible stationary-state stimulus per receptor is $k_3 \cdot k_4/(k_3 + k_4)$. This quantity is entirely analogous to Furchgott's "intrinsic efficacy" (ε). Admittedly it has dimensions of reciprocal time whereas Furchgott's ε (1966) has units of r^{-1} (where r is again the total number of receptors). The latter, however, is an arbitrary convention adopted to yield a dimensionless number for the maximal stimulus ($\varepsilon \cdot r$). The difference in dimensions should not obscure the essential identity of the two concepts. Obviously the classical occupation theory, for which ε was designed, provides no physical basis for efficacy whereas the present model does. Because there is little excuse for introducing a new name or a new symbol, ε will be retained here, but it will now be regarded as having the dimensions $t^{-1} \cdot r^{-1}$.

The interest in ε arises because it provides a useful way to classify drugs. The distinctions can be appreciated by ranking, according to the numerical value of ε, all drugs that are able to compete for the same receptor sites. Based on such a ranking, Table 2 describes various drug types that can be envisaged in terms of the receptor inactivation model. For the full classification it is apparent that k_3 and k_4 must be specified as well as the composite quantity ε. It is also apparent that the boundaries between these drug classes cannot be defined rigorously because a continuous spectrum of reaction patterns is allowed. For the most part the descriptions and relationships outlined in Table 2 can be readily inferred from an examination of the postulated reaction sequence (Fig. 1). A detailed analysis will be offered later (viz. Section VII and Appendices 2–5).

As illustrated in Table 2, the receptor inactivation model encompasses a large variety of drug response patterns. For example, evidence suggests that curare and related antidepolarizers are reversible antagonists of type g (TAYLOR and NEDERGAARD, 1965). The more complex action of the depolarizing agents can be equated to type d. According to this interpretation, such drugs induce transient excitation and sustained depolarization because they generate a weak but prolonged stimulus associated with the slow conversion of R to R'. These events constitute what has been called the phase I block (TAYLOR and NEDERGAARD, 1965). If k_4 is much smaller than k_3, however, R' gradually accumulates at the expense of free R. When the concentration of R is so low that R' can no longer be generated rapidly, the stimulus becomes weak and the preparation repolarizes. Although now fully or nearly fully polarized, the motor endplate is still relatively insensitive to acetylcholine and related

Table 2. A classification of drugs according to the receptor inactivation model

Drug Type	$\varepsilon = \dfrac{k_3 \cdot k_4}{k_3 + k_4}$	k_3	k_4
a) Full agonist	$\varepsilon \geqq s^*$	Large	Very large
b) Partial agonist	$0 \ll \varepsilon < s^*$	Large	Large
c) Agonist producing tachyphylaxis	$0 < \varepsilon < s^*$	Large	Intermediate
d) Antagonist with transient excitatory effect and long persistency	$0 < \varepsilon \ll s^*$	Intermediate	Small
e) "Irreversible" antagonist, subtype I	$\varepsilon = 0$	Small	Zero
f) "Irreversible" antagonist, subtype II	$\varepsilon = 0$	Zero	$k_2 = 0$
g) Reversible antagonist without transient excitatory effect	$\varepsilon = 0$	Zero	$k_2 > 0$

s^* is the stimulus intensity (per r) just sufficient to elicit a maximal response of the effector.

agonists because most of the cholinergic receptors are in the inactivated form R'. According to the inactivation model, however, a few receptor inevitably remain active even in the stationary state. Therefore the block is potentially surmountable, if anticholinesterases or other measures are used to increase the concentration of acetylcholine in the vicinity of the postjunctional receptors.

With respect to irreversible antagonists, there is no difficulty in equating Dibenamine and related alkylhaloamines to category e of Table 2 (NICKERSON, 1957, 1959). According to the inactivation model, the inherent slowness of the alkylation reaction is the only reason why these drugs induce no detectable phase of transient excitation before completion of the blockade. In contrast, antagonists of type f do not inactivate the receptor but merely occupy it to the exclusion of agonist. They differ from reversible, competitive antagonists of type g only in terms of k_2, which must be closer to zero the higher the degree of irreversibility.

The quantity s^* in Table 2 varies in theory from one tissue to another and depends in part upon the total number of available receptors (r). Specifically s^* is defined so that $s^* \cdot r$ represents a stimulus just sufficient to elicit a maximal response of the effector. For any agonist whose ε is greater than s^*, the product $\varepsilon \cdot r$ may exceed this stimulus even if r is reduced, as by the application of an irreversible antagonist. For such an agonist, spare receptors exist; $(\varepsilon - s^*)/\varepsilon$ represents the fraction of the total receptor population that is "spare". Thus the receptor inactivation model is fully consonant with modern concepts about receptor reserve (NICKERSON, 1956; ARIËNS, 1964).

VII. Transient State Behavior with Single Agonists

Because it is the most general model of those listed in Table 1, we shall restrict this analysis to the receptor inactivation theory. As outlined in Figure 1, this theory contains no assumptions that are unrealistic in chemical terms. Indeed, like many other receptor theories, it is patterned after a well-established reaction sequence in enzymology. For example, tetraethylpyrophosphate and many other alkyl phosphate esters are able to phosphorylate the active site of various cholinesterases (O'BRIEN, 1960). Because the phosphorus-to-oxygen covalent bonds formed in this reaction are

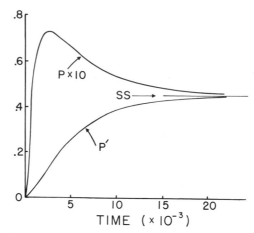

Fig. 2. "On" effect according to receptor inactivation model (see text for explanation). Curves are based on following assigned values: $x = 10^{-3}$; $k_1 = 10^{-1}$; $k_2 = 10^{-4}$; $k_3 = 10^{-3}$; $k_4 = 10^{-4}$. Units of concentration x and of time are arbitrary but same as those implicit in rate constants Symbols p and p' refer to fractional concentrations of DR and R' respectively.

relatively stable, the associated enzyme inhibition is described as "irreversible". These bonds, however, are gradually hydrolyzed by water with consequent reactivation of the enzyme. Experiments by MAIN (1964) established what was long suspected, namely that a reversible combination of enzyme and inhibitor precedes the phosphorylation reaction. Various carbamates and sulfonates are able to engage cholinesterase and some other enzymes in a comparable series of reactions (WILSON, 1967). Indeed the reaction pattern of Figure 1 is a common one.

In all, or essentially all, examples studied by enzymologists, the hydrolysis reaction is so much slower than the other steps in the sequence that it can be ignored or at least isolated. Even a recent theoretical analysis (FILMER et al., 1967) was limited to circumstances in which k_4 (viz. Fig. 1) was much smaller than any of the other three rate constants of the cycle. To appreciate fully the kinetic implications of this reaction scheme, however, no restrictions should be placed on the values of any of the rate constants.

A comprehensive mathematical treatment of this model is contained in Appendices 2–5. We shall examine here graphical representations of the more interesting findings, based on arbitrary values assigned to the four rate constants and to the concentration (x) of uncombined drug. Assume that an agonist (D) is added at zero time to a fully recovered preparation and its concentration x is held constant thereafter. According to the curves of Figure 2, which are based on equations in Appendix 3, the concentration of DR expressed as fractional receptor occupancy ($= p$) rises abruptly and then falls toward a stationary state value, which it approaches asymptotically. In contrast to DR, the concentration of R' ($= p'$) rises monotonically to its stationary-state value. In this stationary state the ratio p/p' is always equal to k_4/k_3.

The receptor inactivation theory asserts that the stimulus intensity (s) is proportional to the rate of formation of R', which in turn is proportional to the concentration of DR ($= p$). Thus the hypothetical stimulus-time curve parallels that for p (viz. Fig. 2). If the effector response E is an increasing function of s, then the effect-

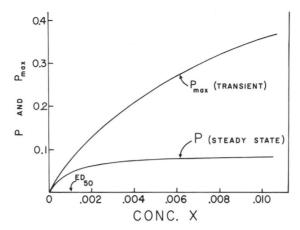

Fig. 3. Hypothetical values of p at transient maximum and in steady (=stationary) state, at various fixed concentrations (x) of agonist. Rate constants have same numerical values as in Figure 2. As used here, "ED_{50}" means that value of x at which stimulus intensity (s) in stationary state is half the sustained maximum generated when x is very large. This x is equal to conventional ED_{50} only if effect E is proportional to s

time curve must also contain a transient maximum, corresponding to that in Figure 2. Such an overshoot has been observed occasionally in the activity of biological effectors, particularly in the responses of guinea pig ileum to some agonists (PATON, 1961). The subsequent decline in the isotonic contraction has been named "fade", and the extent of fade has been defined as the difference between the contraction heights at the transient maximum and stationary state. The receptor inactivation theory provides an explanation of overshoot and fade which differs from that proposed in the original rate theory (PATON, 1961).

Figure 3 further illustrates the receptor inactivation model by depicting p values at the transient maximum and at the stationary state, both as functions of x. In accord with the bottom equation in Table 1, the stationary state curve is a hyperbola. Whereas the p_{max} curve is not hyperbolic, it too rises with x to approach a limiting value of 1 as x approaches infinity. Consequently the stimulus associated with this transient maximum also approaches a limit ($=k_3$). The original rate theory (PATON, 1961) denies any such limit; it specifies that the peak stimulus is proportional to x under all circumstances. In this respect experimental data (e.g., Fig. 15 in Paton's 1961 paper) are in better accord with the inactivation theory than with the rate theory, but the difference is not a crucial one because E cannot be a reliable expression of s once the response capacity of the effector is attained and perhaps not even as it is approached. Both theories agree that the extent of fade is greater the higher the dose, as illustrated in Figure 3.

Based on the inactivation model, Figure 4 depicts two properties of the transient maximum as functions of x, where x is plotted here on a logarithmic scale. The curve labeled "p_{max}" is equivalent to that in Figure 3. The curve labeled "t" represents the time interval between addition of the agonist (at $t=0$) and attainment of the transient maximum in p. At all dose ranges this latency is shorter the higher the value of x. According to the tenets of the receptor inactivation hypothesis, there is a correspond-

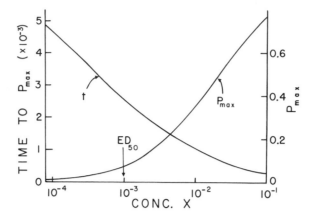

Fig. 4. Properties of transient maximum in $p(=p_{max})$, at various fixed concentrations (x) of agonist. Rate constants have same values as in Figure 2 (see legend of Fig. 3 regarding ED_{50})

ing latency in the peak value of the stimulus, whereas the original rate theory asserts that s is maximal at the moment when exposure to the agonist begins. Similarly the rate theory requires that during washout the stimulus ends abruptly when x reaches zero, but in the inactivation model the stimulus persists until p is reduced to zero by the k_2 and k_3 reactions.

Figure 5 illustrates properties of the drug-receptor stationary state according to the receptor inactivation theory. The curve labeled "t" is a measure of the time required for attainment of the stationary state at fixed concentrations of agonist $(=x)$. Specifically, "t" is a calculated parameter representing elapsed time from the moment when agonist

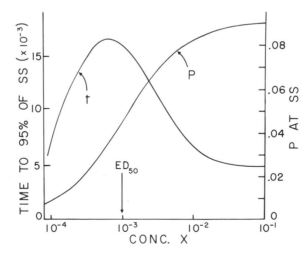

Fig. 5. Properties of stationary state $(=SS)$ at various fixed concentrations (x) of agonist. Curve labeled "t" is a measure of time required for attainment of stationary state, as described in text. Rate constants have same values as in Figure 2 (see legend of Fig. 3 regarding ED_{50})

is introduced to the moment when p and the stationary state value of p differ by exactly 5% for the last time during the "on" response. Figure 5 reveals an unexpected maximum in this parameter. Thus the reaction is inherently faster at low and high doses than at intermediate values of x. The same phenomenon is apparent whatever arbitrary measure one uses to describe the velocity with which the system approaches stationarity after addition of agonist. Of course the postulated stimulus and response curves show a similar temporal dependency on the dose.

Although not described heretofore, implicit in the original rate theory is the same prediction that the stationary state stimulus is reached sooner at high and low doses than at intermediate ones. Conventional occupation theories, however, require that receptor occupation and stimulus generation occur faster the higher the dose in all dose ranges (MACKAY, 1977). Conceivably this distinction might be exploited as a way of testing theory against experiment, but, as noted in Section IX one would first require a biological preparation in which the speed of effector response is limited only by receptor events.

The original rate theory stipulates that the stimulus intensity s is maximal when agonist first comes into contact with receptors. Provided that the agonist concentration does not rise thereafter, s must decline progressively until the stationary state is attained. A parallel decline in E is expected. Fade, however, is not encountered invariably in effector response curves. Indeed, some investigators regard it as exceptional in unloaded isotonic contraction curves (ARIENS, 1964). Various factors have been cited (PATON and WAUD, 1964) to account for this frequent nonconformity between theory and experiment. For example, under some circumstances it is likely that E is a poor reflection of s and may lag behind it. On other occasions x and therefore s may rise slowly rather than abruptly when agonist is introduced, because of permeability barriers that limit the rate at which the receptor compartment can equilibrate with a fixed drug concentration in the organ bath. These factors can indeed mask the kind of overshoot and fade required by the rate theory (PATON and WAUD, 1964). They are also capable of suppressing the overshoot and fade postulated by the receptor inactivation model.

Implicit in the inactivation theory, however, is still another factor that might account for the absence of fade in some cases. In Figure 2–5, values of x and of the rate constants were selected to insure $W > 0$, where by definition $W = (k_1 x + k_2 + k_3 - k_4)^2 - 4k_3 k_1 x$. Under these circumstances p always exhibits a transient maximum, according to the receptor inactivation model (viz. Appendix 3). Whenever W differs only slightly from zero, however, the overshoot is slight, and when $W = 0$, p rises steadily and without overshoot to reach its stationary state value (Appendix 3). Accordingly no overshoot in s or E is then encountered.

Unlike any receptor hypothesis proposed heretofore, the inactivation model is capable of oscillatory behavior in the presence of a fixed concentration of agonist. Thus p and p' may be induced to oscillate by adding drug to a fully recovered preparation. A prerequisite is $k_4 > k_2$. If $k_4 > k_2$, a dose x can always be found such that $W < 0$, which is the necessary and sufficient condition for these oscillations (Appendix 3). For each cyclic fluctuation in p, the theory requires an associated fluctuation in s and in E. Because the oscillations in p are highly damped, one cannot be certain that the corresponding damped oscillations in E are detectable. The question of detectability is analyzed in Appendix 5.

However low the noise level of modern electronic apparatus used to monitor biological signals, the latter invariably contain random noise generated in the biological mechanism itself. On the other hand, receptor events must have somewhat lower noise levels than the effector responses which they control. Thus, oscillations in p should be easier to detect than those in E, even if methods were available for recording both parameters with equal fidelity. It is unlikely that any biological signal of interest to pharmacologists has a signal-to-noise ratio as high as 100. According to the analysis in Appendix 5, a considerably smaller ratio should suffice to reveal the first peak in the oscillatory p curve, but even under optimal conditions the subsequent trough would be hidden by noise unless the signal-to-noise ratio were higher than 700. Therefore it is exceedingly unlikely that an experimentalist could detect even the first trough in the oscillatory response.

Without this evidence, however, it is impossible to distinguish between the oscillatory ($W < 0$) and the nonoscillatory ($W > 0$) case. In both instances the recorded signal rises sharply to a transient maximum, which can be easily recognized even in the presence of considerable noise, and then falls off to a stationary state value. Nothing about the curves is distinctive except for the tails, and the distinctions here cannot be appreciated without a degree of resolution that in practice is unattainable. The problem is illustrated by Figure 6, where numerical values of the rate constants were selected to insure damped oscillations in response to any agonist concentration within the zone marked by the double-headed arrow. Obviously these oscillations would not be even suspected from the parameters plotted here or from any other realistic measure of the speed with which the system attains the stationary state. Similarly, the height and latency of the first peak (i.e., the transient maximum) display no discontinuities or other peculiarities at the boundaries between oscillatory and nonoscillatory zones.

This analysis demonstrates that the oscillatory behavior of the receptor in-activation model is not a useful characteristic for distinguishing between it and

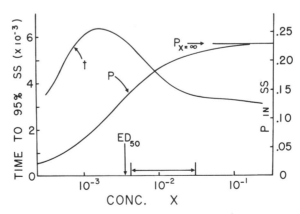

Fig. 6. Properties of stationary state ($=$ SS) at various fixed concentrations (x) of agonist, based on following assigned values: $k_1 = 10^{-1}$; $k_2 = 10^{-4}$; $k_3 = 10^{-3}$; $k_4 = 3 \times 10^{-4}$. *Horizontal double-headed arrow* near abscissa designates zone of x in which damped oscillations of p precede attainment of stationary state. Curve labeled "t" represents elapsed time calculated from moment when p and stationary state p differ by exactly 5 % for last time during "on" response (see legend of Fig. 3 regarding ED_{50})

nonoscillatory models. Because intense damping is inherent in the reaction sequence, it is useless to seek any overt expression of this temporal periodicity except in systems with much higher signal-to-noise ratios than are found in the usual biological effectors.

VIII. Stationary State Behavior with Agonist-Antagonist Mixtures

The measurement of pA_x (SCHILD, 1947, 1957; ROCHA E SILVA, 1959) and dose-ratio analysis (GADDUM et al., 1955) represent the most widely used ways to characterize interactions between agonists and antagonists acting upon the same receptor population. They have been called "null methods" (SCHILD, 1957) because they involve effects of equal intensity in the presence and absence of the antagonist. In operational terms the experimentalist often chooses to determine the concentrations (or doses) of an agonist required to elicit any selected level of effect when tested in the absence and again in the presence of a specified concentration of an antagonist (GADDUM et al., 1955). The two agonist concentrations are usually compared in terms of their ratio (= "dose ratio"). Depending upon the mode of action of the antagonist, this ratio may or may not be a function of the antagonist concentration and of the selected level of effect.

Various interpretations of dose-ratio data are possible, the choice depending upon which theoretic model of drug-receptor action one assumes to be valid. Equations that relate dose-ratio values to hypothetical kinetic constants of receptor-antagonist interaction have been derived in terms of the conventional occupation model (SCHILD, 1947; GADDUM et al., 1955) the rate theory (PATON, 1961), two enzyme activation hypotheses (MACKAY, 1977), and the flux carrier model (MACKAY, 1963). For most of these hypotheses the null equation is independent of the level of response selected, provided that the antagonist is a competitive one. Whereas noncompetitive antagonism has not been neglected (ARIENS, 1964), these theoretic treatments have emphasized competitive antagonism. Almost invariably they have also been restricted to the assumption that receptor, agonist, and antagonist are in equilibrium or in some related stationary state at the time when the pharmacologic response was measured. It is of interest now to extend this type of analysis to the receptor inactivation model.

The mathematic argument is presented in Appendix 6, where Equations (32) and (33) describe competitive antagonism in stationary states. Accordingly, the receptor inactivation theory requires that for any selected intensity of effector response (E) the ratio $y/(\Phi - 1)$ is a constant whose value is independent of the antagonist concentration y and of the agonist dose ratio Φ. This requirement is seen to apply to all stationary states, whether inactivated receptors are generated by agonist, antagonist, neither, or both.

The constancy of this ratio has of course been demonstrated in the laboratory on numerous occasions with various biological preparations (GADDUM et al., 1955; PATON, 1961; ARIËNS, 1964). Such demonstrations, however, are also fully consistent with predictions based on the conventional occupation theory (GADDUM et al., 1955), on variants of the occupation theory such as allosteric models (KARLIN, 1967) and on the rate theory (PATON, 1961), although in the latter instance the theoretic equation is a limiting one restricted to agonist concentrations that are small relative to the agonist-receptor dissociation constant. The constancy of $y/(\Phi - 1)$ is also consonant with steady-state responses predicted by various enzyme activation hypotheses such as the dynamic receptor model (MACKAY, 1977) and with transient peak responses according to the flux carrier model (MACKAY, 1977). Thus it is impossible to distinguish among these theories merely by demonstrating that $y/(\Phi - 1)$ has a fixed value. They differ only in the meaning which they ascribe to this complex constant. Unlike conventional occupation models, the receptor inactivation theory denies that $y/(\Phi - 1)$ is necessarily equal to the antagonist-receptor dissociation constant (K_B).

IX. Transient State Behavior with Agonist-Antagonist Mixtures

Because stationary state responses do not distinguish among available receptor hypotheses, it is necessary to examine transient state behavior. Generalized rate equations for most receptor models, however, tend to be intractable when more than one drug species competes for the same receptor population. For example, the receptor inactivation model requires a pair of differential equations corresponding to (8) and (9) in Appendix 2, for each drug present, whether agonist or competitive antagonist. Given two or more pairs of such simultaneous equations, no explicit solutions are known, except for the stationary state solution described above (see also Appendix 6). It is even difficult to find solutions for a single drug if the preparation starts in any state other than one of full recovery (Appendix 3) or of stationarity (Appendix 4). Admittedly, under some restricted conditions, transient state solutions are possible. With respect to a competitive antagonist B, for example, if $k_{4B} \ll (k_{2B} + k_{3B})$, Equation (22) reduces to a single exponential. If k_{4B} is also much smaller than any of the rate constants for an agonist A, then it is possible to derive an expression for the dose of A required to elicit a standard response as a function of time during recovery from a prior exposure to B.

Of course the mathematical difficulties can be circumvented by numerical integration with the aid of a digital computer. Thus the kinetic scheme of Figure 1 has been programmed for drug pairs by using the convenient and versatile "nets" technique of STIBITZ (1968). With no restrictions on the values of the various rate constants, computer simulation has been employed to study the behavior of the system while the concentrations of A and B were varied at will. The goal of this simulation was to find some dynamic characteristic of the model that might be recognizable in terms of the effector response, whatever the stimulus-effect transform. None of the behavior observed to data, however, was sufficiently bizarre to imply a property that might be exploited as a diagnostic clue. Without such a qualitative characteristic, one is forced to examine more subtle, quantitative distinctions among receptor models (see also Addendum A).

PATON (1961) reported various experiments on guinea pig ileum from the results of which he calculated numerical values for the two rate constants of his model. To accomplish this commendable goal, however, assumptions were required beyond those inherent in the model itself. For example, each procedure required one or both of the following complex conditions to be true: (a) simple proportionality between the stimulus intensity and the response intensity with no temporal lag; (b) identical concentrations (or chemical activities) of the drug in the organ bath and in the receptor compartment at all times (i.e., during transient as well as stationary states). The stimulus concept was not mentioned explicitly by PATON (1961), but the use of an arbitrary system (auxotonic lever) for recording contractile responses in order to insure a hyperbolic dose-response curve is equivalent to having postulated a specific function for the stimulus-effect transform. Alternative ways were suggested for calculating each hypothetical constant from data based on independent experimental observations. The observed agreement, however, does not thoroughly validate the model because an equally good fit exists for at least one other model, namely the receptor inactivation theory described here.

If one is prepared to accept assumptions (a) and (b) listed above, it is possible to devise experiments to secure data from which numerical values could in principle be calculated for most, if not all, the rate constants postulated by other receptor models. In this respect the rate theory provides no unique opportunity, but with more complicated models there are far fewer independent ways to check the validity of the resulting estimates. The reluctance of most pharmacologists to engage in this exercise today appears to stem from a recognition that the two requirements listed above are inherently improbable in the biological systems usually studied.

According to methods recently described (FURCHGOTT, 1966; MACKAY, 1966; VAN ROSSUM, 1966), experimental data can be used to evaluate the ratio of the two rate constants postulated by the occupation theory, i.e., the agonist-receptor dissociation constant. To employ these procedures no information is required about the relationship between stimulus and effect if one is prepared to assume that the external bathing solution, receptor compartment, and receptors are in equilibrium with respect to the agonist at the time when the effect E is measured. Thus requirement (a) but not (b) can be circumvented if a ratio determination is adequate. To ascribe a value to any single rate constant, however, one apparently cannot avoid requirements (a) and (b) or their equivalent.

One acceptable equivalent to (a) is any established relationship between stimulus and effect or between fractional receptor occupancy (p) and effect (E). According to all occupation theories this relationship, which may assume different forms in different biological preparations, can be inferred if the preparation possesses a high receptor reserve. Thus, if a maximal effect utilizes only a small proportion of the receptor population, the $s - E$ transform is essentially identical to the $x - E$ transform, i.e., to the measured dose-response relationship. This property of the classic occupation theory was first recognized by STEPHENSON (1956); it is also characteristic of the receptor inactivation model.

To exploit this property, however, one must still contend with requirement (b). In most biological preparations the drug concentration in the receptor compartment (biophase) cannot be controlled or measured. It cannot even be inferred with any degree of confidence, except perhaps in stationary states when it is commonly assumed to equal the concentration in the external bathing solution. Whether this external solution is the circulating blood or artificial extracellular fluid in an organ bath, it is generally separated from the receptors by various permeability barriers whose dynamic characteristics are unknown. As a result, the agonist concentration in the external compartment is an unreliable measure of that in the internal compartment if either concentration is changing rapidly. The speed of action of atropine and probably of many other drugs appears to be limited in several tissues by the rate at which drug molecules can gain access to their specific receptors (THRON and WAUD, 1968; NICKERSON, 1959).

Barriers to drug transport into the receptor compartment may be insignificant in some biological systems, such as isolated cells in suspension, but such opportunities appear to be rare and not yet adequately exploited in pharmacodynamic studies. In recent trials (GOSSELIN, unpublished) smooth muscle was deaggregated by enzyme treatments to yield healthy looking cells, but they proved to be unresponsive to agonists. A suspension of reactive cells with receptors that are readily accessible because of their location on the external cells surface would be an ideal object of study if it could be established that receptor events and not those inherent in the effector mechanism were responsible for observable time-response curves.

With no certain knowledge about agonist concentrations in the receptor compartment or about the identity of the rate-controlling events, it is doubtful that transient state values of E, however carefully measured, can be used justifiably to calculate rate constants or to distinguish in any other way among alternative receptor models. Even qualitative indices of dynamic receptor activity can be severely distorted by the presence of permeability barriers. As demonstrated by computer simulation (PATON and WAUD, 1964), such transient state phenomena as the overshoot and fade required by the original rate theory disappear if barriers reduce sufficiently the rate of access of agonist to the receptor compartment. The kinds of overshoot and fade predicted by the receptor inactivation theory can also be masked in the same way.

X. General Discussion

None of the receptor models proposed here can be defended as a mechanism by which all or even most drugs act. In such cases as the β-adrenergic actions of catecholamines on glycogenolysis and lipolysis (BUTCHER, 1968), it is likely that the "receptor" is part of a complex with the enzyme adenyl cyclase and that the drug functions as an allosteric effector. Metabolites and antimetabolites are involved in analogous enzymatic mechanisms. For such drugs the occupation theory provides an appropriate basis for kinetic descriptions of the receptor events. There is much less evidence, however, to support the contention that specific agonists also serve as allosteric effectors on membrane-bound receptors, specifically receptors which control the activity of many kinds of muscles and glands. Although membrane phenomena can be interpreted in terms of allosteric models (CHANGEUX et al., 1967), entirely different mechanisms may be operative at these sites. Some of the possibilities have been outlined in Section III above. Among the possibilities is the receptor inactivation theory of Section IV.

Unlike all occupation models, the receptor inactivation theory (viz. Fig. 1) postulates that agonists (and perhaps even some competitive antagonists) alter the structure of the receptor in such a way that it becomes temporarily inactive. Evidence in support of this supposition has appeared recently. Thus, with isolated chick skeletal muscle and leech body wall muscle, RANG and RITTER (1969) found that some competitive antagonists were more effective blockers when applied at the same time or shortly after an exposure to the specific agonists carbachol and suxamethonium. The phenomenon, which was named the "metaphilic effect", appeared to result from an increase in the affinity of the receptors for the antagonist. Thus the effect is the result of an agonist-induced alteration of the receptor structure, an alteration that persists for at least 15 min after washing out a large dose of agonist (see also Addendum B).

Whether right or wrong, the receptor inactivation theory is a more comprehensive hypothesis than any of the other models listed in Table 1. It is also more comprehensive than any conventional occupation theory. Thus several of the reaction patterns included in Table 2 cannot be accounted for by any occupation theory, although real drugs have been observed on many occasions to match these patterns, at least in a superficial way. The phenomenon of tachyphylaxis, for example, finds no explanation in most receptor models, but the inactivation hypothesis provides a promising basis on which to analyze experimental data on specific desensitization (GOSSELIN, unpublished). Indeed the receptor inactivation model appears to encompass all recognized patterns of drug action for which it is reasonable to presume an explanation at the receptor level.

Of course Table 2 includes only drugs that compete for a common site where a uniform kind of stimulus is generated, a target that is often called the "specific" or "active" receptor because its activation leads to a specific observable effect (VAN DEN BRINK, 1969). Other drugs are believed to react only at loci adjacent to the specific receptor; these loci are sometimes called "allosteric" receptors. Like the interaction between allosteric and active sites in enzymology, occupation of the allosteric receptor is believed to alter the properties of the specific receptor. Apparently in this way some compounds are able to modify responses to an agonist without competing with the agonist for a common target. The best established examples are usually called non-competitive antagonists (ARIËNS, 1964), but a wide range of reaction patterns is permitted by this dual receptor mechanism. For such modifier drugs the receptor inactivation model provides no new insights. Although it is conceivable that the allosteric receptor is subject to inactivation like that postulated here for the specific receptor, such an assumption is unwarranted at the present time. Current views about the relationship between specific and allosteric receptors are not inconsistent with the postulates of the receptor inactivation model.

As noted in Section V, on the basis of kinetic criteria the classical occupation theory (ARIËNS, 1964) and the original rate theory (PATON, 1961) are both encompassed by the receptor inactivation model. Thus, whenever the k_3 of Figure 1 is much smaller than the other three rate constants, the new hypothesis is fully equivalent to the occupation theory. When k_3 is much larger than the other constants, it is equivalent to the rate theory. Any conventional pharmacologic data offered in support of either rival theory can inevitably be accounted for by the inactivation model. Any attempt to establish a fit between theory and experiment cannot be less successful with the inactivation theory than with the others. Indeed, with an extra rate constant in the inactivation model, it should be possible to secure an even closer fit. Such a demonstration, however, is not apt to be persuasive unless applied to a body of experimental results that cannot be satisfactorily accounted for by one or both of the simpler theories.

Instead of searching blindly for such a body of information, we have chosen to investigate extensively the kinetic properties of one model itself, in the hope of identifying some characteristic that might be usefully tested against biological data. In this respect dose-response relationships in stationary states are not helpful. The results are inevitably inconclusive, whether agonist is tested alone (Section VI) or together with a competitive antagonist (Section VIII). The transient state behavior of the model is far more distinctive, but one of the more promising features of its dynamic activity, namely drug-induced oscillations, can be dismissed, because the general noise level of biological effectors would almost certainly hide such oscillations (Appendix 5).

Of course experiments could be designed by which dynamic response curves would serve to distinguish conclusively between various pairs of receptor models considered here. Such experiments, however, would require a preparation with attributes not demonstrably true of any known biological receptor-effector system. As minimal requirements the receptor compartment would have to be immediately accessible to drug, and the speed of the effector response would have to be limited only by the speed of receptor events. In the absence of such a preparation there appears to be no possibility of proving or disproving conclusively any of several receptor hypotheses, until a practical and unambiguous way is discovered to measure s or fractional receptor occupancy p without relying on E as an indirect expression of these parameters.

Perhaps some kinds of transient state behavior are so inherently slow that conventional methods may be adequate to investigate them. One such example is the possibility that tachyphylaxis is due to receptor inactivation and recovery to receptor regeneration. The question is now under investigation. Until this issue is clarified, the receptor inactivation hypothesis is presented merely as an alternative to existing theories in providing another way to interpret a large body of experimental data on receptor mechanisms. Furthermore it serves as a unifying hypothesis that encompasses several rival models long regarded as irreconcilable.

XI. Summary

A family of simple drug-receptor models has been formulated on the principle that one step in each postulated reaction sequence generates energy that is coupled in a unique way to the effector and so serves to trigger the pharmacologic effect. The number of quanta of such energy produced per unit time is assumed to be a measure of the stimulus intensity. The original rate theory of PATON (1961) is one member of this family, but it has been reformulated here to remove a thermodynamic objection to the original description.

Of the models considered here, the most general member of this family, named the "receptor inactivation theory", can be depicted as follows:

$$D + R \underset{k_2}{\overset{k_1}{\rightleftharpoons}} DR \xrightarrow{k_3} R' \xrightarrow{k_4} R.$$

In this scheme DR represents the combination of a receptor (R) with a drug (D). The complex (DR) is converted irreversibly to inactive receptor (R'). R' cannot react with D but can be reactivated to generate R. Stimulus for the effector at any moment is assumed to be proportional to the rate of formation of R' $(=k_3[DR])$. Thus, according to kinetic criteria, the model is a modified occupation theory and becomes identical to the classic occupation model whenever $k_2 \gg k_3 \ll k_4$. In contrast, when k_3 is much larger than the other three rate constants, the model becomes formally equivalent to the Paton rate theory. Therefore the occupation and rate theories represent special cases of the present proposal.

In general, this model possesses most of the dynamic (transient state) characteristics of the original rate theory. For example, overshoot and fade are often encountered, but highly damped oscillations are also predicted to occur under some circumstances. In the steady state the intrinsic efficacy (ε) can be represented by $k_3 \cdot k_4/(k_3 + k_4)$. If every drug tends to generate a unique R' with characteristic values of k_3 and k_4, then there must exist two classes of competitive antagonists, one typified by small k_3's and the other by small k_4's. General properties of the new model are examined for agonists, antagonists, and combinations thereof.

Addendum A

Since completion of this manuscript, the "receptor inactivation model" and several more complex models patterned after it have been subjected to extensive computer simulation. Specifically agonist dose-ratios (Φ) have been evaluated at various concentrations of a competitive inhibitor, based on responses at the transient maximum instead of the stationary state. Surprisingly, the ratio $y/(\Phi - 1)$ evaluated from these data are essentially independent of the antagonist concentration (y) for all sets of rate constants selected. Thus, in terms of Schild plots [ARUNLAKSHANA,O., SCHILD,H.O.: Brit. J. Pharmacol. **14**, 48–58 (1959)], linearity does not even require an equilibrium interaction between receptors, agonists, and antagonists. The results of these simulation studies will be reported in more detail elsewhere.

Addendum B

Since completion of the present manuscript, RANG and RITTER have demonstrated experimentally that the apparent alteration in receptor structure induced temporarily by various nicotinic agonists, known as the "metaphilic effect", is indeed associated with specific desensitization of these receptors. At least the ability of agonists to elicit the metaphilic effect parallels their ability to generate specific desensitization in chick, leech and frog muscle [RANG,H.P., RITTER,J,M.: Mol. Pharmacol. **6**, 383–390 (1970)]. Rates of desensitization and recovery, presumably reflecting rates of receptor inactivation and reactivation respectively, have been measured in both chick and frog muscle [RANG,H.P., RITTER,J.M.: Mol. Pharmacol. **6**, 357–382 (1970)].

Whether or not receptor inactivation leading to desensitization is a general phenomenon is not yet known. Except with polypeptide agonists, most attempts to inactivate visceral smooth muscle have led to nonspecific desensitization. Recently, however, R.E.GOSSELIN and R.S.GOSSELIN [J. Pharmacol. Exp. Therap. **184**, 494–505 (1973)] have shown that high doses of histamine impair subsequent responses of guinea pig ileum to histamine more than to muscarinic drugs, whereas high doses of furtrethonium have the opposite effect. Perhaps drug-induced modifications in histaminic and muscarinic receptors are responsible for these differential losses of sensitivity, but no conclusive evidence is likely to be produced until methods are found for preventing nonspecific desensitization in visceral smooth muscle.

Acknowledgement: For invaluable help and advice on mathematic aspects of this project, the author is indebted to Prof. GEORGE STIBITZ of the Physiology Department, Dartmouth Medical School, and to Prof. RICHARD WILLIAMSON of the Mathematics Department, Dartmouth College. The proof of Equation (23) was contributed by Mr. CHARLES FEUSTEL, also of the Mathematics Department. All calculations were made through the time-sharing system operated by the Kiewit Computation Center of Dartmouth College. The manuscript was written during a sabbatical leave in the Department of Pharmacology, University of Nijmegen, Nijmegen, The Netherlands. This project was supported in part by USPHS-NIH Research Grant GM 11598.

Appendices

Appendix 1. Glossary

The following notation is employed in these appendices and in the main part of the text. Only symbols used repeatedly are defined here.

a, a_1, a_2 Arbitrary quantities defined in (11) below.
A   Agonist drug.
b An arbitrary quantity defined in (11) below.
B   A competitive antagonist.
D   A drug, either an agonist (A) or a competitive antagonist (B).
D′   An inactive metabolic of a drug.
E   Intensity of action of a biological effector.
k_i Specific rate constants. In the appendices they are numbered according to Figure 1. A subscript letter indicates the drug involved.
K   Dissociation constant or equivalent stationary state constant of the drug-receptor complex. Sub- or superscript indicates the drug involved.
p, P Fraction of the total receptor population in the form DR (i.e., the amount of DR per r).
$p′, P′$ Fraction of the total receptor population in the form R′ (i.e., the amount of R′ per r).
r Total number of receptors in the population (including free, occupied, and inactivated receptors but excluding any that may be "permanently" inactivated).
R, R′   A free receptor and an inactivated receptor respectively. (A sub- or superscript on R′ designates the drug causing the inactivation.)
s The stimulus intensity per receptor r in the total population.
$s*$ The stimulus intensity per receptor r just sufficient to elicit a maximal response of the effector.
t Elapsed time. For $\hat{t}$, see (14).
V, W Arbitrary quantities defined in (11).
x, x_1, x_2 Concentrations of A in the biophase (receptor compartment).
y Concentration of B in the biophase.
ε The "intrinsic efficacy," defined as the maximal stimulus (per receptor r) that can be generated in the stationary state by any particular drug.
Φ x_{ii}/x_i where x_{ii} and x_i are concentrations of A required to produce a specified stationary-state value of E in the presence and absence of B respectively.

Appendix 2. Generalized Rate Equations for the Receptor Inactivation Model

The kinetic properties of the receptor inactivation model (Fig. 1) are completely characterized by the following pair of differential equations, which are in accord with conventional kinetic postulates:

$$\frac{dp}{dt} = k_1 x(1 - p - p') - k_2 p - k_3 p, \tag{8}$$

$$\frac{dp'}{dt} = k_3 p - k_4 p'. \tag{9}$$

By solving Equation (9) for p and differentiating with respect to t, one obtains an expression for dp/dt which can be equated with (8). Combining terms yields the following second-order differential equation in p':

$$\frac{d^2p'}{dt^2} + \frac{dp'}{dt}(k_1x + k_2 + k_3 + k_4)$$

$$+ p'(k_4k_1x + k_2k_4 + k_3k_4 + k_3k_1x) - k_3k_1x = 0 \quad (10)$$

In solving Equation (10) the following substitutions are useful:

$$J = k_3k_1x/(k_3k_1x + k_4k_1x + k_2k_4 + k_3k_4)$$
$$W = (k_1x + k_2 + k_3 - k_4)^2 - 4k_3k_1x$$
$$a = -(k_1x + k_2 + k_3 + k_4)/2$$
$$a_1 = a + \sqrt{W}/2$$
$$a_2 = a - \sqrt{W}/2$$
$$b = \sqrt{-W}/2$$
$$V = \frac{a}{b} + \frac{a^2}{bk_4} + \frac{b}{k_4}. \quad (11)$$

Appendix 3. "On" Effect

Assume that one starts with a fully recovered preparation (i.e., $p = 0, p' = 0$) and adds an agonist drug at time $t = 0$ and at a fixed concentration x, which is maintained constant thereafter. Based on the receptor inactivation model, Equation (10) yields several different solutions depending upon the value of W.

Subtype 1 — Solution when $W > 0$

If $W > 0$, then a_1 and a_2 are real, negative, and different [see (11) above]. Under these circumstances standard methods yield the following solutions for Equations (8) and (9):

$$p = -\left(\frac{k_4 + a_1}{k_3}\right)\left(\frac{a_2}{a_2 - a_1}\right)J e^{a_1t} + \left(\frac{k_4 + a_2}{k_3}\right)\left(\frac{a_1}{a_2 - a_1}\right)J e^{a_2t} + \frac{k_4}{k_3} \cdot J, \quad (12)$$

$$p' = -\left(\frac{a_2}{a_2 - a_1}\right)J e^{a_1t} + \left(\frac{a_1}{a_2 - a_1}\right)J e^{a_2t} + J. \quad (13)$$

As t becomes very large, it is apparent from (12) that p approaches $\dfrac{k_4}{k_3} \cdot J$, where J is the eventual steady value of p' [see (13)].

Equation (12) can be differentiated with respect to t. Let $t = \hat{t}$ when $dp/dt = 0$. Solving for $\hat{t}$ yields

$$\hat{t} = \frac{1}{a_2 - a_1} \cdot \ln\left(\frac{k_4 + a_2}{k_4 + a_1}\right). \quad (14)$$

If $-a_1 > k_4 < -a_2$, then and only then is $\hat{t} > 0$. Under these conditions t represents the time after addition of the agonist at which p passes through a transient maximum before it falls toward its stationary state value. Under all other conditions p rises monotonically with time and reaches no maximum, although it approaches $\dfrac{k_4}{k_3} J$ asymptotically as t approaches infinity. Whatever the value of k_4 (provided that $W > 0$), Equation (13) reveals that p' always rises monotonically toward its stationary state value J.

Subtype 2 — Solutions when $W = 0$

If $W = 0$, then solutions of (8) and (10) take the form:

$$p = \frac{k_4}{k_3} J[1 - e^{at}(1 - at)]. \tag{15}$$

$$p' = J[1 - e^{at}(1 - at)]. \tag{16}$$

In this rather trivial case, p and p' remain proportional at all times, and each rises monotonically to its stationary state value.

It is of interest to define the circumstances under which W assumes a value of zero. According to (11), W is a quadratic function of the drug concentration x. Therefore, for any drug-receptor system in which the four rate constants are fixed, there exist two and only two values of x at which $W = 0$.

The roots are

$$x_1 = [k_3 + k_4 - k_2 + 2\sqrt{k_3(k_4 - k_2)}]/k_1, \tag{17}$$

$$x_2 = [k_3 + k_4 - k_2 - 2\sqrt{k_3(k_4 - k_2)}]/k_1. \tag{18}$$

Whenever $k_4 > k_2$, x_1 and x_2 are real and different and at least x_1 is positive.

Subtype 3 — Solution when $W < 0$

If $x_1 > x > x_2$, then $W < 0$. Under these circumstances a_1 and a_2 are obviously complex numbers and can be represented as $a + ib$ and $a - ib$ respectively. When the latter expressions are introduced into (12) and (13) and the imaginary terms are removed by substituting trigonometric functions, the following equations are obtained:

$$p = \frac{k_4}{k_3} J[1 - e^{at}(\cos(bt) - V\sin(bt))], \tag{19}$$

$$p' = J\left[1 - e^{at}\left(\cos(bt) - \frac{a}{b}\sin(bt)\right)\right]. \tag{20}$$

Equations (19) and (20) demonstrate that p and p' exhibit temporal periodicity even in the presence of a constant concentration (x) of drug. Because b is a function of x but not of t [see (11)], the oscillatory frequency is constant in time but different for different values of x. The phase difference between p and p' is also a function of x. Because "a" is always negative [see (11)], it is apparent that these oscillations are damped. Appendix 5 below contains an analysis of the circumstances under which this damping effectively hids the oscillatory nature of the "on" effect.

Appendix 4. "Off" Effect

Assume that one starts with a preparation that has already reached a stationary state in the presence of a fixed concentration (x) of an agonist drug. According to the receptor inactivation model, p' and p have then attained values of J and $J \cdot k_4/k_3$ respectively. At time $t = 0$ let the agonist concentration x fall abruptly to zero. Equations (8) and (9) then have the following solutions:

$$p = \frac{k_4}{k_3} \cdot J \cdot e^{-(k_2 + k_3)t} \tag{21}$$

$$p' = \frac{J}{k_4 - k_2 - k_3} [k_4 e^{-(k_2 + k_3)t} - (k_2 + k_3) e^{-k_4 t}] \tag{22}$$

One notes that p declines exponentially, but unless $k_4 \ll (k_2 + k_3)$, a double exponential is required to describe the fall in p'. Under no circumstances do oscillations occur during the "off" effect.

Appendix 5. Analysis of Oscillations

In Appendix 3 above it was shown that under some circumstances $(W < 0)$ p and p' display damped oscillations when an agonist is added to a fully recovered receptor preparation. Because we have assumed that the intensity (E) of the observed pharmacologic effect is some real, single-valued, increasing function of the stimulus and therefore of p, it is obvious that E oscillates at the same frequency as p. For simplicity we shall assume that any oscillation in p with an amplitude in excess of the noise level of the system will be expressed as a detectable oscillation in E. The problem is to define the circumstances under which this might occur.

   According to (19) and (20), when an agonist drug is added to a resting preparation, damping leads eventually to steady levels of p and p', amounting to $J \cdot k_4/k_3$ and J respectively. Each of these levels represents the equivalent of a DC electrical signal upon which the damped oscillations are superimposed. Obviously the AC component can be recognized only while its amplitude exceeds the noise level of the system. Thus the higher the signal-to-noise ratio the longer can the oscillatory character of the response be appreciated. Whatever the signal-to-noise ratio, however, some numerical values of the rate constants lead to more prominent oscillations than do others. The first problem is to determine the circumstances which optimize these oscillations, specifically those of p.

   One obvious approach to this problem is to select values for the four rate constants and for x that minimize the damping constant a. As seen in (11) this condition requires that the rate constants and x be as small as possible. Under these circumstances, however, b and the frequency $(= b/2\pi)$ are also very small, so that the advantage of being able to follow the signal for a longer period of time is at least in part neutralized by a reduction in its information content per unit time. The problem can now be stated more precisely: what are the conditions that maximize the number of cycles that occur before damping reduces the amplitude of the oscillations in p to any stated fraction of the original? In analytical terms the problem is to maximize the ratio b/a.

For the objective it is useful to define a quantity Ψ, where

$$\Psi = \frac{1}{4}\left[\left(\frac{b}{a}\right)^2 - 1\right].$$

To maximize Ψ is obviously equivalent to maximizing b/a. By substituting values of a and b [see (11)],

$$\Psi = \frac{k_3 k_1 x + k_4 k_1 x + k_2 k_4 + k_3 k_4}{(k_1 x + k_2 + k_3 + k_4)^2}.$$

By inspection it is apparent that k_2 must equal zero, and $k_1 x$ and k_3 are seen to be equivalent and so must have the same value, to which we will assign the symbol z. Similarly let

$$C = k_1 x + k_2 + k_3 + k_4$$

where C is understood to be a constant independent of z. By substitution,

$$\Psi = \frac{z^2 + 2z(C - 2z)}{C^2}.$$

By differentation Ψ with respect to z and equating the result to zero, we observe that $z = C/3$. Thus,

$$k_1 x = k_3 = k_4 = C/3 ; \qquad k_2 = 0 \tag{23}$$

represents the condition under which Ψ and therefore b/a are maximal, with peak values of $1/3$ and $7/3$ ($= 1.53$) respectively, whatever the value of C.

If one's ultimate objective, however, is to maximize the number of detectable oscillations associated with the "on" effect, it is not enough to maximize b/a. The amplitude of the predamped oscillation must also be large. This amplitude, which is implicit but not directly expressed in the p response, is represented by V in Equation (19). According to (11), V is also a function of a and b. No analytical solution was found for the problem of making b and V as large as possible while keeping "a" small, in such a way as to maximize the number of detectable oscillations in p. On the assumption, however, that (23) represents at least an approximate solution, a digital computer was employed to make many numerical trials during which each constant was varied systematically. Representative results are summarized in Table 3.

The set of values in the left-hand column of Table 3 represents the best compromise that was found. As seen on the middle column the "approximate" solution [viz. (23)] yields 7% fewer detectable oscillations whatever the detector sensitivity. When the value of k_2 was allowed to approach that of the other constants (right-hand column), the number of detectable oscillations fell sharply. Only the ratios of these constants are important, because identical computer solutions were obtained whenever multiples of these values were employed.

Having defined the optimal conditions for the production of oscillations, we can now ask: what is the maximal number of cycles that can be detected under these idealized circumstances? The answer of course depends upon the signal-to-noise ratio

Table 3. Three sets of rate constants to illustrate their influence on the maximal number of detectable oscillations in p

$k_1 x$	0.403	0.333	0.250
k_2	0	0	0.249
k_3	0.403	0.333	0.250
k_4	0.194	0.333	0.250
No. detectable oscillations	max.	0.93 max.	0.06 max.

of the system. One rather naive, but adequate way to answer this question is to imagine the noise as a random, high frequency signal which can be depicted, as in Figure 7, by a horizontal, shaded zone centered over the stationary state value of p. As p rises from its initial value of zero, it enters the shaded zone. If the zone is sufficiently narrow, as in Figure 7, it reemerges and reenters it several times during its oscillations. Because of damping, however, it must eventually fail to emerge. We may say that p and the effect or response generated from p become indistinguishable from their respective stationary state values at the moment when p enters the shaded zone for the last time. The time interval to this moment divided by the cycle length ($= 2\pi/b$) represents the number of cycles (or fractions thereof) which are "detectable."

This quantity has been calculated for various signal-to-noise ratios, and the results are plotted in Figure 8. To understand the abrupt jumps in the graph, imagine that the shaded area in Figure 7 is so wide that all peaks and troughs are included within it. Without changing the signal, improve the signal-to-noise ratio by letting the shaded zone become progressively narrower. Soon the first peak emerges abruptly from the shaded zone and becomes "detectable," an event represented by the jump in the lower

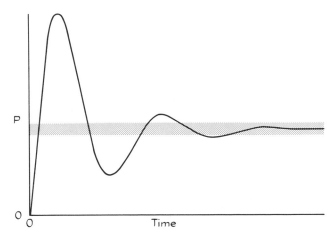

Fig. 7. Hypothetical damped oscillation of constant frequency, assumed to represent p after addition of agonist (but also see text). Because of random noise in biological mechanism and in recording apparatus, it would be more realistic to represent p (and effect generated from p) by wide line or band. For simplicity only stationary-state value is so depicted. *Shaded band* is extrapolated from stationary state back to zero time

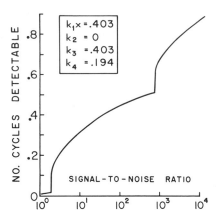

Fig. 8. Number of detectable oscillations induced in p, according to criterion of detectability described in text, as a function of signal-to-noise ratio. Constants enumerated in box are optimal in sense that curve corresponding to any other set of values lies to right

left portion of Figure 8. The next jump is obviously associated with the emergence of the first trough. As seen in Figure 8, however, this second jump does not occur until the signal-to-noise ratio reaches about 720. Because the calculations depicted in Figure 8 are based upon an optimal selection of rate constants (see Table 3), any other set of values requires even higher signal-to-noise ratios. As a representation of p, the curve in Figure 7 is now acknowledged to be a deliberate distortion, since the model requires more intense damping than depicted in the figure.

Appendix 6. Receptor Interactions with Agonist-Antagonist Mixtures

The following analysis is limited to stationary-state responses of the receptor inactivation model to agonist-antagonist mixtures. The antagonist (B) is assumed to compete with the agonist for occupation of the same receptor sites. According to this model, however, there may exist two kinds of such competitive antagonists (viz. Table 2), namely B's that do and those that do not inactivate the receptor by generating R'_B. With respect to reversible antagonism these two types are represented in Table 2 by d and g, respectively. For greater generality we shall examine the former case first and derive stationary state equations for antagonists of this type. For the many kinds of noncompetitive antagonists that have been described as reacting with groups in the vicinity of the active site, the receptor inactivations model contributes no new insights because it is very unlikely that even an irreversible interaction with an allosteric target generates a stimulus for the effector.

Let subscripts i and ii on x, P, P', and s designate two independent stationary states: in state i only an agonist (A) is present whereas in state ii both agonist and a competitive antagonist (B) are present. According to the receptor inactivation hypothesis,

$$s_i = s_{Ai} = k_{3A} \cdot P_{Ai}$$
$$s_{ii} = s_{Aii} + s_{Bii} = k_{3A} \cdot P_{Aii} + k_{3B} \cdot P_{Bii}.$$

Let states i and ii be characterized by equal effector responses ($E_i = E_{ii}$) because of equal stimuli ($s_i = s_{ii}$). Thus,

$$k_{3A} \cdot P_{Ai} = k_{3A} \cdot P_{Aii} + k_{3B} \cdot P_{Bii}. \qquad (24)$$

The problem is to define in terms of rate constants the concentrations of agonist (x_i and x_{ii}) and of antagonist (y) that satisfy the above condition. In practice one selects an antagonist concentration y that, when tested alone, elicits no stationary-state agonistlike effect or one that is trivial compared to the effect of A alone at concentration x_i. Equation (24) thus reduces to

$$k_{3A} \cdot P_{Ai} \simeq k_{3A} \cdot P_{Aii} \quad \text{or} \quad P_{Ai} \simeq P_{Aii}. \qquad (25)$$

When A and B are present together, Equations (8) and (9) must be satisfied for both drugs. In the stationary state, according to (8)

$$\frac{d(P_{Aii})}{dt} = k_{1A} \cdot x_{ii}[1 - P_{Aii} - P'_{Aii} - P_{Bii} - P'_{Bii}] - (k_{2A} + k_{3A}) P_{Aii} = 0, \qquad (26)$$

$$\frac{d(P_{Bii})}{dt} = k_{1B} \cdot y[1 - P_{Aii} - P'_{Aii} - P_{Bii} - P'_{Bii}] - (k_{2B} + k_{3B}) P_{Bii} = 0 \qquad (27)$$

According to (9)

$$P'_{Aii} = P_{Aii}(k_{3A}/k_{4A}), \qquad (28)$$

$$P'_{Bii} = P_{Bii}(k_{3B}/k_{4B}). \qquad (29)$$

When (28) and (29) are substituted into (26) and (27), one obtains a pair of equations from which P_{Bii} can be eliminated. Solving for P_{Aii} yields

$$P_{Aii} = \frac{x_{ii} \cdot K_B}{x_{ii} \cdot K_B \cdot L_A + y \cdot K_A \cdot L_B + K_A \cdot K_B} \qquad (30)$$

where $K = (k_2 + k_3)/k_1$ and $L = (1 + k_3/k_4)$. By similar reasoning,

$$P_{Ai} = x_i/(x_i \cdot L_A + K_A). \qquad (31)$$

Equating (30) and (31) and rearranging yields

$$\frac{y}{(x_{ii}/x_i) - 1} = \frac{k_{2B} + k_{3B}}{k_{1B}} \cdot \frac{k_{4B}}{k_{3B} + k_{4B}} \qquad (32)$$

where (x_{ii}/x_i) is usually called the dose ratio ($= \Phi$). Because the derivation does not require that the response level E be specified, Equation (32) is appropriate for all values of E below E_{max}. (Even the latter restriction disappears if there are no "spare" receptors.)

For competitive antagonists that do *not* generate R'_B, the corresponding equation is

$$\frac{y}{\Phi - 1} = \frac{k_{2B}}{k_{1B}} = K_B \tag{33}$$

where K_B is now the true dissociation constant of the antagonist-receptor complex. Indeed (33) is only a special case of (32), in which $k_{3B} = k_{4B} = 0$.

References

Ariëns, E. J.: Molecular pharmacology, Vol. I. New York: Academic Press 1964.

Ariëns, E. J., Rossum, J. M. van, Simonis, A. M.: Affinity, intrinsic activity, and drug interactions. Pharm. Rev. **9**, 218—236 (1957).

Beckett, A. H., Casy, A. F., Harper, N. J.: Analgesics and their antagonists: some steric and chemical considerations. J. Pharm. Pharmacol. **8**, 874 (1956).

Beidler, L.: Taste receptor stimulation, In: Butler, J. A. V., Huxley, H. E., Zirkle, R. E. (Eds.): Progress in biophysics and biophysical chemistry. Vol. 12, Chap. 4, pp. 107—151. New York: Pergamon Press 1962.

Belleau, B.: A molecular theory of drug action based on induced conformational perturbations of receptors. J. med. Chem. **7**, 776—784 (1964).

Belleau, B., Lacasse, G.: Aspects of the chemical mechanism of complex formation between acetylcholinesterase and acetylcholine-related compounds. J. med. Chem. **7**, 768—775 (1964).

Bloom, B. M., Goldman, I. M.: The nature of catecholamine-adenine mononucleotide interactions in adrenergic mechanisms. In: Harper, N. J., Simonds, A. B. (Eds.): Advances in drug research, Vol. 3, pp. 121—169. London: Academic Press 1966.

Brink, F. G. v. d.: Histamine and antihistamines. Molecular pharmacology structure-activity relations, gastric acid secretion. Ph. D. Thesis, Univ. of Nijmegen, Nijmegen, Netherlands 1969.

Butcher, R. W.: Role of cyclic AMP in hormone actions. New Engl. J. Med. **279**, 1378—1384 (1968).

Castillo, J. del, Katz, B.: Interactions at end-plate receptors between different choline derivatives. Proc. roy. Soc. Lond. B **146**, 369—381 (1957).

Changeux, J., Thiery, J., Tung, Y., Kittel, C.: On the cooperativity of biological membranes. Proc. nat. Acad. Sci. (Wash.) **57**, 335—341 (1967).

Clark, A. J.: The mode of action of drugs on cell. Baltimore: Williams and Wilkins 1933.

Clark, A. J.: General pharmacology. In: Heffter's Handbuch der exper. Pharmakol. IV. Berlin: Springer 1937.

Croxatto, R., Huidobro, F.: Fundamental basis of specificity of pressor and depressor amines in their vascular effects; theoretical fundaments; drug receptor linkage. Arch. int. Pharmacodyn. **106**, 207—243 (1956).

Feher, O., Bokri, E.: Contributions to the kinetics of the acetylcholine-receptor function. Pflügers Arch. ges. Physiol. **272**, 553—561 (1961).

Filmer, D. L., Cannon, J. R., Reiss, N.: A method of determination of rate constants in enzyme reactions. J. theor. Biol. **16**, 280—293 (1967).

Furchgott, R. F.: Receptor mechanisms. Ann. Rev. Pharmacol. **4**, 21—50 (1964).

Furchgott, R. F.: The use of β-haloalkylamines in the differentiation of receptors and in the determination of dissociation constants of receptor-agonist complexes. In: Harper, N. J., Simonds, A. B. (Eds.): Advances in drug research, Vol. 3, pp. 21—55. London: Academic Press 1966.

Gaddum, J. H., Hameed, K. A., Hathway, D. E., Stephens, F. E.: Quantitative studies of antagonists for 5-hydroxytryptamine. Quart. J. exp. Physiol. **40**, 49—74 (1955).

Gosselin, R. E.: Drug receptor kinetics: a new model. Pharmacologist 10, 215 (1968).

Jensen, E. V., Jacobsen, H. L.: Basic guides to one mechanism of estrogen action. Recent Progr. Hormone Res. 18, 387—414 (1962).

Jensen, E. V., Suzuki, T., Kawashima, T., Stumpf, W. E., Jungblut, P. W., de Sombre, E. R.: A two-steps mechanism for the interaction of estradiol with rat uterus. Proc. nat. Acad. Sci. (Wash.) 59, 632—638 (1968).

Karlin, A.: On the application of "a plausible model" of allosteric proteins to the receptor for acetylcholine. J. theor. Biol. 16, 306—320 (1967).

Katz, B., Thesleff, S.: A study of the desensitization produced by acetylcholine at the motor end-plate. J. Physiol. (Lond.) 138, 63—80 (1957).

Knapp, D. E., Mejia, S.: Role of protein synthesis in recovery from local anesthetic-induced conduction blockade. Anesth. Analg. Curr. Res. 48, 189—194 (1969).

Lüllmann, H., Ziegler, A.: Estimation of the cholinergic receptor occupation in guinea pig isolated atria by means of ^{14}C-labelled arecaidine-derivatives. Europ. J. Pharmacol. 5, 71—78 (1968).

Mackay, D.: A flux-carrier hypothesis of drug action. Nature (Lond.) 197, 1171—1173 (1963).

Mackay, D.: A new method for the analysis of drug-receptor interactions. In: Harper, N. J., Simonds, A. B. (Eds.): Advances in drug research, Vol. 3, pp. 1—19. London: Academic Press 1966.

Mackay, D.: A Critical Survey of Receptor Theories of Drug Action. Handbuch der Exper. Pharmakol., Vol. 47, pp. 255—321. Berlin-Heidelberg-New York: Springer 1977.

Main, A. R.: Affinity and phosphorylation constants for the inhibition of esterases by organophosphates. Science 144, 992—993 (1964).

Monod, J., Changeux, J. P., Jacob, F.: Allosteric proteins and cellular control systems. J. molec. Biol. 6, 306—329 (1963).

Monod, J., Wyman, J., Changeux, J. P.: On the nature of allosteric transitions: a plausible model. J. molec. Biol. 12, 88—118 (1965).

Nickerson, M.: Receptor occupancy and tissue response. Nature (Lond.) 178, 697—698 (1956).

Nickerson, M.: Non-equilibrium drug antagonism. Pharmacol. Rev. 9, 246—268 (1957).

Nickerson, M.: Blockade of the actions of adrenaline and noradrenaline. Pharmacol. Rev. 11, 443—461 (1959).

O'Brien, R. D.: Toxic Phosphorus Esters. New York: Academic Press 1960.

Paton, W. D. M.: A theory of drug action based on the rate of drug-receptor combination. Proc. roy. Soc. B 154, 21—69 (1961).

Paton, W. D. M., Rang, H. P.: A kinetic approach to the mechanism of drug action. In: Harper, N. J., Simonds, A. B. (Eds.): Advances in drug research, Vol. 3, pp. 57—80. London: Academic Press 1966.

Paton, W. D. M., Waud, D. R.: A quantitative investigation of the relationship between rate of access of a drug to receptor and the rate of onset or offset of action. Arch. exp. Path. Pharmak. 248, 124—143 (1964).

Rang, H. P., Ritter, J. M.: A new kind of drug antagonism: evidence that agonists cause a molecular change in acetylcholine receptors. Mol. Pharmacol. 5, 394—411 (1969).

Renqvist, Y.: Über den Geschmack. Skand. Arch. Physiol. 38, 97—201 (1919).

Rocha e Silva, M.: Concerning the theory of receptors in pharmacology. A rational estimation of pA_x. Arch. int. Pharmacodyn. 118, 74—94 (1959).

Rossum, J. M. van: Limitations of molecular pharmacology, some implications of the basic assumptions underlying calculations on drug receptor interactions and the significance of biological drug parameters. In: Harper, N. J., Simonds, A. B. (Eds.): Advances in drug research, Vol. 3, pp. 189—234. London: Academic Press 1966.

Rossum, J. M. van: Drug receptor theories. In: Robson, J. M., Stacey, R. S. (Eds.): Recent advances in pharmacology, pp. 99—103. London: J. and A. Churchill 1968.

Schild, H. O.: pA, a new scale for the measurement of drug antagonism. Brit. J. Pharmacol. 2, 189—206 (1947).

Schild, H. O.: Drug antagonism and pA. Pharm. Rev. 9, 242—246 (1957).

Stephenson, R. P.: A modification of receptor theory. Brit. J. Pharmacol. 11, 379—393 (1956).

Stibitz, G.: A model and computer program for biological networks. J. theor. Biol. 19, 116—132 (1968).

Taylor, D. B., Nedergaard, O. A.: Relation between structure and action of quaternary ammonium neuromuscular blocking agents. Physiol. Rev. **45**, 523—554 (1965).

Thron, C. D., Waud, D. R.: The rate of action of atropine. J. Pharmacol. exp. Ther. **160**, 91—105 (1968).

Waud, D. R.: Pharmacological receptors. Pharm. Rev. **20**, 49—88 (1968).

Williams, R. J. P.: Enzymes and drug action. Ciba Foundation Symp., pp. 410—418. London: J. & A. Churchill Ltd. 1962.

Wilson, I. B.: Conformation changes in acetylcholinesterase in cholinergic mechanism. Ann. N. Y. Acad. Sci. **144**, 664—674 (1967).

CHAPTER 7

Kinetics of Drug-Receptor Interaction

C. A. M. van Ginneken

I. Introduction

A. Drug-Receptor Interactions and Pharmacologic Effect

Drugs can exert their pharmacological action in two different ways. First of all some drugs have an effect by virtue of their overall physicochemical characteristics (e.g., osmotic diuretics, antiseptics, antacids, and general anesthetics). Usually these are only effective in rather high concentrations, since they need to bring about changes in the organism by just being present.

The situation is totally different with the other group of drugs, to which this chapter is restricted, namely drugs that can give a very specific effect that is originated by the interaction between the drug and some part of the organism with a special affinity for it. This receptive substance (receptors) was recognized long ago (PARACELSUS, around 1500), and was further elaborated in the beginning of this century (EHRLICH, 1900; LANGLEY, 1905). Typical for this most important group of drugs with specific activity is the fact that they can achieve intensive effects in very low concentrations. For instance, the experiments of DEL CASTILLO and KATZ (1955) on electrophoretic application of acetylcholine to end plates in frog muscle provide very convincing evidence in favor of the actual existence of specific receptors.

The main credit for showing that drug-receptor interactions can be fruitfully described by the law of mass action must go to CLARK (1937). Since publication of his work many pharmacologists have directed their attention to the process occurring between the administration of a drug and the observation of its pharmacologic effect (e.g., ARIENS, 1964). Most of the experimental work has been done on isolated organ preparations of various origins. The reason for this restriction will be obvious from Figure 1, which depicts the long, largely obscure way from administration of a drug to an organism to the ultimately observed effect (cf. van ROSSUM, 1968).

Blocks 1 and 2 (drug transference) refer to the processes of absorption, distribution, and elimination of the drug, preceding and accompanying the events in the biophase or receptor compartment (block 3) where actual interaction between drug and receptor takes place (which is the main topic of this chapter). Only a small fraction of the administered dose will participate in the interaction, while the rest does not react but merely establishes the concentration gradients needed for the achievement of a high enough concentration in the biophase for the effect aimed at. Clearly a much lower dose would suffice if it were administered in or near to the receptor compartment.

The least known steps in drug action are those between drug-receptor interaction and effect: the stimulus-effect relationship. Pharmacologic work may reveal some overall characteristics of the stimulus-effect relationship, but deeper insight can sometimes be gained by a physiologic approach (Werman, 1969). Real progress in the analysis of what happens after a drug has combined with its receptor can only be made after integration of pharmacologic, physiologic, and biochemical concepts and data.

In a Utopian situation, for a certain dose of a certain substance pharmacology would be able to predict not only the nature and intensity of its ultimate activity, but also how fast and for how long it would act on the basis of its chemical structure and its quantity. All the basic steps of Figure 1 would then have been resolved. Unfortunately

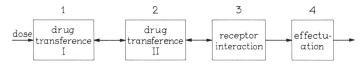

Fig. 1. Block scheme representing the basic steps in drug action. First step includes the relationship between dose and concentration in the central compartment (plasma or bath fluid). Second step gives the link to the concentration in the receptor compartment. Third step implies drug-receptor interaction, leading to a stimulus which is directly proportional to the number of receptors occupied. Finally the fourth step, which as a rule will be rather complicated, gives the relationship between stimulus and eventual effect. (After van Rossum, 1968)

we are still far from this ideal and therefore, for the moment, the whole area has been divided into the separate study of the basic steps of drug action by the various subdisciplines of pharmacokinetics, biochemical pharmacology, molecular pharmacology, neuropharmacology, etc.

Our current knowledge does make some general remarks possible, however. The rate of drug-receptor interaction, which most probably takes place in seconds or less, will usually be very high as compared with the pharmacokinetic processes of absorption, distribution, and elimination (with a time scale of hours or at least minutes).

Furthermore, it is obvious that the significance of pharmacokinetics is largely based on the fact that the concentration of drug in the biophase is somehow related to the plasmaconcentration (and thus to the dose administered), although the relationship may be very complicated, especially by factors like pH differences, protein binding (Krüger-Thiemer et al., this volume) and capacity-limited elimination (van Rossum et al., this volume), which can lead to nonlinear pharmacokinetic phenomena.

Nevertheless, the process of drug-receptor interaction is expected to be a reflection of the pharmacokinetics of the drug rather than determined primarily by the reaction rate constants. There are some clear exceptions for instance in the case of some steroid hormones, with very low dissociation rate constants of the drug-receptor complex, leading to specific retention of the drug-receptor complexes, which however, is still determined by pharmacokinetic parameters since the association rate constant between drug and receptor seems to be very high ($\gg 10^6$ l/mol s).

In general, as long as the rate of effectuation is also fast in comparison to the pharmacokinetic processes, it is possible to obtain pharmacokinetic information from measurement of drug action as a function of time. This indeed has been described for some psychomotor stimulant drugs in rats (van Rossum and van Koppen, 1969) and for succinylcholine in man (Levy, 1967). Of course complications can arise in the study of drugs whose effect is too far removed from the primary interaction with the receptor, for instance the anticoagulant action of coumarin derivatives. But even so, NAGASHIMA et al. (1969) and LEVY et al. (1970) have shown that excellent correlation exists between pharmacokinetics and effect, when the effect is measured as inhibition of the synthesis of blood-clotting factors, instead of the much more delayed prothrombinopenic effect.

B. The Receptor

Although the idea of specific receptors for various kinds of drugs is generally accepted, little direct information concerning the chemical nature of these entities is available. An important factor in this respect is undoubtedly the fact that the receptor is best typified by its ability to initiate an effect after combining with a suitable drug; the effect cannot usually be observed unless a large part of the organism is coupled directly to the receptor. Thus, attempts to isolate the receptor, which are in fact numerous (for a review see EHRENPREIS et al., 1969) and sometimes seem successful (MEUNIER et al., 1972; ELDEFRAWI et al., 1971) are difficult to evaluate because of the loss of the pharmacologic response. Matters are further complicated by any conformational changes occurring during the solubilization and isolation procedure since these will also modify the binding characteristics (KATCHALSKY, 1970; WEBB and JOHNSON, 1969). Another possible way of obtaining direct information about the receptor is chemical or physical modification of the receptor *in situ*. One specific example is found in the work of SILMAN and KARLIN (1969) who described the behavior of the cholinergic receptor of electroplax cells from Electrophorus Electricus after application of reducing and oxidizing agents. Depolarization by receptor activators is strongly inhibited after brief application of low concentrations of reducing agents, and the inhibition can be completely reversed by oxidizing agents. This suggests that disulfide bonds are present near to the active site of the receptor in this case. Another interesting but less successful approach is that of FLEISCH and EHRENPREIS (1968). They heated the isolated rat stomach fundus strip for various times and up to various temperatures, and afterward recorded the dose-response curves for several agonists. Unfortunately their results cannot be interpreted unequivocally. Most of the information available up to now has been gathered via indirect approaches, mainly from the structure-activity relationship for various kinds of agonists and antagonists. Obviously when highly specific interactions are involved some of the characteristics of one reactant can be exposed by an accurate study of the properties of the other reaction partner, in this case the drug which is more easily accessible experimentally. For instance it is a well-established fact that cholinergic drugs need a positively charged group (usually nitrogen) to be fully active (BURGEN, 1965). This most probably means that the receptor contains a negative charge directly involved in drug-receptor interactions. By looking for similar conditions in large series of drugs acting at one receptor it may be possible to construct a hypothetical active site of the receptor. Examples are found in the histaminergic receptor (ROCHA E SILVA, 1966; NAUTA et al., 1968) and the opiate receptor (BECKETT and CASEY, 1965).

However, great care has to be taken in assigning significance to the assumed model, since new findings very often make revisions necessary, and sometimes the value of the model as a working hypothesis becomes very debatable when one is obliged to assume a receptor surface so general and so flexible that almost any structure can be adapted. This seems to be the case for instance with the opiate receptor site (Porthoghese, 1965; Mautner, 1969). For a review of these matters see Korolkovas (1970).

When dealing with the various approaches used for studying drug-receptor interactions we should not overlook the work done with model systems, where instead of interactions between a drug and its receptor the reaction of the drug with a macromolecule thought to share some characteristics with the receptor is followed.

In this sense, the fact that both acetylcholinesterase and the acetylcholine receptor are biosynthetic macromolecules with a more or less specific affinity for acetylcholine led Belleau (1965, 1967) to the use of esterase as a model for the receptor. Indeed he found several remarkable and highly suggestive correlations between the thermodynamics of the binding of alkyltrimethylammonium ions with acetylcholinesterase and their muscarinic activity on the acetylcholine receptor. A more sophisticated model system can best be exemplified by the wotk of Marlow et al. (1969). It is well known that by coupling small molecules (haptens) irreversibly to antigenic proteins, antibodies can be prepared with a more or less specific affinity for the hapten.

Using the nicotinic agonist phenoxycholine as the determinant, Marlow et al. were able to prepare antibodies (from rabbit serum), which, however, exhibited a remarkable lack of specificity in that both muscarinic and nictotinic drugs, both agonists and antagonists were bound and that several unrelated compounds also had a high affinity.

One is forced to conclude that these antibodies have distinct limitations as models for receptors: they have several characteristics differentiating them from receptors.

The same is true of acetylcholinesterase as a model for the cholinergic receptor, since there is fairly good evidence that these two macromolecules are rather different from each other (Karlin, 1967; Bartels, 1968; Mautner et al., 1966; Albuquerque et al., 1968; Webb and Johnson, 1969).

Molecular pharmacologists still find difficulty in defining the receptor, and it seems that the best one can do is to use a fully operational definition, such as: the receptor is that structure in the organism that behaves as R in Equation (1) (Waud, 1968).

$$D + R \rightleftarrows DR \rightarrow Effect \qquad (1)$$

where D = drug and DR = drug-receptor complex.

The purpose of this chapter is a critical exploration of the kinetics of drug-receptor interaction, from the approach of the drug to the receptor to the formation of an active complex and the dissociation of the complex thereafter. From the point of view of reaction kinetics we will try to define the limitations and possibilities of describing the time course of onset and offset of the pharmacologic effect in simple isolated organ preparations. We feel that insight into the kinetics of the interaction can contribute to the clarification of concepts like intrinsic activity, receptor reserve, etc. Our basic assumption is that there are no fundamental differences between the formation of a drug-receptor complex and that of an enzyme-substrate complex.

Encouraging in this respect is the fact that up to now molecular pharmacology and enzymology have successfully applied exactly the same mathematical description for the interactions they study. But whereas the drug-receptor interaction has nearly always been followed in equilibrium or steady state, we would now like to obtain information about the kinetic parameters, which cannot be gained from equilibrium or steady-state data.

A serious limitation of any pharmacologic approach to drug-receptor kinetics is the fact that it is not possible to measure the drug-receptor complex as such, and measurements of higher-order consequences of the interaction have to suffice (WERMAN, 1969). Direct measurements of the drug-receptor complex in intact systems are actually very rare; an interesting approach in this respect is that of FISCHER and JOST (1969), who obtained spectra suggesting a specific interaction between adrenaline and its receptor from nuclear magnetic resonance studies on the binding of adrenaline to isolated mouse liver cells.

II. Diffusion of Drug to Receptor

Before a drug can react with its receptor, it should first reach the receptor-active site by diffusion.

Several equations are relevant to the description of this diffusion process, many of which can be found, together with their appropriate solutions, in the monograph by CRANK (1957). It is clear for instance that the fact that the drug molecule can combine with the receptor once it has reached it will substantially influence the diffusive behavior.

A. Free Diffusion of Drug

We will now outline the approach to the estimation of the rate constant for diffusion-limited reactions, as proposed by SMOLUCHOWSKI (1917) and DEBYE (1942) (cf. also BURGEN, 1966). This seems worthwhile because in general the first step in the interaction between a small molecule (i.e., drug) and a biomacromolecule (i.e., receptor) is assumed to be a diffusion-limited combination, leading to a primary diffusion complex (EIGEN, 1963). It should be noted that this assumption ignores the possible occurrence of perfusion limitation or access limitation by diffusional barriers such as membranes (WAUD, 1968). Only free diffusion is taken into account, and this will be corrected for attraction and repulsion forces.

We consider the scheme:

$$D + R \underset{\overleftarrow{k}_D}{\overset{\overrightarrow{k}_D}{\rightleftharpoons}} D - - - R \underset{\overleftarrow{k}_{tr}}{\overset{\overrightarrow{k}_{tr}}{\rightleftharpoons}} DR \qquad (2)$$

in which   D = drug molecule
R = receptor (active site)
D – – – R = primary diffusion complex
DR = drug receptor complex (after real transformation).

$\overrightarrow{k}_D$ and $\overleftarrow{k}_D$ are the rate constants for diffusive association and dissociation, $\overrightarrow{k}_{tr}$ and $\overleftarrow{k}_{tr}$ are the rate constants describing the actual chemical transformation.

In the case of a drug diffusing to a fixed receptor site we can represent Smoluchowski's equation as:

$$\vec{k}_D = \frac{4\pi N D_D r_R}{1000} \frac{1}{mol/s}$$ (3)

where N = Avogadro's number = $6.02 \cdot 10^{23}$ molecules/mol
  D_D = diffusion coefficient of drug molecule
  r_R = radius of target on receptor.

For the derivation of this equation a spherical molecule is assumed to diffuse into a hemispherical cavity, but when this is not actually the case, the order of magnitude of $\vec{k}_D$ will still be correctly estimated.

Assuming that under the conditions of drug-receptor combination the Stokes-Einstein equation is valid, it is possible with

$$D_D = \frac{\kappa T}{6\pi\eta r_D}$$ (4)

where κ = Boltzmann's constant
  T = absolute temperature
  η = viscosity of the medium
  r_D = radius of diffusing drug molecule
to transform Equation (3) into

$$\vec{k}_D = \frac{2RT}{3000\eta} \frac{r_R}{r_D} \frac{1}{mol/s}$$ (5)

with R = universal gas constant = κN.

Assuming $\frac{r_R}{r_D} = 1$, in other words assuming a rather close spatial correspondence between drug molecule and target, which of course is not necessarily the case, the rate constant becomes

$$\vec{k}_D = \frac{2RT}{3000\eta} \frac{1}{mol/s} .$$ (6)

BURGEN (1966) calculated this constant in water at 37° C to be

$$\vec{k}_D = 2.5 \cdot 10^9 \frac{1}{mol/s}$$

B. Effect of Intermolecular Forces on Diffusion

According to DEBYE (1942), Equation (6) has to be corrected with a function Φ when intermolecular forces occur.

Debye's function is given by:

$$\Phi = \left[a \int_a^\infty e^{u/\kappa T} \frac{dr}{r^2} \right]^{-1} \tag{7}$$

where a = distance of closest approach
$\quad u$ = potential energy of interaction
$\quad r$ = (variable) distance between reactants.

If Coulomb interactions are predominant (as is undoubtedly the case in many drug-receptor interactions) we can write (CALDIN, 1964; CZERLINSKI, 1966)

$$\phi = \left[a \int_a^\infty e^{\left(\frac{Z_R Z_D e_0^2 \beta}{\varepsilon r \kappa T} \right)} \frac{dr}{r^2} \right]^{-1} \tag{8}$$

Z_R and Z_D = valency of receptor and drug molecule
e_0 = electronic charge
ε = dielectric constant of the medium
β = correction factor.

The correction factor $\beta \neq 1$ when the ionic strength of the solution becomes high enough to give shielding by an ionic atmosphere. It is quite possible that this effect plays a role in the drug-receptor interactions, but for a qualitative description of the influence of the operation of intermolecular forces on $\vec{k}_D$ we can assume $\beta = 1$.

Then the solution of Equation (8) is:

$$\Phi = \frac{\delta}{e^\delta - 1} \tag{9}$$

where $\delta = \dfrac{Z_R Z_D e_0^2}{\varepsilon a \kappa T}$.

This leads to:

$$\vec{k}_D = \frac{2RT}{3000\eta} \Phi = \frac{2RT}{3000\eta} \frac{\delta}{e^\delta - 1}. \tag{10}$$

Some calculated values for the factor ϕ as a function of $Z_R Z_D$ and of a can be found in the book by CALDIN (1964). From that it can be concluded that especially when the reactants approach each other closely repulsive forces will have a strong reducing effect on $\vec{k}_D$, whereas attractive forces cannot substantially raise the value of this rate constant. For the estimation of this effect here a particular nature of the intermolecular forces (coulomb interactions) is assumed. That the result is not dependent on this assumption was shown by BURGEN (1966). He demonstrated the same effect by a force field of a more general form, considering that most intermolecular forces depend on distance by a simple inverse power:

$$u = cr^{-p} \tag{11}$$

where c = constant, p = power of inverse relationship.

BURGEN argued that for most practical purposes $p = 3$–9 and he calculated the corrections factors ϕ.

For the diffusion controlled dissociation of the primary drug-receptor complex the rate constant might be given by

$$\bar{k}_D = \bar{k}_{D,0} \, \Phi e^{\delta} = \bar{k}_{D,0} \, \frac{\delta}{e^{\delta} - 1} \, e^{\delta} = \bar{k}_{D,0} \, \frac{\delta}{1 - e^{-\delta}} \tag{12}$$

$\bar{k}_{D,0}$ = diffusion limited rate constant of dissociation in the absence of a force field (EIGEN, 1954).

The maximum value of $\bar{k}_D$ will be in the order $10^9 - 10^{10}\,\mathrm{s}^{-1}$. The effect of the potential energy of interaction here as compared to the case of the association is obvious:

The influence of attractive and repulsive forces on the dissociation rate constants is just opposite to the effect on the association rate constant. Attractive forces can substantially lower the dissociation rate constant (especially when the reactants approach each other closely), whereas the increase of the dissociation rate constant by repulsive forces is much less pronounced.

Since attractive forces as a rule are certain to operate in drug receptor interactions it can be expected that the rate constant for dissociation usually will be decreased far below the limit for diffusion controlled dissociation whereas the corresponding rate constant for association will not be increased substantially. The much larger variability seen in dissociation rate constants than in association rate constants can largely be explained on the basis of these phenomena.

Clearly the simple theory of diffusion-limited reactions which has been successfully applied to interactions between small, well-defined molecules has only limited significance when one is dealing with entities like receptors, the structure of which is still totally unknown.

Several difficulties arise that will profoundly influence the rate of the interaction. Nevertheless, the predictions of the theory are useful in that they give the absolute limits of the rate constants.

The limitations that have to be considered can be roughly divided into two groups: the factors that alter passive diffusion of the drug molecule to the receptive site and those that make the evaluation of intermolecular forces very speculative. We will now discuss some of the problems. An important point is undoubtedly the localization of the receptor and the target site on the receptor. It is quite conceivable that at least part of the way the drug molecule has to go before the actual reaction with the receptor can take place is sterically hindered to such an extent that the diffusive displacements of the drug are no longer random. Furthermore, it has been found in enzyme kinetics (EIGEN and HAMMES, 1963) that the association rate constants for "bad" substrates are in general some orders of magnitude less than those for "good" substrates. So it must be concluded that the fit of the drug on the receptor can play a critical role in the rate of interaction, although several biomacromolecules show a remarkable flexibility in this respect. In the case of drug receptor kinetics it seems plausible that this effect is more outstanding for agonists which interact with the receptor in a very specific way, leading to the perceptible effect, than for antagonists that exert their action solely by blocking the active site. The magnitude of the association rate constant is likely to reflect the specificity of drug-receptor interaction. Another questionable assumption is the fact that the medium in which diffusion and interaction take place is regarded as a continuous solvent. This may be a valid approximation as far as hydrophobic molecules are concerned, but hydrophilic molecules or groups within molecules are definitely at least partially surrounded by water molecules that are rather tightly bound and organized in a structure that is totally different from the watery environment. This fact has far-reaching consequences for the estimation of the rate constants governing drug-receptor interaction.

Hydration of the drug molecule will increase its effective radius and thereby reduce its diffusion coefficient. Hydration of the receptor makes the size of the target site uncertain, but what is even more important, it will alter viscosity and dielectric constant in the neighborhood of the receptor. Since the rate constant for diffusion-limited reactions is inversely proportional to the viscosity of the medium and the magnitude of electrostatic interactions is highly influenced by variations in the dielectric constant, it is clear that the uncertainty in these parameters may give immensely wide deviations from theoretical behavior. Structural organization of water molecules will probably result in a considerable increase in effective viscosity and thus a possibly strong reduction of diffusion rate of the drug molecule in the neighborhood of the receptor. Some experimental support for this idea can be found in the work of CROTHERS (1964) on DNA helix-random coil transition (see also HAMMES, 1968). Another aspect of hydration is that charges on drug and receptor are screened to some (uncertain) extent. For instance, the net charge on proteins in a plane layer can be expected to lead to extremely high electrical fields (up to about 1000000 V/cm^2, SETLOW and POLLARD, 1962).

It is clear that in normal systems these fields are highly reduced by effective shielding of the charges. Of course, the magnitude of the ionic strength of the medium plays a major role in this. The effect of the pH of the solvent is also obvious, but this will be considered in more detail in connexion with another point. Furthermore, we should not overlook the fact that most probably the actual transformation process requires solution of the hydration layers surrounding drug and receptor. There is experimental evidence in favor of the view that alterations in the solvation mantle of macromolecules can result in dramatic conformational changes (cf. HIRSCHFELDER, 1965). The significance of these modifications for drug-receptor interactions will be discussed in more detail later. The next topic to be considered is the nature of the forces that constitute the energy of interaction between drug and receptor. Obviously we can only account for them in qualitative terms, since too many uncertain factors are prevalent.

III. Intermolecular Forces in Drug-Receptor Reactions

Numerous reviews on the intermolecular forces have appeared in the literature (see, for instance, the excellent concise survey by HIRSCHFELDER, 1965). A full examination of all the forces that might occur is beyond the scope of this chapter, so we will restrict ourselves to some main points.

In general, *covalent* bonding is not very important for drug-receptor interactions. The binding energy for this type of bonding is high (20–200 kcal/mol) which results in extremely low dissociation rate constants. Only in the case of irreversible antagonists do we have to reckon with the occurrence of covalent bonds. Usually these antagonists are alkylating agents and the order of magnitude (10^{-6} s^{-1} at 37° C) of the dissociation rate constant found with benzilylcholine mustard and some of its homologues on the muscarinic receptor is interesting in this connexion (Young et al., 1972). It should be noted that although strong interaction evidently occurs, the blockade produced by these antagonists is not totally irreversible.

Electrostatic interactions are undoubtedly much more important. Several types should be distinguished. The most important in the sense of binding energy contributed are *direct electrostatic interactions*, i.e., interactions between oppositely charged groups. These are the least dependent on intermolecular distance: in the absence of double layers they are proportional to the reciprocal of the distance, but shielding effects make the range of the force shorter. The interaction energy is in the order of 4–6 kcal/mol. Since of all the forces involved direct electrostatic interactions are the most long-range in character, an attractive hypothesis seems that they will be material to the first orientation of the drug, so that afterward binding can be completed in the right way. There is substantial evidence in favor of the importance of ionic interaction at the muscarinic receptor. On guinea-pig ileum, measurements of the activity of arecoline are consistent with the view that nonprotonated arecoline has less than 2% of the activity of protonated arecoline, the difference being due largely to a difference in affinity for the receptor (Burgen, 1965). Presumably the same holds true for several other systems. On the other hand, the results of Rocha e Silva (1960), suggesting that the activity of histamine is dependent on a group with a *pKa* of about 7, while the *pKa*'s of histamine are 5.9 and 9.7, are in favor of the idea that the observed dependence on pH is due to a change in the charge on the receptor. Here we touch a fundamental difficulty in studying the mechanism of drug-receptor interaction by changes in pH, which can influence the activity of the drug in at least three ways: by modifying the state of the drug, by transforming the receptor or by varying the chain of events that leads to the effect ultimately measured. The changes brought about can be diverse: alterations in charge or solvation are likely to be the primary effect. However, it is still not known at what level this occurs and exactly what consequences can be expected of it; the same is true with other variations that can be imposed, for instance in temperature.

Before any conclusion is possible it is necessary to elucidate the elementary steps that constitute the whole of the drug-receptor interaction and then find out which part of the mechanism is affected by the variations imposed.

In some enzyme-substrate interactions where the kinetic mechanism is better understood it has turned out that changes, for instance in pH, that have a profound influence on one step leave another totally unaffected. In the same way, some parts of the chain of events appear to be wholly independent of the concentration of the substrate, and so on. Furthermore, one should realize that nonspecific binding, which certainly occurs as a rule in biological systems, can be strongly favored in a certain pH traject, while of course the opposite is also possible. A last reason to be careful in ascribing special effects to changes in the external conditions lies in the sensitivity of the conformation of biomacromolecules, e.g., the receptor, to pH, temperature, solvation, etc.

In general, electrostatic interaction is the resultant of all forces existing between the di- or multipole moments and dependent on intermolecular distance, dielectric constant of the medium, ionic strength, solvation, and often the orientation of the reactants.

Ion-dipole and dipole-dipole interactions are more sensitive to distance than purely ionic forces, and furthermore their energy contribution is much less (strongly dependent on correct orientation of dipoles).

Induced electrostatic interaction is still less important, although the fact that in biomacromolecules very large dipole moments may be induced under certain circumstances, which can definitely strengthen the complexes formed, should not be overlooked.

Dispersion interaction (between transient dipoles and induced dipoles) is as a rule only important when rather large groups are concerned, so that the energy can cumulate to a considerable amount.

Undoubtedly of much more interest in drug-receptor interactions is the energy contribution provided by *hydrophobic forces*. These forces originate from the free energy of transfer of nonpolar groups from an aqueous phase to nonpolar environments. BELLEAU and LACASSE (1964) pointed out that the effect of extra CH_2 groups in a drug molecule on its affinity for the receptor is entirely accountable on the basis of hydrophobic interactions (and certainly not due to dispersion forces). This implies that at least part of the receptor surface has a nonpolar character. Discontinuities in affinity in a series of homologues most probably arise from irregularities in the nature of the receptor surface, where a variable pattern of polar and nonpolar moieties exists. Hydrophobic forces are not specific by nature, and an attractive hypothesis that could be used to estimate their energy on the basis of loss of water-surface free energy has been proposed (LEWIN, 1971). However, a major driving force appears to originate from entropy gain, mainly by changes in the water structure in the neighborhood of the drug-receptor complex that is formed and in the macromolecular structure of the receptor itself (cf. NEMETHY and LAIKEN, 1970). Two remarks must be made at this point. In the first place affinity is only affected by net changes in free energy. This means that electrostatic interactions in general will not contribute very much to increasing affinity since their net energy contribution is limited by the fact that the interaction actually stands for a replacement of counterions and water molecules already present on drug and receptor. On the other hand, hydrophobic interactions with net energies amounting to 0.7 kcal per one-carbon fragment can increase affinity substantially (BELLEAU and LACASSE, 1964). Secondly it is quite possible that in this respect there are large differences between agonists and antagonists. Agonists must give a very specific interaction with the receptor, so presumably a close structural fit prevails, where several electrostatic interactions can sum up to an appreciable amount. Hydrophobic interactions can contribute something to affinity, but only as long as specificity of the structure of the complex formed is retained.

On the other hand, for antagonists to be effective it is sufficient that other drugs (agonists) are prevented from forming the specific complex with the receptor. PATON

(1961), in proposing his rate theory, presented evidence that the dissociation rate constant is much lower for competitive antagonists than for agonists.

This is totally in line with the reflexions on the nature and the specificity of the forces between drug and receptor discussed here. For, since the antagonist only needs to block the receptor's "active site" in some way, quite non-specific hydrophobic interactions may contribute to the intermolecular energy, whereas the necessarily specific agonist-receptor interaction will be strongly limiting in this regard.

Furthermore, it is plausible that even if they possess an ionic group analogous to the corresponding agonists, most antagonists do not show an ionic interaction as intimate as that seen with agonists, because strong hydrophobic interaction in one part of the molecule will prevent optimal orientation of another (ionic) part.

Indeed, comparative calculations for acetylcholine and benzilylcholine suggest equilibrium distances, between the quaternary nitrogen of the drugs and a negatively charged group on the receptor, of about 3.3 Å for the agonist and about 5 Å for the antagonist (Burgen, 1965). In this context the terms actophoric and haptophoric groups (Ehrlich, 1900) also acquire a special meaning, in that the former are presumably largely ionic in nature, while the latter are usually hydrophobic groups, since these above all can contribute to affinity. Inherent in the kind of intermolecular forces that constitute the overall affinity is undoubtedly the fact that structural resemblance is much greater among agonists on a receptor than among antagonists on the same receptor. This in fact is generally encountered in pharmacology: it is easier to transform an agonist into an antagonist (for instance, by coupling large hydrophobic groups to it) than to do the reverse.

IV. Kinetics of Drug-Receptor Association and Dissociation

So far we have discussed several factors which make the estimation of the velocity of associative and dissociative diffusion inaccurate. We have to return to Scheme 2, however, in order to see the actual significance of what we have said for drug-receptor interactions. Assuming that the stationary-state approximation is valid for D ... R, it is obvious that the overall rate constant for association is given by:

$$k_1 = \frac{\vec{k}_D \vec{k}_{tr}}{\vec{k}_D + \vec{k}_{tr}} . \tag{13}$$

It is very credible that this approximation is valid, for the intermediate D ... R complex must necessarily be rather short-lived, since if it is not very rapidly transformed into the chemical complex DR it quickly dissociates again. Of course, an induction period is required before the steady state is established. During this period the rate of appearance of the drug-receptor complex is necessarily smaller. This implies that receptor occupation by a drug as a function of time is always expected to follow a sigmoid curve.

The duration of the induction period is dependent mainly on the amount of primary diffusion complex once the steady state is reached, and on the rate of formation of the diffusion complex $k_D [D] [R]$, and can very well be in a measurable range when the initial rate is low enough. An expression analogous to (13) is valid for the rate constant of dissociation:

$$k_{-1} = \frac{\overleftarrow{k}_D \overleftarrow{k}_{tr}}{\overleftarrow{k}_D + \overleftarrow{k}_{tr}} \,. \tag{14}$$

On the basis of the foregoing account it is reasonable to assume that $\overleftarrow{k}_D$ will be rather small and in general will be actually much smaller than $\overleftarrow{k}_{tr}$, in other words the actual transformation of D...R to DR will take place before D and R escape from their intermolecular force field. In fact this means nothing less than a diffusion-limited reaction between drug and receptor, and Equations (13) and (14) reduce to:

$$k_1 = \overrightarrow{k}_D \,, \tag{15}$$

$$k_{-1} = \overleftarrow{k}_D \, \frac{\overleftarrow{k}_{tr}}{\overrightarrow{k}_{tr}} \tag{16}$$

(cf. EIGEN and HAMMES, 1963).

With the differences in $\overleftarrow{k}_D$ and $\overrightarrow{k}_D$ these equations show still another reason why k_{-1} will be much more variable than k_1 and eventually much smaller. The factor $\dfrac{\overleftarrow{k}_{tr}}{\overrightarrow{k}_{tr}}$, the equilibrium constant for the reversible rearrangement of D...R to DR, will be specific for every drug-receptor combination, whereas this specific aspect is lacking in k_1. Apart from the plausibility of the detailed fundamentals of the rate theory (PATON, 1961) a comparison seems pertinent, since PATON suggests that the dissociation rate constant is the primary determinant of the activity of a drug. It should be clear, however, that this probably valid approximation is not bound to Paton's general approach. As will be pointed out later, it is very probable that a drug's activity (or part of it) can be expressed by a function consisting of several rate constants. We should notice that diffusion limitation formally does not necessarily mean a very high association rate constant, for $k_1 = \overrightarrow{k}_D$ may be some orders of magnitude below the expected upper limit, provided that $\overleftarrow{k}_D \ll \overleftarrow{k}_{tr}$ is still valid. This may be the case, for instance, when the access to the receptive site is hindered, which often decreases not only $\overrightarrow{k}_D$ but obviously also $\overleftarrow{k}_D$.

We can assume that once the drug has come near to the receptor, it will only escape from the intermolecular force field with difficulty, so that every encounter will last long enough to allow several collisions before dissociation occurs. Thus correct orientation and breaking of solvation mantles will probably not impose too serious restrictions, although they can definitely reduce the actual rate of complex formation.

Table 1 shows some rate constants concerning enzyme-substrate and hapten-antibody association and dissociation as studied by fast reaction techniques. Most association rate constants actually are high, but nevertheless definitely below the limiting value for diffusion-controlled reactions. The dissociation rate constants are much lower, as expected, and vary within the range from 10^{-4} up to $10^4 \, s^{-1}$.

From the foregoing discussion it is clear that great care has to be taken in comparing affinities of drugs for a receptor and deriving general features concerning the structure of the receptor and the forces that constitute the interaction.

Table 1. Association and dissociation rate constants for some enzyme-substrate and hapten-antibody reactions

System	k_{ass} ($M^{-1}s^{-1}$)	k_{diss} (s^{-1})	References
ribonuclease + cytidine 3′phosphate	$6.0 \cdot 10^7$	$4.0 \cdot 10^3$	CATHOU and HAMMES (1965)
ribonuclease + cytidine 2′3′phosphate	$1.2 \cdot 10^8$	$6.0 \cdot 10^3$	ERMAN and HAMMES (1966)
lactate dehydrogenase + NADH	$1.7 \cdot 10^9$	$1.0 \cdot 10^4$	CZERLINSKI and SCHRECK (1964)
malate dehydrogenase + NADH	$5.0 \cdot 10^8$	50.0	CZERLINSKI and SCHRECK (1963)
ribonuclease + uridine 3′phosphate	$6.0 \cdot 10^6$	$1.6 \cdot 10^4$	HAMMES and WALTZ (1969)
ribonuclease + uridine 2′3′phosphate	$1.1 \cdot 10^7$	$2.1 \cdot 10^4$	DEL ROSARIO and HAMMES (1970)
aspartate transcarbamylase subunit + succinate	$1.6 \cdot 10^6$		HAMMES et al. (1971)
aspartate transcarbamylase subunit + carbamylphosphate	$2.4 \cdot 10^8$	$9.5 \cdot 10^3$	
aspartate transcarbamylase (native) + carbamylphosphate	$1.3 \cdot 10^7$	$3.8 \cdot 10^2$	HAMMES and WU (1971)
ribonuclease $A + 2′$deoxyuridine 3′phosphate	$5.2 \cdot 10^7$	$5.0 \cdot 10^3$	WALTZ (1971)
hemoglobin $(O_2)_3 + O_2$	$2.0 \cdot 10^7$	36.0	ROUGHTON (1960)
BSA + (naphthol 3 sulfonic acid 4(4′azobenzene) azo)phenylarsonic acid	$3.5 \cdot 10^5$	2.5	FROESE et al. (1962)
BSA + (naphthol 4(4′azobenzene azophenyl)arsonic acid	$2.0 \cdot 10^6$	35.0	FROESE et al. (1962)
aspartate aminotransferase + ketoglutarate	$2.1 \cdot 10^7$	70.0	HAMMES and FASELLA (1962)
aspartate aminotransferase + oxalacetate	$7.0 \cdot 10^7$	$1.4 \cdot 10^2$	HAMMES and FASELLA (1962)
aspartate aminotransferase + glutamate	$3.3 \cdot 10^7$	$2.8 \cdot 10^3$	HAMMES and FASELLA (1962)
aspartate aminotransferase + NH_2OH	$3.7 \cdot 10^6$	38.0	HAMMES and FASELLA (1963)
aspartate aminotransferase + β-hydroxyaspartate	$1.6 \cdot 10^5$	72.0	CZERLINSKI and MALKEWITZ (1965)
peroxidase + H_2O_2	$9.0 \cdot 10^6$	< 1.4	CHANCE (1949)
old yellow enzyme + flavin mononucleotide	$1.5 \cdot 10^6$	$\sim 1.0 \cdot 10^{-4}$	THEORELL and NYGAARD (1954)
liver alcohol dehydrogenase + DPN	$5.3 \cdot 10^5$	74.0	BLOOMFIELD et al. (1962) and THEORELL and MCKINLEY (1961)
liver alcohol dehydrogenase + DPNH	$1.1 \cdot 10^7$	3.1	BLOOMFIELD et al. (1962) and THEORELL and MCKINLEY (1961)
hexokinase + glucose	$3.7 \cdot 10^6$	$1.5 \cdot 10^3$	HAMMES and KOCHAVI (1962)
Hapten – Antibody reactions			
4(4′aminophenylazo)phenylarsonic acid	$\geqq \quad 10^6$	$\geqq 1.0$	SCHNEIDER and SEHON (1961)
2(2,4-dinitrophenylazo)1 naphtol-3,6--disulfonic acid	$8.0 \cdot 10^7$	1.4	DAY et al. (1963)
2,4-dinitrophenyllysine	$8.0 \cdot 10^7$	1.0	DAY et al. (1963)
2,4-dinitrophenylaminocaproate	10^8	1.1	DAY et al. (1963)
1 naphtol 4,4(4′azobenzene azo)--phenylarsonic acid	$2.0 \cdot 10^7$	50.0	FROESE et al. (1962)
4,5-dihydroxy 3(4′nitrophenylazo)2,7--naphthalene disulfonic acid	$1.8 \cdot 10^8$	$7.6 \cdot 10^2$	FROESE and SEHON (1964)
4(4′-dimethylaminophenylazo) benzene arsonic acid	$1.1 \cdot 10^7$	$1.4 \cdot 10^3$	FERBER (1965)

The rate of association will probably not vary too much for most, whereas the rate constant for dissociation is a priori very uncertain, so that in order to study structure-activity relationships among a series of drugs it is desirable to correlate the structure of the drugs not with an overall equilibrium constant but with the single rate constants. Unfortunately, only a few rate constants for drug-receptor interaction are available in the literature. Table 2 shows some of the most reliable data. These values have been selected because they are measured quite directly from uptake of the labeled substances by suitable tissue, while the rate constants obtained are compatible with the equilibrium constant that can be derived from enhancement of glucose oxidation (in the case of insulin) or from antagonism on the muscarinic receptor (atropine, N-methylatropine and lachesine).

Table 2. Some association and dissociation rate constants for drug-receptor interactions

Drug	k_{ass} $(M^{-1}\,s^{-1})$	k_{diss} (s^{-1})	T $(°C)$	References
atropine	$1.8 \cdot 10^6$	$1.8 \cdot 10^{-3}$	37	PATON and RANG (1966)
N-methylatropine	$3.5 \cdot 10^6$	$1.7 \cdot 10^{-3}$	37	PATON and RANG (1966)
lachesine	$1.0 \cdot 10^6$	$1.0 \cdot 10^{-3}$	30.5	PATON and RANG (1966)
	$2.6 \cdot 10^6$	$3.7 \cdot 10^{-3}$	37	
benzilylcholine	$5.8 \cdot 10^5$	$1.1 \cdot 10^{-3}$	30	REASBECK and YOUNG (1973)
insulin	$1.5 \cdot 10^7$	$7.4 \cdot 10^{-4}$	24	CUATRECASAS (1971)
HFurMe$_3$ (furtrethonium)	$0.9 \cdot 10^7$	$3.7 \cdot 10^{-1}$	37	
MeFurMe$_3$	$1.5 \cdot 10^6$	$3.5 \cdot 10^{-1}$	37	
MeFurMe$_2$Pr	$2.0 \cdot 10^4$	$1.8 \cdot 10^{-1}$	37	determined from dose-depen-
histamine	$5.1 \cdot 10^5$	$9.5 \cdot 10^{-1}$	37	dent time-effect curves as
N-methylhistamine	$1.9 \cdot 10^5$	$8.2 \cdot 10^{-1}$	37	described in the text
betazole	$7.2 \cdot 10^2$	$7.6 \cdot 10^{-1}$	37	
4(β-aminoethylpyrazole)	$1.8 \cdot 10^2$	$4.5 \cdot 10^{-1}$	37	
benzilylcholine mustard	$1.8 \cdot 10^5$	irreversible	30	
propyl-benzilylcholine mustard	$1.7 \cdot 10^5$	irreversible	30	
butyl-benzilylcholine mustard	$2.7 \cdot 10^4$	irreversible	30	YOUNG et al. (1972)
pentyl-benzilylcholine mustard	$1.2 \cdot 10^4$	irreversible	30	
cyclohexyl-benzilylcholine mustard	$7.2 \cdot 10^4$	irreversible	30	

Clearly these data fit very well within the range expected for small molecule-biomacromolecule interactions. As far as agonists are concerned we can expect k_1 to be in the same order of magnitude as given for the antagonists, whereas k_{-1} for agonists will be some orders of magnitude higher than for antagonists: exact values are rare.

V. Possibilities for Measuring Rate Constants in Drug-Receptor Interaction

So far we have simplified the original fundamental scheme (2) to

$$D + R \underset{k_{-1}}{\overset{k_1}{\rightleftharpoons}} DR \qquad (17)$$

and the anticipated range for k_1 and k_{-1} has been considered. It can be assumed that the complex formation is a fast reaction and the question arises as to whether or not the rate of the reaction is measurable by classic techniques. Apart from the special difficulties in drug-receptor kinetics, which can generally only be followed by making use of some effect that is generated by the basic interaction, it may be helpful to consider the first approach of chemical kinetics. When dealing with fast reactions one actually refers to high reaction rate constants. One way to follow the reaction kinetics is to minimize the smallest time interval that can be solved by a fast reaction technique. Although these techniques have been successfully applied to several types of ligand macromolecule interactions (Eigen and Hammes, 1963; Hammes, 1968) it is unlikely that they could be utilized for such inhomogeneous and complex systems as are usually encountered in drug-receptor kinetics. The other possibility lies in lowering the reaction rate in order to bring it into a range that can be measured by classic techniques. For instance, rate constants are temperature-dependent according to the Arrhenius equation: when a positive activation energy exists (which is usually the case), the rate constant will become smaller when temperature is decreased. In drug-receptor kinetics, where the reaction between drug and receptor is generally measured on the basis of the effect that ultimately arises (or is blocked), it is impossible, however, to change the temperature, pH, etc. without affecting several other components or steps in the chain of events involved in the process of measurement. When we take the half-life $t_{1/2}$ as a measure for the velocity of a reaction, it is obvious that for a first-order reversible reaction of the general form

$$A \underset{k_{-1}}{\overset{k_1}{\rightleftharpoons}} B \tag{18}$$

we find

$$t_{1/2} = \frac{\ln 2}{k_1 + k_{-1}}, \tag{19}$$

which means that it will hardly be possible to determine the kinetics of, for instance, a reversible conformational change in a receptor, unless both k_1 and k_{-1} are below a limit of, say $1\,\mathrm{s}^{-1}$. Of course, the same is true for an irreversible reaction

$$A \xrightarrow{k_1} B, \tag{20}$$

$$t_{1/2} = \frac{\ln 2}{k_1}. \tag{21}$$

A totally different situation, however, arises with second-order reactions, as will be shown for the drug-receptor interaction in the simple form:

$$D + R \underset{k_{-1}}{\overset{k_1}{\rightleftharpoons}} DR. \tag{17}$$

The rate of this reaction is given by

$$\frac{d[DR]}{dt} = k_1[D][R] - k_{-1}[DR]. \tag{22}$$

Assuming that the concentration of the drug [D] remains unaffected by its reaction with the receptor, and substituting $[R] = [R_T] - [DR]$ with $[R_T] = $ total concentration of the receptor population, we obtain

$$d \frac{\dfrac{[DR]}{[R_T]}}{dt} = k_1[D] - (k_1[D] + k_{-1}) \frac{[DR]}{[R_T]} . \tag{23}$$

The rate equation for receptor occupation is derived by integrating Equation (17) and inserting the correct boundary condition, namely on $t = 0$, $\dfrac{[DR]}{[R_T]} = 0$

$$\frac{[DR]}{[R_T]} = \frac{1}{1 + \dfrac{k_{-1}}{k_1} \dfrac{1}{[D]}} \left\{ 1 - e^{-(k_1[D] + k_{-1})t} \right\} . \tag{24}$$

Thus it can be easily seen that in this case

$$t_{1/2} = \frac{\ln 2}{k_1[D] + k_{-1}} . \tag{25}$$

It should be noted that the denominator is made up by the terms $k_1[D]$ and k_{-1}.

When we suppose k_1 to be in the order of 10^6 l/mol s, it is clear that for [D] $\leq 10^{-6}$ mol/l the term $k_1[D]$ will be ≤ 1 s^{-1}. This situation prevails for most natural full agonists, e.g., acetylcholine, histamine, adrenaline when applied to suitable isolated organ preparations, since then the whole dose-response curve for these drugs is completed when a bath concentration of about 10^{-6} mol/l is reached.

For several synthetic analogues higher bath concentrations are required, but it is quite conceivable that for these substances k_1 is lower than 10^{+6} l/mol s, in analogy with "bad" substrates in enzyme kinetics.

In general it can be stated that isolated organ preparations provide very sensitive systems for measuring drug receptor interactions, so that in many cases it will be possible to record an effect (which is thought to be some function of drug receptor complexes formed), while the product $k_1[D]$ is smaller than 1 s^{-1}. The second term in the denominator of the equation for the half-life (25) is k_{-1}. This term is independent of the drug concentration. For antagonists k_{-1} is probably very small (in the order of 10^{-3} s^{-1} as argued before), but for agonists it can be several orders of magnitude higher. According to BURGEN (1966) the rate constant for *free* diffusion away from a plane source into an infinite medium is $2.3 \cdot 10^9$ s^{-1} for atropine. It is likely that this value also for other drugs with approximately the same molecular radius presents an upper limit for the dissociation rate constant. However, there are undoubtedly several factors that can depress this limit substantially. Formally all those factors can be reduced to the same denominator, namely the overall activation energy for dissociation. Then the Maxwell-Boltzmann distribution law states that in order to obtain the actual rate constant, the tentative estimate has to be multiplied by a probability factor

$$f = e^{-E/RT} \tag{26}$$

(for most practical purposes E is equal to the energy of activation), indicating the fraction of molecules with an energy high enough to surpass the transition state. Some evidence in favor of this approach can be found in the data of Paton and Rang (1966) concerning the acetylcholine antagonism of lachesine at different temperatures. Insertion of their value of 17 kcal/mol for the activation enthalpy into Equation (26) gives the factor $f = 1.5 \cdot 10^{-12}$ at 37° C. So, for lachesine, a k_{-1} of about $3.5 \cdot 10^{-3} \, \mathrm{s}^{-1}$ would be predicted, which is quite close to the experimental value of $3.7 \cdot 10^{-3} \, \mathrm{s}^{-1}$.

As long as k_{-1} is also below $1 \, \mathrm{s}^{-1}$ (activation energy for dissociation 12 kcal/mol or more, which will in all likelihood be the case for any antagonist) clearly the half-life for receptor occupation will always be longer than half a second, which means that the reaction takes place on a time scale that in principle is measurable by fast recording of the effect that originates, assuming that the response in time is a real reflection of the degree of receptor occupation. Some information about the rate constants determining the reaction with the receptor for agonists might be obtained by the use of dissociation constants, regardless of their inaccuracy and uncertainty, and rough estimates of the association rate constant. The most reliable data for the dissociation constant probably are those from Furchgott and Bursztijn (1967). For acetylcholine, carbamylcholine, methacholine, and pilocarpine they propose dissociation constants of $2.1 \cdot 10^{-6}$, $1.6 \cdot 10^{-5}$, $2.5 \cdot 10^{-6}$, $6.9 \cdot 10^{-6}$ respectively. Assuming k_1 to be in the range $10^5 - 10^7 \, \mathrm{l/mol} \, \mathrm{s}$, and the dissociation constant for agonists to be not higher than about $10^{-5} \, \mathrm{mol/l}$, we can expect values below $1 \, \mathrm{s}^{-1}$ for k_{-1} in certain cases. On the basis of this rough estimate it seems quite possible that agonists can also fulfil the criterium mentioned.

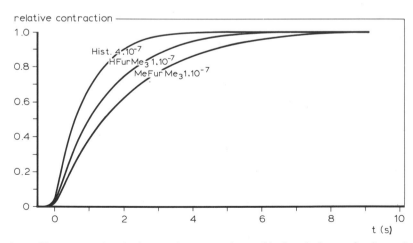

Fig. 2. Time-effect curves for the isometric contractions of isolated pieces of guinea pig ileum, induced by the indicated concentration (in mol/l) of histamine, furtrethonium and methylfurtrethonium. Each curve represents the time-dependent contraction relative to the equilibrium value of that contraction for a certain dose of a certain drug. It should be noted that the effectuation is a very rapid process, equilibrium being obtained within 10 s

It is known, that the guinea-pig ileum for instance can give a very fast response to administered cholinergic or histaminergic drugs. Reaction times of well-prepared organs are fractions of seconds (Fig. 2). For other organs the reaction time amounts to minutes or more, as is the case with frog rectus abdominis muscle (Fig. 3). In the latter example it is unlikely that the drug-receptor occupation is the rate-limiting step for effectuation; much more probably one has to consider diffusional barriers that slow down the rate of reaction, or some other limiting step in the chain of events leading from receptor occupation to the ultimate effect, i.e. the contraction of the muscle.

We saw that the observed rate constant k_{obs} for a simple reversible bimolecular drug-receptor interaction is $k_{obs} = k_1[D] + k_{-1} \, s^{-1}$. Two extremes are very interesting:

1. $k_1[D] \ll k_{-1}$, e.g., when [D] is very small. Then:

$$k_{obs} = k_{-1} \tag{27}$$

and

$$t_{1/2} = \frac{\ln 2}{k_{-1}}. \tag{27a}$$

Thus the reaction rate is independent of concentration and determined exclusively by the dissociation rate constant.

2. $k_1[D] \gg k_{-1}$, e.g., when [D] is large or k_{-1} very small (antagonists). Then:

$$k_{obs} = k_1[D] \tag{27b}$$

and

$$t_{1/2} = \frac{\ln 2}{k_1[D]} \tag{27c}$$

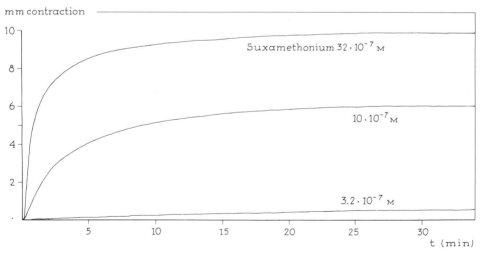

Fig. 3. The isotonic contractions produced by suxamethonium on the isolated rectus abdominis of the frog. Whereas Figure 2 shows a time scale of seconds, here equilibrium takes some 20 min. (From van Rossum, 1968)

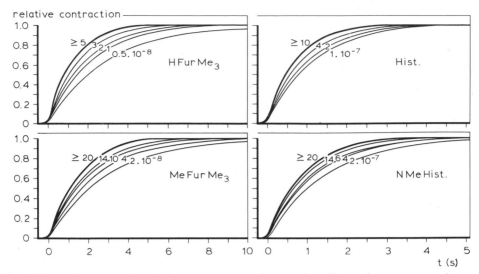

Fig. 4. Time-effect curves for the isometric contractions produced by various concentrations of furtrethonium, methylfurtrethonium, histamine, and N-methyl-histamine on isolated guinea pig ileum. With increasing concentrations, the rate of effectuation increases up to a certain maximum, which is different for the different drugs. This phenomenon may indicate the occurrence of conformational changes in the drug-receptor complex, as discussed in the text (page 383). The time-dependent effects for each dose are given as a function of the ultimate contraction maximally attainable by that dose (relative contraction). For each agonist the various doses have been applied to the same organ preparation

In this case the rate continues to increase with increasing drug concentration and other factors will become limiting for the rate of effectuation.

This shows that only relatively low drug concentrations can give information about the kinetics of drug receptor interactions, because with higher concentrations limitations arise from the nature of the tested organ. Preliminary experiments with several cholinergic and histaminergic agonists and partial agonists on guinea pig ileum (van Ginneken and van Rossum, 1971) demonstrate some striking features (Fig. 4). Firstly a concentration dependence of the rate of effectuation is observed with intermediate concentrations. This dependence vanishes with very low and supramaximal concentrations, as expected from the foregoing discussion. Secondly, the rate is clearly different for the various agonists and partial agonists. These facts suggest that the rate of effectuation genuinely is at least partly determined by the kinetic parameters of the drugs with regard to their receptor.

With high, supramaximal concentrations a transient maximum of effect is sometimes reached, which decreases afterwards to a lower steady value. The possible significance of this phenomenon will be discussed later.

When we assume that the half-life of the generation of the effect corresponds to the half-life of receptor occupation, it is possible to obtain k_1 and k_{-1} separately from a series of time-effect curves at different drug concentrations.

For this purpose Equation (25) can be modified to

$$t_{1/2}k_1[D] + t_{1/2}k_{-1} = \ln 2 \tag{28}$$

or

$$t_{1/2} = \frac{\ln 2}{k_{-1}} - t_{1/2}[D]\frac{k_1}{k_{-1}}. \tag{29}$$

Thus when $t_{1/2}$ is plotted against $t_{1/2}[D]$, a straight line should appear with intercept on the $t_{1/2}$ axis of $\dfrac{\ln 2}{k_{-1}}$ and a slope of $\dfrac{k_1}{k_{-1}}$.

Evidently rather far-reaching assumptions have been made up to now. However, it should be noted that the shape of the time-effect curves obtained with the guinea pig ileum is approximately the same as that expected for the curve describing receptor occupation as a function of time and that no matter how complex the relationship between stimulus (a linear function of receptor occupation) and effect may be, it is to be expected that at least parts of this relationship may be approximated by straight lines.

The latter seems most likely to be the case as long as the concentration of drugs used is kept within a limited range under as standardized conditions as possible.

Unfortunately, the experimental results are not straightforward. Some examples are given in Figure 5 and the values found for k_1 and k_{-1} are in the order of 10^5–

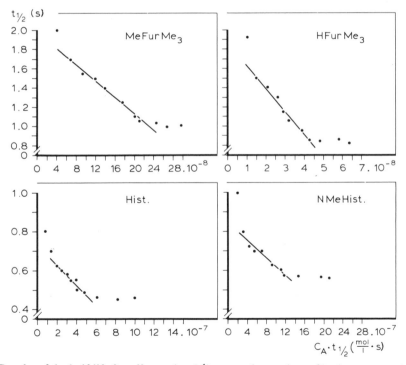

Fig. 5. Graphs of the half-life for effectuation ($t\frac{1}{2}$) versus the product of bath concentration (C_A) and half-life for some agonists on isolated pieces of guinea pig ileum (cf. Fig. 4). As discussed in the text part of these graphs obeys a linear relationship, whereas deviations occur at very high and very low bath concentrations. From the linear part of the curves, estimates can be made of the time constants for drug-receptor interactions

10^6 l/mol s and 10^{-1}–10^0 s^{-1} respectively. The order of magnitude of these parameters may be right, but serious problems are encountered with regard to reproducibility and adaptation to theoretical relations of the observed kinetic parameters.

For the moment, the only admissible conclusion might be that in principle it does seem possible to study drug-receptor kinetics by means of analyzing time-effect curves, since the time scale in which effectuation takes place is not in fact contradictory to that expected for the process of receptor occupation.

Two more remarks must be made at this point. It appears that different organ preparations can exhibit different kinetic behaviour in that the estimated rate constants for effectuation (and so, by assumption, of receptor occupation) are variable (compare for instance frog rectus addominis muscle and guinea pig ileum). An attractive hypothesis for the explanation of this phenomenon can be found in the biophase model proposed by Furchgott (1964) and elaborated by Rang (1966). The variability can be fully understood on the basis of differences in potential barriers between the medium in the organ bath and the compartment in the tissue where the receptors are located. Such barriers could give rise to effective concentrations of the drug in the receptor compartment that are substantially different from the applied bath concentrations. As a first approach the difference can be taken as a fixed factor, at least when the passage of the barrier is not rate-limiting. Obviously, complications show up when the passage is not fast as compared with the drug-receptor interaction. Another explanation could be a major difference in the nature of the receptors in the various preparations which, however, would be expected to result not only in different rates but also in different selectivity with respect to drugs.

The second remark concerns the experimental possibilities. It is clear that by means of other limiting conditions, namely at $t=0$, $[DR]=[DR]_0$ and $[D]=0$, the differential Equation (22) can be integrated to

$$[DR]=[DR]_0\, e^{-k_{-1}t}, \tag{30}$$

which describes the rate of dissociation of the drug-receptor complex on wash-out of the drug. The rate constant for this process is of course smaller than that for receptor occupation, but, whereas a wash-out procedure can very well be applied to antagonists (cf. Paton, 1961), insurmountable practical problems arise in the case of agonists, with their much higher dissociation rate constants: very rapid injection of drugs into and equilibration with the bathing solution is possible, but refreshing of the bathing solution cannot be performed within a fraction of a second.

VI. Conformational Changes in the Drug-Receptor Complex

The drug-receptor interaction has so far been considered as a one-step mechanism. This, however, seems hardly tenable in view of the overwhelming evidence from the field of enzyme kinetics that the interaction between enzyme and substrate in general is at least a two-step mechanism (cf. Hammes, 1968).

Of course such a complex reaction cannot be revealed by steady-state measurements, but only by kinetic observation at several different temperatures and/or concentrations. For the moment this is still impossible in molecular pharmacology, but obviously the occurrence of a multi-step mechanism strongly influences the meaning of the kinetic parameters measured.

Taking into account that after formation of a complex between drug and receptor one or more conformational changes in the complex take place, the least complicated scheme necessary becomes:

$$D + R \underset{k_{-1}}{\overset{k_1}{\rightleftarrows}} DR_1 \underset{k_{-2}}{\overset{k_2}{\rightleftarrows}} DR_2. \tag{31}$$

It should be borne in mind that k_1 and k_{-1} are not actually elementary rate constants, but are made up from $\bar{k}_D$, $\bar{\bar{k}}_D$, $\bar{k}_{tr}$, and $\bar{\bar{k}}_{tr}$, as outlined above. Inherent in the Scheme (31) is the assumption of only one conformational change of the drug-receptor complex to a special form. In the case of agonists this will be the active form, leading to the ultimately perceptible effect (thus the stimulus is thought to be linearly related to $[DR_2]$).

Antagonists, on the other hand, could show a DR_2 form, which is inactive, but in which a more stable complex exists than in DR_1. On the other hand, it is obvious that for an antagonist the form DR_1 also contributes to the antagonistic action. A discrepancy encountered in several studies (cf. RANG, 1967) is that the rate of onset of acetylcholine antagonism by atropine is much faster than the rate of uptake of atropine. This anomaly might be explained on the basis of scheme (31) by proposing for the rate of onset of antagonism:

$$\frac{d(DR_1 + DR_2)}{dt} = k_1 [D][R] - k_{-1}[DR_1], \tag{32}$$

whereas the rate of uptake may be better approximated by

$$\frac{d[DR_2]}{dt} = k_2 [DR_1] - k_{-2}[DR_2], \tag{33}$$

which is of course much slower than the former. This approach seems logical since as soon as atropine is in interaction with the receptor, antagonism takes place and real uptake is more or less confined to formation of DR_2 which is not as readily reversible as DR_1.

According to occupation theory, the equilibrium stimulus S caused by a concentration $[D]$ of agonist is given by:

$$\frac{S}{S_M} = \frac{[DR]}{[R_T]} = \frac{\alpha}{1 + \dfrac{K_{diss}}{[D]}} \tag{34}$$

where S_M = maximal attainable stimulus

        α = intrinsic activity

$$K_{diss} = \frac{k_{-1}}{k_1}.$$

Scheme (31) can be analyzed in an analogous way to yield the equilibrium value (assuming only DR_2 to be the active receptor conformation)

$$\frac{S}{S_M} = \frac{[DR_2]}{[R_T]} = \frac{\beta \dfrac{k_2}{k_2 + k_{-2}}}{1 + \dfrac{k_2}{k_2 + k_{-2}} \dfrac{K_{0.diss}}{[D]}} \tag{35}$$

where $\beta =$ a constant (analogous to intrinsic activity), $K_{0.diss} = \dfrac{k_{-1}k_{-2}}{k_1 k_2}$ (overall thermodynamic dissociation constant).

Obviously it is impossible to distinguish Schemes (17) and (31) on the basis of steady-state observations. The main differences would reside in the meaning of the parameters that are experimentally determined. From Equation (35) one may derive that the apparent dissociation constant estimated is actually a composite of the overall dissociation constant $\dfrac{k_{-1}k_{-2}}{k_1 k_2}$ multiplied by a factor $\dfrac{k_2}{k_2 + k_{-2}}$ representing the drug-specific part of the classic concept intrinsic activity. For the assumption that only one receptor conformation is effective implies that β is a factor independent of the drug and totally defined by the nature of the receptor-containing effector organ. So an attractive characteristic of the mechanism depicted in Scheme (31) would be that at least part of the intrinsic activity can be accounted for at a molecular level, namely by drug-dependent – induced conformational changes in the receptor. The "classical" intrinsic activity can thus be represented by

$$\alpha = \beta \frac{k_2}{k_2 + k_{-2}}. \tag{36}$$

The maximal attainable value of α would be reached when $k_2 \gg k_{-2}$. Then $\alpha = \beta$, which might be the case for strong, full *agonists*.

Partial agonists could then behave in two quite different ways:

1. k_{-2} is not very small as compared to k_2, or
2. both an active and an inactive DR_2 conformation occur (cf. Belleau, 1965), which means that the maximal attainable stimulus is reduced since part of the receptor population is complexed in a noneffective manner. Antagonists, of course, would only give nonspecific (or noneffective) isomerizations of the receptor molecule or no isomerization at all. It should be noted that formation of the DR_2 complex (and so eventually the effect), as a function of time, is now predicted to follow a sigmoid curve. The unequivocal demonstration of this could, however, never be an argument exclusively in favor of the model of Scheme (31), for several other explanations are possible, e.g., the inherent complexity of k_1 (as discussed above), the occurrence of cooperative processes or the existence of a diffusion barrier, causing a rate-limiting step before actual drug-receptor interaction takes place.

Under the assumption that [D] remains unchanged during the process of drug-receptor interaction, the model of Scheme (31) can be fully described in terms of a linear second-order differential equation with suitable boundary conditions (see Appendix).

GOSSELIN (this volume) has given a thorough mathematical treatment of this kind of equation in connection with his receptor-inactivation theory.

However, since it is rather difficult to obtain any deeper insight into the general consequences of the unabridged models of this sort (as becomes clear in the appendix), in this context we will restrict ourselves to the broad outlines of some interesting extreme cases.

VII. Kinetics of Drug-Receptor Interaction, Including Conformational Changes

A. Conformational Changes that are Fast in Comparison with Association and Dissociation

The first extreme that has to be considered is the case where the isomerization step $DR_1 \rightleftharpoons DR_2$ is very fast in comparison with the bimolecular association. Then we may assume that $k_2[DR_1] = k_{-2}[DR_2]$ is valid at any moment, and we obtain

$$\frac{[DR_2]}{[R_T]} = \frac{\dfrac{k_2}{k_2 + k_{-2}}}{1 + \dfrac{k_2}{k_2 + k_{-2}} \dfrac{k_{-1}k_{-2}}{k_1 k_2} \dfrac{1}{[D]}} \left\{ 1 - e^{-\left(\frac{k_2 + k_{-2}}{k_{-2}} k_1[D] + k_{-1} \right)t} \right\}, \qquad (37)$$

which means that formation of DR_2 is governed by the observable rate constant

$$k_{obs} = \frac{k_2 + k_{-2}}{k_{-2}} k_1[D] + k_{-1} \qquad (38)$$

and so

$$t_{1/2} = \frac{\ln 2}{\dfrac{k_2 + k_{-2}}{k_{-2}} k_1[D] + k_{-1}}. \qquad (39)$$

Clearly it will be practically impossible to distinguish this relationship experimentally from the simple Equation (25) resulting from Scheme (17).

Before describing the other limiting case of the model, we have to make some general remarks. It will be obvious that different kinetic behaviour in a certain mechanism cannot be distinguished experimentally from steady-state or equilibrium measurements, but what is more, even kinetic observations are often not sufficient for this aim (see also Appendix).

So in general, but especially in drug-receptor kinetics, as well as the ability and necessity to explain experimental results, chemical and physiological plausibility is strongly required for a model to be acceptable.

In the last respect the mechanism pictured with a very rapid receptor isomerization step seems to be wanting.

For instance, in biochemistry it is generally found that the rate of conformational changes in enzymes and enzyme substrate complexes is relatively low compared with

Table 3. Isomerisation rate constants

System	$k_{12}(s^{-1})$	$k_{21}(s^{-1})$	References
ribonuclease	$7.8\cdot10^2$	$2.5\cdot10^3$	French and Hammes (1965)
ribonuclease-cytidine 2'3' phosphate	$1.1\cdot10^4$	$2.0\cdot10^3$	Erman and Hammes (1966)
lactate dehydrogenase-NADH	10^3	$3.0\cdot10^2$	Czerlinski and Schreck (1964)
aspartate aminotransferase-β-hydroxy aspartate	$3.0\cdot10^3$	$2.0\cdot10^4$	Czerlinski and Malkewitz (1965)
	1.7	0.4	
LADH-red. diphosphopyridine nucleotide-imidazole	$1.5\cdot10^2$	$2.5\cdot10^2$	Czerlinski (1962)
haemoglobin (activated)	$2.0\cdot10^2$		Gibson (1959)
cytochrome C (activated)	7		Ebert (1973)
furylacryloyl tryptophanamide--chymotrypsin	1.5	30	Hess et al. (1970)
ribonuclease-uridine 3' phosphate	$9.4\cdot10^2$	$1.65\cdot10^2$	Hammes and Waltz (1969)
ribonuclease-uridine 2'3' phosphate	$9.0\cdot10^3$	$2.6\cdot10^4$	del Rosario and Hammes (1970)
aspartate transcarbamylase			
-succinate	$4.6\cdot10^3$	$6.2\cdot10^2$	Hammes et al. (1971)
-malate	$3.6\cdot10^3$	$5.6\cdot10^3$	
aspartate transcarbamylase-carbamylphosphate	$3.0\cdot10^3$	$1.2\cdot10^3$	Hammes and Wu (1971)
ribonuclease A-2'deoxyuridine 3'phosphate	$1.2\cdot10^3$	$1.0\cdot10^3$	Waltz (1971)
α-chymotrypsin	1.4		Sturtevant (1962)
chymotrypsin	0.7	0.3	Kim and Lumry (1971)
lysozyme-N-acetylglucosamine dimer	$1.5\cdot10^4$	$2.0\cdot10^3$	Holler et al. (1969)
lysozyme-N-acetylglucosamine trimer	$4.0\cdot10^2$	50	Holler et al. (1969)
lysozyme-N-acetylglucosamine hexamer	11.0	3.5	Holler et al. (1970)
lysozyme-N-acetylglucosamine hexamer	$2.4\cdot10^2$	10	Holler et al. (1970)

the bimolecular association of substrate and enzyme (cf. Hammes, 1968). This restriction is not a fundamental one, for the isomerization rate constant can easily rise to about $10^7\,s^{-1}$, for instance when the conformational change is based on rupture and rearrangement of a number of hydrogen bonds (Eigen and Hammes, 1963). Mostly, however, the rate constants are definitely far below this value (see Table 3).

B. Conformational Changes that are Slow in Comparision with Association and Dissociation

In enzymology it appears that several conformational changes occur in the process of enzyme-substrate interaction, where in each step the conformation of the enzyme is adapted in order to divide the activation energy of the substrate modification into a set of various much lower successive activation energies. In molecular pharmacology, however, one could think of a primary association between drug and receptor, largely based on electrostatic interactions, followed by a conformational change in receptor or drug-receptor complex, whereby the drug is critically positioned with respect to the receptor so that other (short-range) intermolecular forces can also contribute to the overall affinity.

Some typical examples of a very fast association process followed by a much slower isomerization step are given in the references of the Tables 1 and 3. Since fast reaction techniques have become available, the evidence in favor of this type of mechanism in biochemical reactions, including interactions between small molecules and macromolecules, is ever increasing.

A mathematical description of such systems can easily be given if

$$k_1[D][R] = k_{-1}[DR_1]$$

is assumed to be valid at any moment during the interaction.

Then we obtain

$$\frac{[DR_2]}{[R_T]} = \frac{\dfrac{k_2}{k_2 + k_{-2}}}{1 + \dfrac{k_2}{k_2 + k_{-2}} \dfrac{k_{-1}k_{-2}}{k_1 k_2} \dfrac{1}{[D]}} \left[1 - e^{-\left(k_2 \frac{[D]}{[D] + \frac{k_{-1}}{k_1}} + k_{-2}\right)t}\right] \qquad (40)$$

so that

$$k_{obs} = k_2 \frac{[D]}{[D] + \dfrac{k_{-1}}{k_1}} + k_{-2} \qquad (41)$$

and

$$t_{1/2} = \frac{\ln 2}{k_{obs}}. \qquad (42)$$

It is clear that the crucial point in the kinetics of this type is the relative magnitudes of [D] and $\dfrac{k_{-1}}{k_1}$. Whenever $[D] \ll \dfrac{k_{-1}}{k_1}$ the observed rate constant will be

$$k_{obs} = k_2 \frac{k_1}{k_{-1}} [D] + k_{-2}, \qquad (43)$$

which is indistinguishable from the other rate constants considered [Eqs. (25), (38), and (39)].

A totally different situation arises when $[D] \gg \dfrac{k_{-1}}{k_1}$, for then

$$k_{obs} = k_2 + k_{-2}, \qquad (44)$$

which means that at high drug concentrations the observed rate constant is no longer dependent on the drug concentration, but merely on the drug and the receptor preparation used.

This last phenomenon indeed is observed experimentally (Fig. 4; cf. also CUTHBERT and DUNANT, 1970), but only when supramaximal concentrations of agonists are used.

Since for most agonists $\dfrac{k_{-1}}{k_1}$ can be expected to be rather high (about 10^{-5} mol/l) as follows from the facts above, the submaximal concentration of D used is usually low compared with $\dfrac{k_{-1}}{k_1}$. A larger part of the time-effect curves can thus be analyzed according to the simplified Equation (43), which means that from the intercepts in the linearized graph ($t_{1/2}$ versus $[D]t_{1/2}$, cf. Fig. 5) instead of k_1 and $k_{-1}, k_2 \dfrac{k_1}{k_{-1}}$ and k_{-2} respectively are obtained. In this way reasonable values for all rate constants arise, but clearly the only argument exclusively in favor of the last mechanism lies in the limitation of $t_{1/2}$, ultimately reached by increasing $[D]$.

C. Conformational Changes and Irreversible Antagonists

If part of the receptor pool is blocked with the irreversible antagonist Dibenamine, the effect of an agonist is substantially decreased but is generated more rapidly (Fig. 6). If the effect of this irreversible noncompetitive antagonist were only blockade of part of the receptor pool, it could hardly be expected that the rate of receptor occupation by an agonist after application of the antagonist would change, since this rate only depends upon the magnitude of the several rate constants (which would not change) and of the drug concentrations. Experimentally, however, the same drug concentration is found to exhibit a higher k_{obs} after Dibenamine has been used than without this treatment. There seems to be only one logical way to account for this finding, namely the assumption that Dibenamine (and probably other irreversible antagonists) somehow brings about changes in (some of) the rate constants involved in drug-receptor

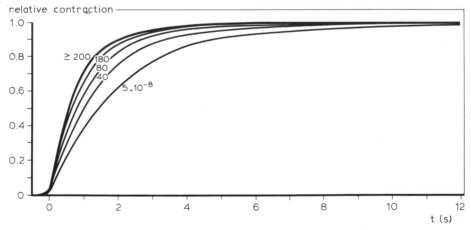

Fig. 6. Relative contractions (isometric) as a function of time produced by various concentrations of methylfurtrethonium on the same piece of guinea pig ileum, after treatment of the organ with dibenamine. The maximally attainable effect was reduced to about 10% of the control. On the other hand comparison with Figure 4 indicates that the rate of effectuation is increased by treatment with dibenamine. As is discussed in the text, this effect may be related to some nonspecific influence of dibenamine on the conformation of the receptors

interaction. What kinds of changes we might expect can be found by reverting to Equations (40) and (41). The observed rate constant given in Equation (41) increases with Dibenamine treatment.

Increasing k_2 or k_{-2} or decreasing $\dfrac{k_{-1}}{k_1}$ are obviously possible explanations.

The equilibrium value of

$$\frac{[DR_2]}{[R_T]} = \frac{1}{1 + \dfrac{k_{-2}}{k_2} + \dfrac{k_{-1}k_{-2}}{k_1 k_2}\dfrac{1}{[D]}} = \frac{\dfrac{k_2}{k_2 + k_{-2}}}{1 + \dfrac{k_2}{k_2 + k_{-2}}\dfrac{k_{-1}k_{-2}}{k_1 k_2}\dfrac{1}{[D]}} \quad (45)$$

decreases, which can be caused by increase in $\dfrac{k_{-2}}{k_2}$ or in $\dfrac{k_{-1}}{k_1}$. Naturally, all kinds of combinations can be thought of, but it is clear that the full effect of the antagonists could very well be explained on the basis of a change in a single parameter: an increase of $\dfrac{k_{-2}}{k_2}$.

The central point in this discussion is the fact that the irreversible antagonist would not block the receptor as such but would alter the equilibrium constant of the isomerization step (a destabilization of the active drug-receptor complex). From this point of view it is unlikely that the antagonist would actually react with the receptor-active site.

Irreversible antagonists are usually alkylating agents which attach a small group to the receptor molecule. There seems to be no a priori argument for a specific interaction with the site on the receptor with which agonists in fact do interact.

The well-known observation that a substance like Dibenamine antagonizes cholinergic, histaminergic and adrenergic agents which act on different receptors is also illuminating. On the other hand, it seems very credible that the covalent attachment of small groups to the receptor molecules causes pronounced changes in the structure of these entities, which most probably lead to changes in the observed rate constants.

This implies that the observable apparent dissociation constant for the agonist also changes after treatment of the receptor pool with the irreversible antagonist. On the basis of the model of Scheme (31) the apparent dissociation is represented by

$$K_{app} = \frac{k_2}{k_2 + k_{-2}}\frac{k_{-2}}{k_2}\frac{k_{-1}}{k_1} = \frac{\dfrac{k_{-2}}{k_2}}{1 + \dfrac{k_{-2}}{k_2}}\frac{k_{-1}}{k_1}. \quad (46)$$

It is evident that with increasing $\dfrac{k_{-2}}{k_2}$, K_{app} is also increased to a degree dependent upon the magnitude of $\dfrac{k_{-2}}{k_2}$ relative to 1.

When $\dfrac{k_{-2}}{k_2}$ is much smaller than unity x-fold increase in $\dfrac{k_{-2}}{k_2}$ will lead to an approximately x-fold higher K_{app} value. This idea actually seems to be supported by experimental evidence published by Waud (1969). Comparing K values for agonists determined in different ways, he finds that the values he obtains when using irreversible antagonists tend to be higher than the others. It should be noted that the allosteric receptor model also predicts these K values will be different, but differences in the opposite direction are expected (Thron, 1973).

Another interesting aspect has to be mentioned. Equation (36) gives the following expresseion for the "intrinsic activity" α:

$$\alpha = \beta \frac{k_2}{k_2 + k_{-2}} = \frac{\beta}{1 + \dfrac{k_{-2}}{k_2}}. \tag{36}$$

This means that a larger $\dfrac{k_{-2}}{k_2}$ will result in a smaller apparent intrinsic activity although the reduction is hardly worthwhile as long as $\dfrac{k_{-2}}{k_2} \ll 1$, as it seems to be for full agonists. Unfortunately no further experimental evidence in favor of the above-mentioned hypothesis is available. It is clear, however, that the mechanism of blockade by nonselective irreversible antagonists like Dibenamine needs to be studied in more detail.

VIII. Some Other Notions in Molecular Pharmacology

A. Desensitization and Fade

So far no attention has been paid to other, probably important conformations in which the receptor (or the drug-receptor complex) can exist. For instance, desensitization is a phenomenon not accounted for by the models considered. The reason for this is that our aim was to give the simplest kinetic description of the process of drug-receptor interaction. The place of desensitization in this context is uncertain, since at least some of the desensitization phenomena that are encountered in typical experiments with isolated organs seem to arise from other influences than the drug used. However, desensitization sometimes seems to be caused by receptor mechanisms and as early as 1957 Katz and Thesleff proposed a kinetic model involving an isomerization step of the receptor (drug-receptor complex) to an inactive conformation, which only slowly reversed to a receptor able to participate in the activation process by agonists. As Rang (1973) pointed out, this assumed that conformational change would exhibit strikingly low time constants for protein isomerizations: namely minutes instead of the seconds or less usual for this kind of isomerization reaction.

Nevertheless, some types of specific desensitization can be described very well with the use of such a slow protein isomerization step (Rang, 1973; Katz and Thesleff, 1957).

It appears reasonable, however, to treat the kinetics of drug-receptor interaction in typical short-term experiments by applying the model of Scheme (31), so neglecting the much slower desensitization steps. Of course a kinetic model able to describe qualitatively all the experimental results reported can be constructed. The problem with such a model, however, is the lack of quantitative insight yielded by conventional kinetic methods and the impossibility of discriminating between several models.

We feel that several parts of the undoubtedly complex system we are dealing with can be treated and explored separately (also in a quantitative respect) because of the very different time scales on which they proceed (e.g., receptor activation versus receptor desensitization).

We therefore outlined the kinetic aspects of the first events in drug-receptor interaction and tried to define the minimum requirements for a model to be acceptable. In a similar way, only after very careful analysis including the available data on the other parts of the chain of events can a scheme fulfilling the minimum requirements be constructed. It should be noted that classic equilibrium or steady-state measurements in molecular pharmacology are inappropriate for discrimination between various proposed kinetic mechanisms. On the other hand, the simple occupation theory accounts so well for most equilibrium measurements that any kinetic model in equilibrium circumstances might be expected to reduce to equations that are formally indiscernable from the simple occupation equation.

In the appendix some alternative mechanisms are described, and the conclusion that it will be extremely difficult to discriminate experimentally between the various theoretical possibilities seems inevitable.

A phenomenon that may be similar to desensitization and that is sometimes encountered in drug-receptor interaction is the so-called fade. This means that the effect of a certain dose of drug as a function of time rises to a transient maximum and thereafter drops to a lower steady value. With his rate theory, PATON (1961) gives a specific explanation for this phenomenon. In view of severe criticism, however (e.g., BELLEAU, 1964) the rate theory seems hardly tenable, so that fade has to be accounted for in other ways. Furthermore, fade is usually only observed when high (supramaximal) doses of agonists are applied to isolated organs (whereas rate theory expects it to be a general phenomenon), and one cannot help but wonder whether it is a specific part of the drug-response process or just a symptom of fatigue of the organ due to overloading.

If nevertheless specific fading does occur, it is easy to explain on the basis of "occupational" models with receptor isomerization steps. For instance, if in Scheme (31) DR_1 were the active receptor conformation and DR_2 an inactive one or DR_2, as the active conformation, could isomerize to a third but inactive conformation, it is obvious that under certain circumstances fade would occur (see also the Appendix). It should be noted that any second-order differential equation gives as one of the possible solutions an oscillatory function, which, provided that it is damped enough, can explain fading (GOSSELIN, this volume). On the other hand, it seems that oscillatory processes are very common in biological systems considered at a molecular level, so that a fadelike phenomenon could occur at several different levels (DESHCHEREVSKII et al., 1970).

B. Receptor Reserve

It has often been observed that only a fraction of the total receptor population in an organ preparation needs to be available for the maximal effect to be obtained with agonists. The overcapacity is reflected in the concept of receptor reserve, but has only relative significance, since it is derived from indirect measurements of a higher-order result of drug-receptor interaction (Werman, 1969). It is probable that the "over-capacity" very often arises from limitations in the capacity of some step following the activation of the receptor. A clear experimental demonstration of such a process can be found in the work of Seelig and Sayers (1973) on corticosterone production by isolated adrenal cortex cells under the influence of several ACTH analogues. Corticosterone production is mediated by cyclic AMP, which is released under the influence of the interaction of ACTH and its analogues with their receptor (of course several other steps may occur in between). Seelig and Sayers found that as little as about 15% of maximal cyclic AMP release was sufficient for maximal attainable corticosterone production; if the mechanisms were less well known this would lead to the conclusion of a large receptor reserve. Obviously the experimental determination of intrinsic activity is also affected by these processes, since drugs that are different in potency at the level of the primary effect may turn out to be equipotent when higher-order effects are considered. From these facts it is obvious that only submaximal concentrations should be applied in the study of the kinetics of drug-receptor interaction, since only in this way can limitations other than those at the drug-receptor level be avoided.

C. Homogeneity of Receptor Preparations

Some authors (Furchgott, 1955, 1964; Rang, 1966) have considered the possibility of diffusional barriers affecting the kinetics of drug-receptor interaction. As Furchgott and Bursztyn (1967) pointed out, the measured equilibrium constants for drug-receptor combination are of thermodynamic significance even if barriers do exist, provided that real equilibrium has been reached. From a kinetic point of view the question of which would be the rate-limiting step is more important. If diffusion through some barrier were rate-limiting, the rate of onset of action of a drug would presumably be equal to the rate of offset after washout. This is not found, however (Rang, 1966), but Thron and Waud (1968) offered an explanation for this by assuming that the biophase can exhibit a large virtual space. However, on the basis of the very high, concentration-dependent and drug-specific rate of effectuation observed in time-effect curves recorded for guinea pig ileum it does not seem plausible that effective diffusional barriers exist in this organ preparation. Another point is the homogeneity of the receptor population. It should be borne in mind that differences in the receptor will not be experimentally accessible unless they are rather large. A theoretical discussion published by Weber (1965) shows that differences in binding between a small molecule and macromolecules practically cannot be measured unless more than 20% difference in equilibrium constants exists, even when very precise techniques can be applied. Katchalsky (1970) demonstrated the dependence of equilibrium constants on the manner in which the macromolecule is placed in its surroundings. Inhomogeneities in the receptor population can certainly be expected, but for the moment it would be impossible to measure binding characteristics precisely enough to provide experimental evidence for this.

D. Allosteric Models

CHANGEUX (1967, 1970) and CHANGEUX and PODLESKI (1968) proposed a simplified allosteric model for drug-receptor interactions. The model resembles that discussed above in that great importance is attached to conformational changes, but differs from it in the concept of a preexisting equilibrium between active and inactive receptor conformations. The allosteric models certainly exhibit attractive features, but for the moment the experimental evidence is scarce (WERMAN, 1969; THRON, 1973).

IX. Activation Parameters

A. Arrhenius' Equation and Transition-State Theory

In Section III the forces and energies involved in drug-receptor interaction were briefly discussed. Knowledge of these makes it possible to predict whether or not a certain interaction *can* take place, but it must be borne in mind that even if the reaction is thermodynamically favored, there is no need for it to take place in fact. The rate of a reaction is not determined by the difference in thermodynamic state functions between beginning and end, but by other, kinetic, parameters.

This can be seen from Arrhenius' familiar equation:

$$k = A e^{-E_a/RT} \qquad (47)$$

where k = rate constant of a reaction

A = Arrhenius' preexponential factor (a constant for a certain reaction)

E_a = Arrhenius' activation energy

R = universal gas constant

T = absolute temperature.

Thus $e^{-E_a/RT}$ represents the fraction of encounters that are effective, i.e., that lead to product(s); E_a is the minimum energy required for effective collision. Since, for the preexponential factor A, values in the order of $10^{11} \, l \, mol^{-1} \, s^{-1}$ are to be expected in case of bimolecular reactions, it is easy to see that reactions with activation energies $E_a \leq 10$ kcal/mol are so fast that special techniques are required for following them (rate constant $k \geq 10^4 \, l \, mol^{-1} \, s^{-1}$, at 25° C; CALDIN, 1964).

For the fastest reaction, however, the applicability of the Arrhenius' equation is limited, since in this case the rate of reaction is practically equal to the rate of molecular encounter. The rate constant can then be calculated according to the theory of diffusion-limited reactions (Section II), but even so the rate constant appears to increase with rising temperature. The reason for this is the dependence of the diffusion process on the viscosity of the medium, and the viscosity can be represented as a function of temperature as

$$\eta = \eta_0 e^{B/RT} \qquad (48)$$

where η = viscosity

η_0 = constant

B = temperature coefficient of viscosity; usually 1–4 kcal/mol.

Substitution in Equation (5) gives:

$$\vec{k}_D = k_{D,0}\, T e^{-B/RT}\ ; \qquad (49)$$

compare

$$\vec{k}_D = A e^{-E_a/RT} \qquad (50)$$

$k_{D,0}$ is the part of the diffusional rate constant that is not temperature-dependent. It will be clear that in the case of hindered diffusion Ea for "diffusion-limited" reactions can be higher than the expected value for B, but general statements are hardly possible, since the preexponential factor should also be considered.

Insight into the meaning of the preexponential factor (and also of Ea) can best be obtained from the transition-state theory (see for instance Benson, 1960; Amdur and Hammes, 1966; Frost and Pearson, 1953). In this theory the reaction is assumed to proceed via a transition state (or activated complex) and the reaction rate constant is expressed as a function of the difference in entropy and enthalpy between the transition state and the reactant(s), the so-called activation entropy and activation enthalpy, according to the following equation:

$$k = \frac{\kappa T}{h} e^{+\Delta S^{\ddagger}/R}\, e^{-\Delta H^{\ddagger}/RT}, \qquad (51)$$

where κ = Boltzmann's constant

h = Planck's constant

$\Delta S^{\ddagger}$ = activation entropy

$\Delta H^{\ddagger}$ = activation enthalpy.

This relation is valid for constant volume and constant pressure and has been derived for ideal cases, but it appears to be a fundamental one, valid under several different sets of circumstances (Amdur and Hammes, 1966).

For constant pressure systems, as solutions usually are, the following relation between the Arrhenius' activation energy and the activation enthalpy holds: $E_a = \Delta H^{\ddagger} + RT$.

As a rule the contribution of $RT (\approx 0.6$ kcal/mol at room temperature) is negligible, so for most practical purposes E_a can be set equal to $\Delta H^{\ddagger}$. Replacing $\Delta H^{\ddagger}$ by E_a in Equation (51) gives:

$$k = e\frac{kT}{h} e^{+\Delta S^{\ast}/R}\, e^{-E_a/RT}. \qquad (52)$$

Comparison with Equation (47) leads to the expression for A

$$A = e \frac{kT}{h} e^{\Delta S^* / R}. \tag{53}$$

Thus it can be seen that the magnitude of the preexponential factor is determined by the activation entropy: entropy gain on the way to the transition state increases A, and thus k, while entropy loss has the opposite effect.

Comparison of Equation (49) with a form analogous to Equation (52) shows $B = E_a$, and reaction rates will not usually be adequately predicted from the theory of diffusion-limited reactions when the value of E_a exceeds plausible values of B.

Obviously Arrhenius' and transition-state theory are only applicable insofar as elementary noncomplex rate constants are concerned. Nearly always, however, a chemical reaction appears to be complex in nature and then the estimated rate constants are some function of the elementary rate constants, which can be simplified to a relationship that allows quantitative elaboration with the use of transition-state theory or Arrhenius' equation only in extreme cases.

For instance, in Section IV we saw that the rate constant for a bimolecular association is generally given by:

$$k_1 = \frac{\vec{k}_D \vec{k}_{tr}}{\vec{k}_D + \vec{k}_{tr}}. \tag{13}$$

When the reaction is diffusion-limited ($\vec{k}_{tr} \gg \vec{k}_D$) the expression reduces to:

$$k_1 = \vec{k}_D \tag{15}$$

and the rate constant can be handled according to the principles described above.

A totally different situation arises, however, when k cannot be simplified in this way. Calculation of the activation energy (after measurement of k at several different temperatures) then leads to an apparent activation energy which is related to the real activation energies of the elementary rate constants involved.

The relationship can be derived by the use of the Arrhenius' equation in the form

$$\frac{d \ln k_1}{dT} = \frac{E_a}{RT^2} \tag{54}$$

$$\ln k_1 = \ln \vec{k}_D + \ln \vec{k}_{tr} - \ln(\vec{k}_D + \vec{k}_{tr}), \tag{55}$$

$$\frac{d \ln k_1}{dT} = \frac{d \ln \vec{k}_D}{dT} + \frac{d \ln \vec{k}_{tr}}{dT} - \frac{1}{\vec{k}_D + \vec{k}_{tr}} \left(\vec{k}_D \frac{d \ln \vec{k}_D}{dT} + \vec{k}_{tr} \frac{d \ln \vec{k}_{tr}}{dT} \right) \tag{56}$$

so:

$$E_{a_{k_1}} = E_{a_{\overleftarrow{k}_D}} + E_{a_{\overleftarrow{k}_{tr}}} - \frac{\overleftarrow{k}_D E_{a_{\overleftarrow{k}_D}} + \overleftarrow{k}_{tr} E_{a_{\overleftarrow{k}_{tr}}}}{\overleftarrow{k}_D + \overleftarrow{k}_{tr}} \tag{57}$$

where the suffix to E_a denotes the rate constant to which E_a is related.

It will be obvious that transition-state theory predicts an equation different from the Arrhenius' form, namely:

$$\frac{d \ln k_1}{dT} = \frac{1}{T} + \frac{E_a}{RT^2} = \frac{RT + E_a}{RT^2}. \tag{58}$$

As already mentioned, however, the term RT is generally negligible with respect to E_a.

It is clear that since $\overleftarrow{k}_D$, $\overrightarrow{k}_D$, and $\overleftarrow{k}_{tr}$ are temperature-dependent, this will also be true of $E_{a_{k_1}}$. In fact, the temperature-dependence of the activation energy (leading to a nonlinear Arrhenius' plot) is an indication of a complex reaction mechanism. Unfortunately, however, the temperature range that can be studied by kinetic methods is usually too narrow for this effect to be clearly demonstrable. The same is true of dependence on the concentration of the reactants, which, as we will see, is also often encountered in complex kinetics.

With respect to the preexponential factor (and thus also the activation entropy), matters are even more complicated. For example, if the same suffixes as were used in Equation (57), the preexponential factor of the rate constant under consideration would be represented by the following impractical equation:

$$A_{k_1} = \frac{A_{\overleftarrow{k}_D} A_{\overleftarrow{k}_{tr}} e^{(E_{a_{k_1}} - E_{a_{\overleftarrow{k}_D}} - E_{a_{\overleftarrow{k}_{tr}}})/RT}}{A_{\overleftarrow{k}_D} e^{-E_{a_{\overleftarrow{k}_D}}/RT} + A_{\overleftarrow{k}_{tr}} e^{-E_{a_{\overleftarrow{k}_{tr}}}/RT}}. \tag{59}$$

B. Energetics of Drug-Receptor Interaction

For drug-receptor interaction we assumed a first reversible diffusion-limited step followed by a much slower conformational change in the drug-receptor complex according to

$$D + R \underset{k_{-1}}{\overset{k_1}{\rightleftharpoons}} DR_1 \underset{k_{-2}}{\overset{k_2}{\rightleftharpoons}} DR_2. \tag{31}$$
$$\quad\quad \text{fast} \quad\quad\quad \text{slow}$$

The rate constants as estimated on the basis of this model by uptake or time-effect studies can be derived from a comparison of Equations (25), (26), and (41).

$$\overleftarrow{k}_{obs} = \frac{k_1 k_2}{k_1 [D] + k_{-1}} \tag{60}$$

and

$$\overleftarrow{k}_{obs} = k_{-2}, \tag{61}$$

which lead to

$$\vec{E}_a = E_{a_1} + E_{a_2} - \frac{k_1[D]E_{a_1} + k_{-1}E_{a-1}}{k_1[D] + k_{-1}},$$ (62)

$$\overleftarrow{E}_a = E_{a-2},$$ (63)

$$\vec{A} = \frac{A_1 A_2 e^{(\vec{E}_a - E_{a_1} - E_{a_2})/RT}}{A_1[D]e^{-E_{a_1}/RT} + A_{-1}e^{-E_{a-1}/RT}},$$ (64)

$$\overleftarrow{A} = A_{-2}.$$ (65)

Since $\overleftarrow{k}$ is an elementary rate constant under the experimental conditions, we can thus expect the energetics to exhibit straightforward behavior for the dissociation. For the association, however, the observed activation parameters can be related to real, elementary constants only with some additional assumptions. Normally both $\vec{E}_a$ and $\vec{A}$ are subject to temperature and concentration influences, although in the necessarily narrow ranges that are experimentally accessible this fundamental inconstancy can be obscured by the unfavorable relation between the experimental errors and the (small) observable changes. Nevertheless, it should be realized that treating the rate constant of association as a noncomplex one involves severe inaccuracies in the estimated activation parameters.

Unfortunately practically no data are available on the temperature-dependence of the rate constants involved in drug-receptor interaction. Only the interaction between the cholinergic antagonist lachesine and its receptor has been the subject of a preliminary study in this respect (PATON and RANG, 1966). Paton's uptake experiments at two different temperatures yield

$\vec{E}_a = 10\,\text{kcal/mol}$

$\overleftarrow{E}_a = 17\,\text{kcal/mol}$

$\vec{A} = 1.35\cdot 10^{14}$

$\overleftarrow{A} = 1.84\cdot 10^9.$

To start with the parameters for the backward reaction: the activation energy $\overleftarrow{E}_a$ of 17 kcal/mol is fully compatible with the idea that $\overleftarrow{k} = k_{-2}$, the rate constant of a conformational change (HAMMES, 1968; MORAWETZ, 1972).

The preexponential factor $\overleftarrow{A}$ can be analyzed according to transition-state theory to give a $\overleftarrow{\Delta S}^{\ddagger}$ (activation entropy) of -18.4 entropy units (EU), which also seems a reasonable value indicating that the transition state between DR_1 and DR_2 has a lower entropy content than the complex DR_2.

Problems arise with the assignation of a specific meaning to the observed, apparent parameters for the forward reaction. The apparent $\vec{E}_a$ of 10 kcal/mol is definitely higher than expected for a simple diffusion-controlled reaction, but could certainly be formed by the various contributions, as described in Equation (62). However, it has to be noted that the $\vec{E}_a$ of 10 kcal/mol has only limited significance, because of temperature and concentration restrictions. This is also true of the observed $\vec{A}$ value

$(1.35 \cdot 10^{14})$. The apparent $\vec{\Delta S}$ would be $+4$ EU, which would mean that going through the transition state the entropy would rise, which would certainly be strange for a simple bimolecular association (that is normally accompanied by loss of entropy). So we might conclude that also these parameters are more in line with the model of Scheme (31) than that of Scheme (17).

In extreme cases the expressions for the parameters of the forward reaction might also be reduced to much simpler equations.

1. When $k_1 D \gg k_{-1}$ the Equations (60), (62), and (64) become respectively:

$$\vec{k}_{obs} = \frac{k_2}{[D]}, \tag{66}$$

$$\vec{E}_a = E_{a_2}, \tag{67}$$

$$\vec{A} = \frac{A_2}{[D]}. \tag{68}$$

2. When $k_1 D \ll k_{-1}$ we get:

$$\vec{k}_{obs} = \frac{k_1 k_2}{k_{-1}}, \tag{69}$$

$$\vec{E}_a = E_{a_1} + E_{a_2} - E_{a_{-1}}, \tag{70}$$

$$\vec{A} = \frac{A_1 A_2}{A_{-1}}, \tag{71}$$

$$\text{or} \quad \vec{\Delta S}^{\ddagger} = \Delta S_1^{\ddagger} + \Delta S_2^{\ddagger} - \Delta S_{-1}^{\ddagger}. \tag{72}$$

The first extreme case can be expected to prevail at very high concentrations of the drug, which as has been shown actually implies that the observed reaction rate has become independent of the applied drug concentration. However, this is certainly not applicable to the data under consideration, since if it were the kinetics could not have been analyzed according to the bimolecular association model as it was by Paton and Rang (1966).

On the basis of the model of Scheme (31) such an analysis is only fruitful if it is confined strictly to cases in which extreme 2 prevails. It is quite conceivable that on the basis of Equation (70) an apparent activation energy of about 10 kcal/mol would arise. But the apparent entropy of activation, estimated at 4 EU, promises to be more interesting, though we can only speculate about it.

Equation (72) can also be written:

$$\vec{\Delta S}^{\ddagger} = \Delta S_1^0 + \Delta S_2^{\ddagger} \tag{73}$$

where ΔS_1^0 denotes the standard entropy difference between DR_1 and $D + R$.

We should assume that ΔS_1^0 was negative unless a rather high entropy gain were obtained by changes in solvation etc., and thus that $\Delta S_2^{\ddagger}$ was positive. The value of 4

EU is certainly not inconsistent with the mechanism. Whereas the assumption $k_1[D] \ll k_{-1}$ can be somewhat doubtful in the case of antagonists (for which k_{-1} is presumably rather small, cf. Sect. II), for agonists in normal concentration ranges it seems very plausible. At this point a comparison with Belleau's ideas (BELLEAU, 1965, 1967) seems pertinent. Belleau emphasizes the importance of entropy changes in drug-receptor interaction. According to his macromolecular-perturbation theory, antagonists give a nonspecific complex with the receptor characterized by a high degree of disorder (ΔS^0 is positive), whereas agonists do the opposite and partial agonists exhibit $\Delta S^0 \approx 0$.

It will be obvious that for the overall reaction as depicted in Scheme (31) the following expression is most significant:

$$\Delta S^0 = \overleftarrow{\Delta S}^{\ddagger} - \overrightarrow{\Delta S}^{\ddagger}. \tag{74}$$

For lachesine one can calculate from this that $\Delta S^0 = 22.4\,\mathrm{EU}$, which means that in this case the result is indeed consistent with Belleau's theory. Unfortunately, no data are available for agonists or partial agonists so that no further arguments can be obtained. In our denotation, macromolecular-perturbation theory predicts for agonists

$$\overrightarrow{\Delta S}^{\ddagger} < \overleftarrow{\Delta S}^{\ddagger}. \tag{75}$$

Since

$$\overrightarrow{\Delta S}^{\ddagger} = \frac{\left(\ln \overrightarrow{k} - \ln \dfrac{kT}{h}\right)RT + \overrightarrow{\Delta H}^{\ddagger}}{T} \tag{76}$$

and

$$\overleftarrow{\Delta S}^{\ddagger} = \frac{\left(\ln \overleftarrow{k} - \ln \dfrac{kT}{h}\right)RT + \overleftarrow{\Delta H}^{\ddagger}}{T} \tag{77}$$

we can write

$$RT\ln\overrightarrow{k} + \overrightarrow{\Delta H}^{\ddagger} < RT\ln\overleftarrow{k} + \overleftarrow{\Delta H}^{\ddagger} \quad \text{or} \quad RT\ln\frac{\overrightarrow{k}}{\overleftarrow{k}} < \overleftarrow{\Delta H}^{\ddagger} - \overrightarrow{\Delta H}^{\ddagger}. \tag{78}$$

Note that $\overleftarrow{\Delta H}^{\ddagger} - \overrightarrow{\Delta H}^{\ddagger} = \Delta H^0_{\mathrm{DR_2}} =$ standard enthalpy difference between $\mathrm{DR_2}$ and $\mathrm{D + R}$.

By substitution of Equations (60) and (61) into Equation (78) and rearrangement we obtain:

$$\frac{k_2}{k_{-2}} \frac{k_1}{k_1[D] + k_{-1}} < e^{(\overleftarrow{\Delta H}^{\ddagger} - \overrightarrow{\Delta H}^{\ddagger})/RT} \tag{79}$$

and thus for antagonists

$$\frac{k_2}{k_{-2}} \frac{k_1}{k_1[D] + k_{-1}} > e^{(\overleftarrow{\Delta H}^{\ddagger} - \overrightarrow{\Delta H}^{\ddagger})/RT}. \tag{80}$$

This means that according to Belleau's theory, the terms $\dfrac{k_2}{k_{-2}}\dfrac{k_1}{k_1[D]+k_{-1}}$ for agonists cannot exceed a certain maximum value whereas for antagonists the ratio cannot be smaller than a certain minimum. This is highly interesting especially since presumably the factor $\dfrac{k_1}{k_1[D]+k_{-1}}$ does not differ greatly for agonist and antagonist as argued before on the basis of the kinetics of the elementary steps. Therefore the difference in the limitations of the kinetic constants for agonists and antagonists as given by Equation (79) should reside largely in the equilibrium constant $\dfrac{k_2}{k_{-2}}$ for the isomerization step $DR_1 \rightleftharpoons DR_2$. One possible explanation is that antagonists have a larger k_2 and/or a smaller k_{-2} than agonists which is quite conceivable on the basis of the differences in chemical structure between agonists and antagonists and thus in the nature of the complex formed. One might even expect this difference to occur since only then the common idea that the agonistic complex is more easily reversible than the antagonistic can be incorporated in the kind of model where the rate limiting steps are on the level of conformational changes.

This discussion is quite straightforward if $\Delta H^0_{DR_2}$ for agonists and antagonists is about the same, but it should be realized that differences in this state function have profound influences on the argumentation.

When we consider, for instance, two equilibria with equilibrium constants K_1 and K_2, then the following relationship is obvious from simple thermodynamics

$$\Delta S^0_1 - \Delta S^0_2 = \frac{\Delta H^0_1 - \Delta H^0_2}{T} + R \ln \frac{K_1}{K_2}. \tag{81}$$

This means that a difference in ΔS^0 of, e.g., 20 EU in the case of equal ΔH^0 means that the ratio $K_1/K_2 \approx 2.2 \cdot 10^4$ whereas the same difference in ΔS^0 is obtained at a ratio $K_1/K_2 = 1$, when $\Delta H^0_1 - \Delta H^0_2 = 6$ kcal/mol ($T = 300$ K).

In conclusion it should be stated that for the moment this type of analysis is highly speculative and that extreme caution is necessary. When more and reliable data become available, however, study of the energetics of drug receptor interaction can give deeper insight in the underlying mechanisms. Three more remarks can be made:

1. The above considerations can also be applied to the drug-receptor mechanism with a very rapid isomerization step. It would be very difficult to obtain arguments in favor of Equation (38) or Equation (41) in this way, but as we have seen, the last mechanism is much less plausible on other grounds. With the simplest model, ignoring conformational changes in the drug-receptor complex, difficulties would certainly be encountered in attempts to give a suitable basis for the energetics as proposed by Belleau's macromolecular-perturbation theory and for the data that have been reported by Paton.

2. It will be very difficult, if not impossible, to study the energetics of drug-receptor interaction (which could give actual insight in the mechanism of the reaction) adequately in the necessarily narrow temperature and concentration ranges that are experimentally accessible. Totally wrong conclusions may be drawn regarding the

kinetic mechanism on the basis of measurements in this narrow range of circumstances where the data will nearly always fit one simple model or another.

3. Although there may be no a priori reason why interactions between small molecules and macromolecules could not be well described by transition-state theory, it seems questionable whether the estimated parameters actually bear significance from the thermodynamic point of view. It is well known that the structure of biomacromolecules is very sensitive to changes in temperature (and other external variables).

BLYUMENFELD (1971) therefore discussed the possibility that the energetic parameters measured in enzymology are actually artefacts. According to this theory, the following relation is valid in the narrow temperature interval that can be studied:

$$E_{a,a} = E_{a,r} + bT, \tag{82}$$

where $E_{a,a}$ = apparent (measured) activation energy
$E_{a,r}$ = real activation energy
b = temperature-sensitivity factor.

The expression for the rate constant in terms of transition-state theory then becomes:

$$k = \frac{e\kappa T}{h} e^{\Delta S^{\ddagger}/R} e^{b/R} e^{-E_{a,a}/RT}. \tag{83}$$

In other words, the measured activation energy is higher than the real one by the amount bT, but on the other hand the apparent activation entropy also becomes higher than the real value $(\Delta S^{\ddagger}_{app} = \Delta S^{\ddagger} + b)$.

This would be some artificial compensation effect (in contrast to real compensation, which is encountered in several series of allied chemical reactions). It is evident that such complications greatly reduce the thermodynamic meaning of the estimated parameters, although it is certainly still possible that the reactions in question can be formally described by transition-state theory (see also SIDORENKO, 1972).

Finally, it should be borne in mind that the the discussion of the energetics is not restricted to the specific mechanism to which it has been applied. There are several other mechanisms taking receptor-isomerizations that cannot be discriminated from a kinetic or energetic point of view (see also Appendix) into account.

Appendix

The general solution of a kinetic receptor model proceeds as follows (see for instance RESCIGNO and SEGRE, 1961).

Suppose the system:

$$D + R_1 \underset{k_2}{\overset{k_1}{\rightleftharpoons}} DR_2 \ldots \underset{k_{2i-2}}{\overset{k_{2i-3}}{\rightleftharpoons}} DR_i \underset{k_{2i}}{\overset{k_{2i-1}}{\rightleftharpoons}} \ldots \underset{k_{2n-2}}{\overset{k_{2n-3}}{\rightleftharpoons}} DR_n \overset{k_{2n-1}}{\rightarrow} D + R_1 . \quad (A.1)$$

$$\frac{d[R_1]}{dt} = -k_1[DR_1] + k_2[DR_2] + k_{2n-1}[DR_n]$$

$$\frac{d[DR_2]}{dt} = k_1[DR_1] - (k_2 + k_3)[DR_2] + k_4[DR_3]$$

$$\frac{d[DR_i]}{dt} = k_{2i-3}[DR_{i-1}] - (k_{2i-2} + k_{2i-1})[DR_i] + k_{2i}[DR_{i+1}]$$

$$\frac{d[DR_n]}{dt} = k_{2n-3}[DR_{n-1}] - (k_{2n-2} + k_{2n-1})[DR_n]$$

$$(A.2)$$

with the boundary condition

$$t = 0, \quad [R_1] = [R_T], \quad [DR_i] = 0,$$

where $[R_1]$ = concentration of free receptors
$[DR_i]$ = concentration of drug-receptor complex DR_i
$[R_T]$ = total receptor concentration.

Assuming that during the process of drug-receptor interaction the concentration $[D]$ remains unchanged, this set of equations is most easily solvable by use of Laplace transformation. Upon Laplace transformation (with the transform of $[R_1] = x_1$, of $[DR_i] = x_i$ and of $[R_T] = x_0$) one obtains:

$$Sx_1 - x_0 = -k_1[D]x_1 + k_2 x_2 + k_{2n-1}x_n$$
$$Sx_2 = k_1[D]x_1 - (k_2 + k_3)x_2 + k_4 x_3$$
$$\ldots \ldots$$
$$Sx_i = k_{2i-3}x_{i-1} - (k_{2i-2} + k_{2i-1})x_i + k_{2i}x_{i+1}$$
$$\ldots \ldots$$
$$Sx_n = k_{2n-3}x_{n-1} - (k_{2n-2} + k_{2n-1})x_n , \quad (A.3)$$

where S is a real or complex number according to Laplace's theory. According to Cramer's rule the solution of such a set of equations becomes:

$$\frac{x_i}{x_0} = (-1)^{i+1} \frac{\Delta_{1,i}}{\Delta} , \quad (A.4)$$

where Δ is the determinant of the set of Equations (A.3) and $\Delta_{1,i}$ is the determinant which is obtained from Δ by deleting the first row and the ith column.

It can easily be shown that this general solution here takes the form:

$$\frac{x_i}{x_0} = \frac{\lambda_i S^{n-i} + \lambda_{i+1} S^{n-(i+1)} + \lambda_{i+2} S^{n-(i+2)} + \ldots + \lambda_n}{S(S^{n-1} + \mu_2 S^{n-2} + \mu_3 S^{n-3} + \mu_4 S^{n-4} + \ldots + \mu_n)}, \quad (A.5)$$

where the λ's and μ's are constants.

The solution for $\dfrac{[DR_i]}{[R_T]}$ is the antitransform of this equation and can be very complex but will often be a series of n exponential terms. For large systems, the mathematics becomes very complicated. Relatively small systems, however, can easily be described this way, as will be shown in the rest of this appendix.

General kinetic description of Scheme (31)

$$D + R \underset{k_{-1}}{\overset{k_1}{\rightleftarrows}} DR_1 \underset{k_{-2}}{\overset{k_2}{\rightleftarrows}} DR_2. \quad (A.6)$$

The kinetic behaviour in this system is governed by the following simultaneous differential equations:

$$\frac{d[DR_1]}{dt} = k_1[D][R] + k_{-2}[DR_2] - (k_{-1} + k_2)[DR_1], \quad (A.7)$$

$$\frac{d[DR_2]}{dt} = k_2[DR_1] - k_{-2}[DR_2] \quad (A.8)$$

By substituting $[R] = [R_T] - [DR_1] - [DR_2]$ and by indicating the Laplace transforms of $[DR_1]$ and $[DR_2]$ with x_1 and x_2 we obtain:

$$Sx_1 = \frac{k_1[D][R_T]}{S} - (k_{-1} + k_2 + k_1[D])x_1 + (k_{-2} - k_1[D])x_2 \quad (A.9)$$

$$Sx_2 = k_2 x_1 - k_{-2} x_2. \quad (A.10)$$

The solution of this system in the form of its Laplace transform becomes:

$$x_1 = \frac{Sk_1[D][R_T] + k_1 k_{-2}[D][R_T]}{S[S^2 + S(k_{-1} + k_{-2} + k_2 + k_1[D]) + k_{-1}k_{-2} + k_1 k_{-2}[D] + k_1 k_2[D]]} \quad (A.11)$$

and

$$x_2 = \frac{k_1 k_2[D][R_T]}{S[S^2 + S(k_{-1} + k_{-2} + k_2 + k_1[D]) + k_{-1}k_{-2} + k_1 k_{-2}[D] + k_1 k_2[D]]} \quad (A.12)$$

The form of the antitransforms of Equations (A.11) and (A.12) depends upon the value of the discriminant of the quadratic equation between the brackets in the denominator.

This discriminant, which is given by $(k_{-1}+k_{-2}+k_2+k_1[D])^2 - 4(k_{-1}k_{-2}+k_1k_{-2}[D]+k_1k_2[D]) = (k_{-1}+k_1[D]-k_2-k_{-2})^2 + 4k_{-1}k_2$, will always be ≥ 0.

The case that the discriminant is equal to 0 is not relevant here, since that would require that at least k_{-1} or k_2 be 0.

Therefore the general solutions can be written as:

$$\frac{[DR_1]}{[R_T]} = \frac{\dfrac{k_{-2}}{k_2+k_{-2}}}{1+\dfrac{k_{-2}}{k_2+k_{-2}}\cdot\dfrac{k_{-1}}{k_1}\dfrac{1}{[D]}} + k_1[D]\left\{\frac{b-k_{-2}}{b(a-b)}e^{-bt} - \frac{a-k_{-2}}{a(a-b)}e^{-at}\right\}$$

(A.13)

and

$$\frac{[DR_2]}{[R_T]} = \frac{\dfrac{k_2}{k_2+k_{-2}}}{1+\dfrac{k_{-2}}{k_2+k_{-2}}\dfrac{k_{-1}}{k_1}\dfrac{1}{[D]}} + k_1k_2[D]\left\{\frac{1}{a(a-b)}e^{-at} - \frac{1}{b(a-b)}e^{-bt}\right\}$$

(A.14)

where

$$(S+a)(S+b) = S^2 + S(k_{-1}+k_{-2}+k_2+k_1[D]) + k_{-1}k_{-2}+k_1k_{-2}[D] + k_1k_2[D].$$

(A.15)

It can easily be derived that the expression for $\dfrac{[DR_2]}{[R_T]}$ is always a gradually increasing function, without a transient maximum or minum, ultimately reaching an equilibrium value.

This is not always the case for $\dfrac{[DR_1]}{[R_T]}$: as long as $k_{-2} < k_1[D]$ here at a time t

$= \dfrac{1}{a-b}\ln\dfrac{a-k_{-2}}{b-k_{-2}}$ a maximum is reached after which the concentration $[DR_1]$ declines to an equilibrium value, in other words $[DR_1]$ shows a "fade" phenomenon.

It should be noticed that Equations (A.13) and (A.14) have a very similar form, and that it will be extremely difficult to diffentiate between these two. The most important difference, which might be revealed only by kinetic measurements, is the occurrence of a transient maximum in $[DR_1]$ which is absent in $[DR_2]$, but which only will be found when $k_{-2} < k_1[D]$.

The extreme cases which are discussed in the text obviously do not show this fading.

Starting from the model with a very rapid association followed by a much slower conformational change to an active receptor, it is interesting to see what the implications are of assuming a second conformational change or a dissociation of DR_2 directly.

1. $D+R \underset{k_{-1}}{\overset{k_1}{\rightleftarrows}} DR_1 \underset{k_{-2}}{\overset{k_2}{\rightleftarrows}} DR_2 \underset{k_{-3}}{\overset{k_3}{\rightleftarrows}} DR_3$. $\qquad\qquad$ (A.16)

$\qquad\qquad$ fast $\quad$ inactive $\;$ slow $\;$ active $\;$ slow $\;$ inactive

Assuming that the first equilibrium is very fast with regard to the second and third one, it can easily be shown, analogously to the above, that receptor activation in this model proceeds as:

$$\frac{[DR_2]}{[R_T]} = \frac{\dfrac{k_2 k_{-3}}{k_{-2}k_{-3}+k_2 k_{-3}+k_2 k_3}}{1+\dfrac{k_2 k_{-3}}{k_{-2}k_{-3}+k_2 k_{-3}+k_2 k_3}\ \dfrac{k_{-1}k_{-2}}{k_1 k_2}\ \dfrac{1}{[D]}}$$
$$+\frac{k_2}{1+\dfrac{k_{-1}}{k_1}\ \dfrac{1}{[D]}}\left\{\frac{d-k_{-3}}{d(c-d)}\,e^{-dt}-\frac{c-k_{-3}}{c(c-d)}\,e^{-ct}\right\}$$

(A.17)

with

$$(S+c)(S+d)=S^2+S\left(k_3+k_{-2}+k_{-3}+\frac{k_1 k_2[D]}{k_{-1}+k_1[D]}\right)$$

(A.18)

$$+k_{-2}k_{-3}+\frac{k_1 k_2 k_{-3}[D]+k_1 k_2 k_3[D]}{k_{-1}+k_1[D]}\ .$$

Now, $[DR_2]$ also shows a transient maximum at $t=\dfrac{1}{c-d}\ \ln\dfrac{c-k_{-3}}{d-k_{-3}}$ $\Big($ provided that $k_{-3}<\dfrac{k_1 k_2[D]}{k_{-1}+k_1[D]}\Big)$ whereas $[DR_3]$ in this case increases gradually to its equilibrium value. Clearly this model is very attractive in combining the features discussed in the text with a plausible explanation of possible fade phenomena.

2. $D+R\underset{k_{-1}}{\overset{k_1}{\rightleftharpoons}}DR_1\underset{k_{-2}}{\overset{k_2}{\rightleftharpoons}}\underset{\text{active}}{DR_2}\overset{k_3}{\to}D+R\ .$ (A.19)

The Laplace transform $f(S)$ for the general solution of the time dependence of $[DR_2]$ in this system becomes:

$$f(S)=\frac{k_1 k_2[D][R_T]}{S[S^2+(k_1[D]+k_{-1}+k_2+k_{-2}+k_3)S+k_1 k_2[D]+k_1 k_{-2}[D]+k_1 k_3[D]+k_{-1}k_{-2}+k_{-1}k_3+k_2 k_3]}$$

(A.20)

Here the discriminant of the quadratic equation in the denominator is:

$$(k_1[D]+k_{-1}+k_2+k_{-2}+k_3)^2-4(k_1 k_2[D]+k_1 k_{-2}[D]+k_1 k_3[D]+k_{-1}k_{-2}$$
$$+k_{-1}k_3+k_2 k_3)$$

(A.21)

$$=(k_1[D]+k_{-1}-k_2-k_{-2}-k_3)^2+4k_2(k_{-1}-k_{-3})\ .$$

Therefore the solution for $[DR_2]$ can have three different forms:

a) When the discriminant >0, which will be the case when $k_3<k_{-1}+\dfrac{1}{4k_2}(k_1[D]$ $+k_{-1}-k_2-k_{-2}-k_3)^2$:

$$\frac{[DR_2]}{[R_T]}=\frac{\dfrac{k_2}{k_2+k_{-2}+k_3}}{1+\dfrac{k_{-1}k_{-2}+k_{-1}k_3+k_2 k_3}{k_1 k_2+k_1 k_{-2}+k_1 k_3}\ \dfrac{1}{[D]}}+k_1 k_2[D]\left[\frac{1}{a(a-b)}e^{-at}-\frac{1}{b(a-b)}e^{-bt}\right]$$

(A.22)

where

$$(S+a)(S+b)=S^2+S(k_1[D]+k_{-1}+k_2+k_{-2}+k_3)+k_1k_2[D]$$
$$+k_1k_{-2}[D]+k_1k_3[D]+k_{-1}k_{-2}+k_{-1}k_3+k_2k_3. \tag{A.23}$$

Clearly this solution cannot easily be differentiated from Equation (A.14).

b) When the discriminant $=0$, so when $k_3=k_{-1}+\dfrac{1}{4k_2}(k_1[D]+k_{-1}-k_2-k_{-2}-k_3)^2$

$$\frac{[DR_2]}{[R_T]}=\frac{\dfrac{k_2}{k_2+k_{-2}+k_3}}{1+\dfrac{k_{-1}k_{-2}+k_{-1}k_3+k_2k_3}{k_1k_2+k_1k_{-2}+k_1k_3}\dfrac{1}{[D]}}[1-e^{-at}-at\,e^{-at}] \tag{A.24}$$

where

$$a=\sqrt{k_1k_2[D]+k_1k_{-2}[D]+k_1k_3[D]+k_{-1}k_{-2}+k_{-1}k_3+k_2k_3} \tag{A.25}$$

c) When the discriminant <0, an oscillatory function will arise for $[DR_2]$. Obviously this would require $k_3>k_{-1}+\dfrac{1}{4k_2}(k_1[D]+k_{-1}-k_2-k_{-2}-k_3)^2$.

The general solution then will be:

$$\frac{[DR_2]}{[R_T]}=\frac{\dfrac{k_2}{k_2+k_{-2}+k_3}}{1+\dfrac{k_{-1}k_{-2}+k_{-1}k_3+k_2k_3}{k_1k_2+k_1k_{-2}+k_1k_3}\dfrac{1}{[D]}}\left[1-e^{-at}\cos bt-\frac{a}{b}e^{-at}\sin bt\right] \tag{A.26}$$

where $a=1/2(k_1[D]+k_{-1}+k_2+k_{-2}+k_3)$

$$a^2+b^2=k_1k_2[D]+k_1k_{-2}[D]+k_1k_3[D]+k_{-1}k_{-2}+k_{-1}k_3+k_2k_3. \tag{A.27}$$

This type of solution is analysed in detail elsewhere in this volume (Chap. 6, Gosselin).

It should be noted that when, for instance, k_{-2} is set equal to 0 (as in Gosselin's model), the same solutions arise, which cannot be experimentally differentiated. On the other hand it is obvious that somewhat more complicated models also will lead to solutions that are formally indiscernable from the ones given here. Damped oscillatory behaviour can only arise when a model contains a cyclic process where the activated receptor can be regenerated directly by another way than that which activation occurs.

Recently Ariëns (1974) referred to this type of model to explain semiquantitatively the contribution of different parameters to a drug's intrinsic activity. It will be obvious from the equations given here and in the text that in most models the kinetic parameters, drug-dependent or -independent, governing the conformational changes in the receptor, contribute to its so-called intrinsic activity. On the other hand in most cases the apparent affinity includes a factor which is very similar to the "kinetic" part of the intrinsic activity. True differentiation between "affinity" and "intrinsic activity" will not be possible in most cases.

It is interesting to see what will happen when the association equilibrium $D + R \rightleftharpoons DR_1$ is assumed to be very fast with respect to the other steps in Scheme (A.16).

The assumption that during the reaction, $k_1[D][R] = k_{-1}[DR_1]$ is always valid leads very simply to the following expression:

$$\frac{[DR_2]}{[R_T]} = \frac{\dfrac{k_2}{k_2 + k_{-2} + k_3}}{1 + \dfrac{k_{-1}k_{-2} + k_{-1}k_3}{k_1k_2 + k_1k_{-2} + k_1k_3} \dfrac{1}{[D]}} \left(1 - e^{-\left(k_2 \frac{[D]}{\frac{k_{-1}}{k_1} + [D]} + k_{-2} + k_3\right)t}\right). \tag{A.28}$$

As could be expected, this equation is formally equal to Equation (40) in the text, which means that under the assumption of a fast first association-dissociation step, this model would only explain "fade" if yet another intermediate receptor form between the activated and regenerated one is enclosed.

One might argue about the necessity of explaining this fade phenomenon, but it is clear that occupation models can very easily give a mathematical basis for it, by predicting both transient maxima and damped oscillations in certain cases (cf. GOSSELIN, this volume Chap. 6).

If now, instead of DR_2, DR_1 is taken as the active receptor form, one obtains the following solution (in Laplace form):

$$f(S) = \frac{k_1[D][R_T]S + (k_1k_{-2}[D] + k_1k_3[D])R_T}{S[S^2 + (k_1[D] + k_{-1} + k_2 + k_{-2} + k_3)S + k_1k_2[D] + k_1k_{-2}[D] + k_1k_3[D] + k_{-1}k_{-2} + k_{-1}k_3 + k_2k_3]} \tag{A.29}$$

which leads to

a) when $k_3 < k_{-1} + \dfrac{1}{4k_2}(k_1[D] + k_{-1} - k_2 - k_{-2} - k_3)^2$

$$\frac{[DR_1]}{[R_T]} = \frac{k_{-2} + \dfrac{k_3}{k_2 + k_{-2} + k_3}}{1 + \dfrac{k_{-1}k_{-2} + k_{-1}k_3 + k_2k_3}{k_1k_2 + k_1k_{-2} + k_1k_3} \dfrac{1}{[D]}}$$

$$+ k_1[D]\left[\frac{b - k_{-2} - k_3}{b(a-b)} e^{-bt} - \frac{a - k_{-2} - k_3}{a(a-b)} e^{-at}\right] \tag{A.30}$$

where a and b are the same as in Equation (A.23).

This function is formally indiscernable from Equation (A.13), and shows also a transient maximum when $k_{-2} + k_3 < k_1[D]$;

b) when $k_3 = k_{-1} + \dfrac{1}{4k_2}(k_1[D] + k_{-1} - k_2 - k_{-2} - k_3)^2$

$$\frac{[DR_1]}{[R_T]} = \frac{k_{-2} + \dfrac{k_3}{k_2 + k_{-2} + k_3}}{1 + \dfrac{k_{-1}k_{-2} + k_{-1}k_3 + k_2k_3}{k_1k_2 + k_1k_{-2} + k_1k_3} \dfrac{1}{[D]}} (1 - e^{-at}) + \frac{k_1[D](a - k_{-2} - k_3)}{a} t e^{-at} \tag{A.31}$$

where a has the same meaning as in Equation (A.25).

c) When $k_3 > k_{-1} + \dfrac{1}{4k_2}(k_1[D] + k_{-1} - k_2 - k_{-2} - k_3)^2$

$$\frac{[DR_1]}{[R_T]} = \frac{k_{-2} + \dfrac{k_3}{k_2 + k_{-2} + k_3}}{1 + \dfrac{k_{-1}k_{-2} + k_{-1}k_3 + k_2 k_3}{k_1 k_2 + k_1 k_{-2} + k_1 k_3}\dfrac{1}{[D]}}(1 - e^{-at}\cos bt)$$
$$+ \frac{k_1[D]}{b}\left(1 - \frac{a(k_{-2} + k_3)}{b(a^2 + b^2)}\ e^{-at}\sin bt\right) \tag{A.32}$$

where a and b have the same definition as in Equation (A.27).

Del Castillo and Katz (1957) and Katz and Thesleff (1957) proposed several possible models for drug receptor interaction. The kinetics of some of these models, viz., those with successive isomerisation steps, have already been discussed in this appendix. They also mentioned a model with two simultaneous drug receptor interactions

$$D + R \underset{\searrow DR_2}{\overset{\nearrow DR_1}{\rightleftarrows}} \tag{A.33}$$

where one of the two complexes is active and the other inactive, thus accounting for desensitization phenomena, when the active one is formed in a fast and the inactive one in a slower equilibration step. This model can easily be elaborated mathematically, and one obtains:

$$\frac{[DR_1]}{[R_T]} = \frac{\dfrac{k_1 k_{-2}}{k_{-1}k_2 + k_1 k_{-2}}}{1 + \dfrac{k_{-1}k_2}{k_{-1}k_2 + k_1 k_{-2}}\dfrac{1}{[D]}} + k_1[D]\left[\frac{b - k_{-2}}{b(a - b)}e^{-bt} - \frac{a - k_{-2}}{a(a - b)}e^{-at}\right], \tag{A.34}$$

$$\frac{[DR_2]}{[R_T]} = \frac{\dfrac{k_{-1}k_2}{k_{-1}k_2 + k_1 k_{-2}}}{1 + \dfrac{k_{-1}k_2}{k_{-1}k_2 + k_1 k_{-2}}\dfrac{1}{[D]}} + k_2[D]\left[\frac{b - k_{-1}}{b(a - b)}e^{-bt} - \frac{a - k_{-1}}{a(a - b)}e^{-at}\right] \tag{A.35}$$

where

$$(S + a)(S + b) = S^2 + S(k_1[D] + k_{-1} + k_2[D] + k_{-2}) + k_1 k_{-2}[D] + k_{-1}k_2[D] \tag{A.36}$$
$$+ k_{-1}k_{-2}.$$

The form of these equations is the same as that of Equations (A.13–14) so that this model can hardly be distinguished from model (A.6), even by kinetic measurements.

Indeed these equations predict transient maxima. $[DR_1]$ will show a transient maximum as long as $k_{-2} < k_{-1}$, $[DR_2]$ when $k_{-2} > k_{-1}$. So a transient maximum in one of the complexes implies that the other one exhibits a gradually increasing concentration. Therefore when for instance DR_1 is the active receptor conformation k_{-2} must be smaller than k_{-1} to account for fade, etc., while the relative magnitudes of k_1 and k_2 are not relevant in this respect.

When a direct isomerisation between DR_1 and DR_2 is allowed, so that we get

$$D + R \underset{\displaystyle DR_2}{\overset{\displaystyle DR_1}{\rightleftharpoons}} \qquad (A.37)$$

the same kinetic behaviour is predicted, only the overall rate constants and the equilibrium value become more complex, since the isomerisation rate constants also have to be incorporated.

A more complex kinetic behaviour arises when the free receptor is assumed to exist in two different conformational states, each of which can combine with the drug.

Two such models have been proposed and elaborated to some extent in the literature. KATZ and THESLEFF (1957), on the basis of thermodynamic considerations and to explain desensitization and S-shaped dose-effect curves, regarded the following scheme as an acceptable alternative:

$$D + \quad \begin{array}{c} R_1 \rightleftharpoons DR_1 \\ \updownarrow \qquad \updownarrow \\ R_2 \rightleftharpoons DR_2 \end{array} \qquad (A.38)$$

Changeux (1967) proposed an allosteric model

$$D + \quad \begin{array}{c} R_1 \rightleftharpoons DR_1 \\ \updownarrow \\ R_2 \rightleftharpoons DR_2 \end{array} \qquad (A.39)$$

in which the stimulus to the ultimate effect is dependent upon the shift in receptor conformation.

These two models are very similar, and have the same complexity and the same possibilities. It is very easy to calculate all equilibrium values for each of the reactants or combinations of reactants in these schemes, but a full kinetic analysis is difficult. Of course, the general procedure of Appendix I can be applied and one can predict that mostly three exponential time-dependent terms plus a fourth constant term are needed.

However, it will be very difficult if not impossible to express the overall kinetic parameters like the rate constants in terms of the 8 and 6 respective elementary rate constants of Schemes (A.38) and (A.39).

Furchgott (1964) tried to account for the existence of diffusional barriers on the way of the drug to its receptor and assuming first-order diffusion kinetics he formulated the scheme

$$D_0 \underset{k_{i0}}{\overset{k_{0i}}{\rightleftharpoons}} D_i + R \underset{k_{-1}}{\overset{k_1}{\rightleftharpoons}} DR \tag{A.40}$$

where D_0 = drug in the bath

D_i = drug in the receptor compartment.

In general this model cannot be solved analytically, since it requires nonlinear differential equations. Two extreme cases, however, can readily be described (Furchgott, 1964).

1. When $D_0 \rightleftharpoons D_i$ is very fast with respect to receptor combination $[D_i]$ $= \dfrac{k_{0i}}{k_{i0}} [D_0]$ will always be valid, so that we may write

$$\frac{d[DR]}{dt} = k_1 \frac{k_{0i}}{k_{i0}} [D_0]([R_T] - [DR]) - k_{-1}[DR] . \tag{A.41}$$

Assuming that $[D_0]$ is equal to the applied bath concentration $[D]$ (so not altered by distribution), one arrives at

$$\frac{[DR]}{[R_T]} = \frac{1}{1 + \dfrac{k_{i0}}{k_{0i}} \dfrac{k_{-1}}{k_1} \dfrac{1}{[D]}} \left[1 - e^{-\left(k_1 \frac{k_{0i}}{k_{i0}} [D] + k_{-1} \right)} \right] \tag{A.42}$$

which is very similar to Equation (24) in the text, the only difference being that the apparent association rate constant k_1 and the apparent association constant $\dfrac{k_1}{k_{-1}}$ are a factor $\dfrac{k_{0i}}{k_{i0}}$ higher.

2. When drug receptor combination is very fast with respect to the barrier passage, $k_1[D_1][R] = k_{-1}[DR]$ is always valid and one obtains

$$[D_i] = \frac{k_{i0}}{k_{0i}} [D_0] (1 - e^{-k_{i0}t}) \tag{A.43}$$

and assuming $[D_0] = [D]$ this leads to

$$\frac{[DR]}{[R_T]} = \frac{1}{1 - e^{-k_{i0}t} + \dfrac{k_{i0}}{k_{0i}} \dfrac{k_{-1}}{k_1} \dfrac{1}{[D]}} (1 - e^{-k_{i0}t}) . \tag{A.44}$$

This relationship shows that when diffusion of the drug through a barrier is rate limiting, it would be primarily the rate constant of back-diffusion which determines the time course of receptor occupation.

References

Albuquerque, E. X., Sokoll, M. D., Sonesson, B., Thesleff, S.: Studies on the nature of the cholinergic receptor. Europ. J. Pharmacol. **4**, 40—46 (1968).

Amdur, I., Hammes, G. G.: Chemical kinetics. Principles and selected topics. New York-St. Louis-San Francisco-Toronto-London-Sidney: McGraw-Hill Book Comp., Inc. 1966.

Ariëns, E. J.: Molecular Pharmacology, Vol. I. New York: Academic Press 1964.

Ariëns, E. J.: Drug levels in the target tissue and effect. Clin. Pharmacol. Ther. **16**, 155—176 (1974).

Bartels, E.: Reactions of the acetylcholine receptor and esterase studies on the electroplax. Biochem. Pharm. **17**, 945—966 (1968).

Beckett, A. H., Casey, A. F.: Analgesics and Their Antagonists: Biochemical aspects and structure activity relationships. In: Ellis, G. P., West, G. B. (Eds.): Progress in Medicinal Chemistry, 4. London: Butterworths 1965, pp. 171—218.

Belleau, B.: A molecular theory of drug action based on induced conformational perturbations of receptors. J. med. Chem. **7**, 776—784 (1964).

Belleau, B.: Conformational perturbation in relation to the regulation of enzyme receptor behaviour. In: Harper, N. J., Simmonds, A. B. (Eds.): Advances in Drug Research Vol. 2. London: Academic Press 1965, pp. 89—126.

Belleau, B.: Water as the determinant of thermodynamic transitions in the interaction of aliphatic chains with acetylcholinesterase and the cholinergic receptors. Ann. N. Y. Acad. Sci. **144**, 705—719 (1967).

Belleau, B., Lacasse, G.: Aspects of the chemical mechanism of complex formation between acetylcholinesterase and acetylcholine-related compounds. J. med. Chem. **7**, 768—775 (1964).

Benson, S. W.: The foundations of chemical kinetics. New York-Toronto-London: McGraw-Hill Book Comp. Inc. 1960.

Bloomfield, V., Peller, L., Alberty, R. A.: Multiple intermediates in steady-state enzyme kinetics. III. Analysis of the kinetics of some reactions catalyzed by dehydrogenases. J. Amer. chem. Soc. **84**, 4375—4381 (1962).

Blumenfeld, L. A.: Activation parameters of enzymatic reactions (applicability of the theory of the activated complex in enzymology). Biofizika **16**, 724—727 (1971).

Burgen, A. S. V.: The role of ionic interaction at the muscarinic receptor. Brit. J. Pharmacol. **25**, 4—17 (1965).

Burgen, A. S. V.: The drug-receptor complex. J. Pharm. Pharmacol. **18**, 137—149 (1966).

Caldin, E. F.: Fast reactions in solution. New York: Wiley 1964.

Castillo, J. del., Katz, B.: On the localization of acetylcholine receptors. J. Physiol. (Lond.) **128**, 157—181 (1955).

Cathou, R. E., Hammes, G. G.: Relaxation spectra of ribonuclease. III. J. Amer. chem. Soc. **87**, 4674—4680 (1965).

Chance, B.: The enzyme-substrate compounds of horseradish peroxidase and peroxides. II. Kinetics of formation and decomposition of the primary and secondary complexes. Arch. Biochem. **22**, 224—252 (1949).

Changeux, J.-P.: Remarks on the symmetry and cooperative properties of biological membranes. Proc. 11th Nobel Symposium, Stockholm 1968, pp. 235—256. New York: Wiley Interscience Div. 1970

Changeux, J.-P., Podleski, T. R.: On the excitability and cooperativity of the electroplax membrane. Biochemistry **59**, 944—950 (1968).

Changeux, J.-P., Thiéry, J., Tung, Y., Kittel, C.: On the cooperativity of biological membranes. Proc. nat. Acad. Sci. (Wash.) **57**, 335—341 (1967).

Clark, A. J.: General Pharmacology. In: Heubner, W., Schüller, J. (Eds.): Heffters Handbuch der Experimentelle Pharmakologie. Berlin: Springer 1937.

Crank, J.: The Mathematics of Diffusion. London: Oxford University Press 1957.

Crothers, D. M.: The kinetics of DNA denaturation. J. molec. Biol. **9**, 712—733 (1964).

Cuatrecasas, P.: Insulin-receptor interactions in adipose tissue cells: direct measurement and properties. Proc. nat. Acad. Sci. (Wash.) **68**, 1264—1268 (1971).

Cuthbert, A. W., Dunant, Y.: Diffusion of drugs through stationary water layers as the rate limiting process in their action at membrane receptors. Brit. J. Pharmacol. **40**, 508—521 (1970).

Czerlinski, G. H.: Two ternary complexes of liver alcohol dehydrogenase with reduced diphosphopyridine nucleotide and the inhibitor imidazole. Biochem. Biophys. Acta (Amst.) **64**, 199—201 (1962).

Czerlinski, G. H.: Chemical Relaxation. New York: Marcel Dekker Inc. 1966.

Czerlinski, G. H., Malkewitz, J.: Chemical relaxation spectrum of glutamac aspartic aminotransferase/erythro-β-hydroxyaspartate. Biochemistry **4**, 1127—1131 (1965).

Czerlinski, G. H., Schreck, G.: Fluorescence detection of the chemical relaxation of the reaction of lactate dehydrogenase with reduced nicotinamide adeninedinucleotide. J. biol. Chem. **239**, 913—918 (1964).

Day, L. A., Sturtevant, J. M., Singer, S. J.: The kinetics of the reactions between antibodies to the 2,4-dinitrophenol group and specific haptens. Ann. N. Y. Acad. Sci. **103**, 611—625 (1963).

Debye, P.: Reaction rates in ionic solutions. Trans. Amer. Electrochem. Soc. **82**, 265—272 (1942).

Deshcherevskii, V. I., Zhabotinskii, A. M., Sel'kov, Ye. Ye., Sidorenko, N. P., Shnol', S. E.: Oscillatory biological processes at the molecular level. Biofizika **15**, 225—234 (1970).

Ebert, M.: Molecular radiobiology. Brit. med. Bull. **29**, 12—15 (1973).

Ehrenpreis, S., Fleisch, J. H., Mittag, T. W.: Approach to the molecular nature of pharmacological receptors. Pharmacol. Rev. **21**, 131—181 (1969).

Ehrlich, P.: From the collected papers of P. Ehrlich (1900), F. Himmelweit (Ed.), pp. 3, 443 and 505. London: Pergamon Press 1960.

Eigen, M.: Über die Kinetik sehr schnell verlaufender Ionenreaktionen in wässeriger Lösung. Z. physik. Chem. (N. F.) **1**, 176—200 (1954).

Eigen, M., Hammes, G. G.: Elementary steps in enzyme reactions. In: Nord, F. F. (Ed.): Advances in Enzymology, Vol. 25, pp. 1—38. New York: Interscience 1963.

Eldefrawi, M. E., Britten, A. G., Eldefrawi, A. T.: Acetylcholine binding to torpedo electroplax: relationship to acetylcholine receptors. Science **173**, 338—340 (1971).

Eldefrawi, M. E., Eldefrawi, A. T., O'Brien, R. D.: Binding sites for cholinergic ligands in a particulate fraction of *Electrophorus* electroplax. Proc. nat. Acad. Sci. (Wash.) **68**, 1047—1050 (1971).

Erman, J., Hammes, G. G.: Relaxation spectra of ribonuclease IV. J. Amer. chem. Soc. **88**, 5607—5614 (1966).

Erman, J., Hammes, G. G.: Relaxation spectra of ribonuclease V. J. Amer. chem. Soc. **88**, 5614—5617 (1966).

Fischer, J. J., Jost, M. C.: Nuclear magnetic resonance studies of drug-receptor interactions. Molec. Pharmacol. **5**, 420—431 (1969).

Fleisch, J. H., Ehrenpreis, S.: Thermal alteration in receptor activity of the rat fundal strip. J. Pharmacol. exp. Ther. **162**, 21—29 (1968).

French, T. C., Hammes, G. G.: Relaxation spectra of ribonuclease II. J. Amer. chem. Soc. **87**, 4669—4673 (1965).

Froese, A., Eigen, M., Sehon, A. H.: Kinetic studies of protein-dye and antibody-hapten interactions with the temperature-jump method. J. Canad. Chem. **40**, 1786—1797 (1962).

Froese, A., Sehon, A. H.: Kinetics of antibody-hapten reactions. Ber. Bunsenges.-Physik. Chem. **68**, 863—864 (1964).

Frost, A. A., Pearson, R. G.: Kinetics and mechanisms (A study of homogeneous chemical reactions). New York-London: John Wiley and Sons, Inc. 1953.

Furchgott, R. F.: Pharmacology of the vascular smooth muscle. Pharmacol. Rev. **7**, 183—265 (1955).

Furchgott, R. F.: Receptor mechanisms. Ann. Rev. Pharmacol. **4**, 21—50 (1964).

Furchgott, R. F., Bursztyn, P.: Comparison of disssociation constants and of relative efficacies of selected agonists acting on parasympathetic receptors. Ann. N. Y. Acad. Sci. **144**, 882—899 (1967).

Gibson, Q. H.: The photochemical formation of a quickly reacting form of haemoglobin. Biochem. J. **71**, 293—303 (1959).

Ginneken, C. A. M. van, Rossum, J. M. van: Unpublished Results. (1971).

Hammes, G. G.: Relaxation spectrometry of biological systems. In: Anfinsen, C. B. Jr., Anson, M. L., Edsall, J. T., Richards, F. M. (Eds.): Advances in Protein Chemistry, Vol. 23, pp. 1—57. New York: Academic Press 1968.

Hammes, G. G., Fasella, P.: A kinetic study of glutamic-aspartic transaminase. J. Amer. chem. Soc. **84**, 4644—4650 (1962).

Hammes, G. G., Fasella, P.: The interaction of glutamic-aspartic transaminase with pseudo substrates. J. Amer. chem. Soc. **85**, 3929—3932 (1963).

Hammes, G. G., Kochavi, D.: Studies of the enzyme hexokinase. I. Steady-state kinetics at pH 8. J. Amer. chem. Soc. **84**, 2069—2073 (1962).

Hammes, G. G., Kochavi, D.: Studies of the enzyme hexokinase. II. Kinetic inhibition by products. J. Amer. chem. Soc. **84**, 2073—2076 (1962).

Hammes, G. G., Kochavi, D.: Studies of the enzyme hexokinase. III. The role of the metal ion. J. Amer. chem. Soc. **84**, 2076—2079 (1962).

Hammes, G. G., Porter, R. W., Stark, G. R.: Relaxation spectra of aspartate transcarbamylase. Interaction of the catalytic subunit with carbamyl phosphate, succinate and L-malate. Biochemistry **10**, 1046—1050 (1971).

Hammes, G. G., Waltz, F. G.: Relaxation spectra of ribonuclease VI. J. Amer. chem. Soc. **91**, 7179—7186 (1969).

Hammes, G. G., Wu, C. W.: Relaxation spectra of aspartate transcarbamylase. Interaction of the native enzyme with carbamyl phosphate. Biochemistry **10**, 2150—2156 (1971).

Hess, G. P., Conn, J. Mc., Ku, E., McCosskey, G.: Studies of the activity of chymotrypsin. Phil. Trans. B **257**, 89 (1970).

Hirschfelder, J. O.: Intermolecular forces. In: Pullman, B., Weissbluth, M. (Eds.): Molecular Biophysics, pp. 325—342. New York: Academic Press 1965.

Holler, E., Rupley, J. A., Hess, G. P.: Kinetics of lysozyme-substrate interactions. Biochem. Biophys. Res. Commun. **37**, 423—429 (1969).

Holler, E., Rupley, J. A., Hess, G. P.: Kinetics of lysozyme-substrate interactions. Biochem. Biophys. Res. Commun. **40**, 166—170 (1970).

Karlin, A.: Chemical distinctions between acetylcholinesterase and the acetylcholine receptor. Biochem. Biophys. Acta (Amst.) **139**, 358—362 (1967).

Katchalski, E.: Preparation and properties of enzymes immobilized in artificial membranes. Proc. 11th Nobel Symposium, Symmetry and function of biological systems at the macromolecular level. A. Engström and B. Strandberg, Eds., pp. 283—304. New York: Wiley Interscience Div. 1970.

Katz, B., Thesleff, S.: A study of the desensitization produced by acetylcholine at the motor endplate. J. Physiol. (Lond.) **138**, 63—80 (1957).

Kim, Y. D., Lumry, R.: Studies of the chymotrypsinogen family. XII. "A" type substrates of α-chymotrypsin at neutral and alkaline pH values. J. Amer. chem. Soc. **93**, 1003—1013 (1971).

Korolkovas, A.: Essentials of Molecular Pharmacology. New York: Wiley Interscience Div. 1970.

Langley, J. N.: On the physiology of the salivary excretion. Part 2: on the mutual antagonism of atropin and pilocarpine having especial reference to their relations in the sub-maxillary gland of the cat. J. Physiol. (Lond.) **1**, 339—369 (1905).

Levy, G.: Kinetics of pharmacologic activity of succinylcholine in man. J. pharm. Sci. **56**, 1687—1688 (1967).

Levy, G., O'Reilly, R. A., Apgeler, P. M., Keech, G. M.: Pharmacokinetic analysis of the effect of barbiturates on the anticoagulant action of warfarin in man. Clin. Pharmacol. Ther. **11**, 372—377 (1970).

Lewin, S.: Water surface energy contribution to adherence of hydrophobic groups in relation to stability of protein conformation. Nature (Lond.) New Biol. **231**, 80—81 (1971).

Marlow, H. F., Metcalfe, J. C., Burgen, A. S. V.: The specificity of drug receptors. An immunochemical model for cholinergic receptors. Molec. Pharmacol. **5**, 156—165 (1969).

Mautner, H. G.: Molecular basis of drug action. Ann. Rep. Med. Chem. **4**, 230—245 (1969).

Mautner, H. G., Bartels, E., Webb, G. D.: Sulfur and selenium isotops related to acetylcholine and choline. IV. Activity in the electroplax preparation. Biochem. Pharmacol. **15**, 187—193 (1966).

Meunier, J. C., Olsen, R. W., Menez, A., Fromageot, P., Bouquet, P., Changeux, J. P.: Some physical properties of the cholinergic receptor protein from electrophorus electricus revealed by a tritiated α-toxin from Naja Nigricollis Venom. Biochemistry **11**, 1200—1210 (1972).

Morawetz, H.: Rate of conformational transitions in biological macromolecules and their analogs. In: Anfinsen, C. B., Jr., Edsall, J. T., Richards, F. M. (Eds.): Advances in Protein Chemistry, Vol. 26, pp. 243—277. New York: Academic Press 1972.

Nagashima, R., O'Reilly, R. A., Levy, G.: Kinetics of pharmacologic effects in man: the anticoagulant action of warfarin. Clin. Pharmacol. Ther. **10**, 22—35 (1969).

Nauta, W. Th., Rekker, R. F., Harms, A. F.: Diarylcarbinol ethers: Structure activity relationships—A physicochemical approach. In: Ariëns, E. J. (Ed.): Physicochemical Aspects of Drug Action, pp. 305—325. Oxford: Pergamon Press 1968.

Némethy, G., Laiken, N.: Intermolecular forces and conformational changes in protein-ligand interactions. Il Farmaco — Ed. Sci. **25**, 999—1018 (1970).

Paton, W. D. M.: A theory of drug action based on the rate of drug-receptor combination. Proc. Roy. Soc. B. **154**, 21—69 (1961).

Paton, W. D. M., Rang, H. P.: A kinetic approach to the mechanism of drug action. In: Harper, N. J., Simmonds, A. B. (Eds.): Advances in Drug Research, Vol. 3, pp. 57—80. London: Academic Press 1966.

Porthoghese, P. S.: A new concept on the mode of interaction of narcotic analgesics with receptors. J. med. Chem. **8**, 609—616 (1965).

Rang, H. P.: The kinetics of action of acetylcholine antagonists in smooth muscle. Proc. Roy. Soc. B. **164**, 488 — 510 (1966).

Rang, H. P.: The uptake of atropine and related compounds by smooth muscle. Ann. N. Y. Acad. Sci. **144**, 756—765 (1967).

Rang, H. P.: Receptor mechanisms. Brit. J. Pharmacol. **48**, 475—495 (1973).

Reasbeck, P. G., Young, J. M.: Interaction of benzilylcholine mustard, benzilylcholine and lachesine with the histamine receptor in the longitudinal muscle of guinea-pig ileum. Brit. J. Pharmacol. **48**, 148—155 (1973).

Rescigno, A., Segre, G.: La Cinetica dei Farmaci e dei Traccanti radioattivi. Torino: Ed. Boringhieri 1961.

Rocha e Silva, M.: Influence of pH on the interaction of histamine with its receptors in the guinea pig ileum. Arch. int. Pharmacodyn. **128**, 355—375 (1960).

Rocha e Silva, M.: Action of histamine on the smooth muscle. Handb. Exp. Pharmakol. Vol. XVIII/1, pp. 225—237. Berlin-Heidelberg-New York: Springer 1966.

Rosario, E. J., del, Hammes, G. G.: Relaxation spectra of ribonuclease VII. J. Amer. chem. Soc. **92**, 1750—1753 (1970).

Rossum, J. M. van: The relation between chemical structure and biological activity. J. Pharm. Pharmacol. **15**, 285—316 (1963).

Rossum, J. M. van: Drug-Receptor Theories. In: Robson, J. M., Stacey, R. S. (Eds.): Recent Advances in Pharmacology. IVth Ed., pp. 99—133. London: J. & A. Churchill 1968.

Rossum, J. M. van, Koppen, A. Th. J. van: Kinetics of psycho-motor stimulant drug action. Europ. J. Pharmacol. **2**, 405—408 (1968).

Roughton, F. J. W.: The origin of the Hartridge-Roughton rapid reaction method and its application to the reactions of haemoglobin in the intact red blood corpuscule. Z. Elektrochem. **64**, 3—4 (1960).

Schneider, H., Sehon, A. H.: Determination of lower limits for the rate constants of a hapten-antibody reaction by polarography. Trans. N. Y. Acad. Sci. **24**, 15—22 (1961).

Seelig, S., Sayers, G.: Isolated adrenal cortex cells: ACTH agonists, partial agonists, antagonists, cyclic AMP and corticosterone production. Arch. Biochem. Biophys. **154**, 230—239 (1973).

Setlow, R. B., Pollard, E. C.: Molecular Biophysics. Reading-Massachusetts-London: Addison-Wesley Publishing Comp., Inc.; London-Paris: Pergamon Press 1962.

Sidorenko, N. P.: Does an enzyme reduce the activation energy? Biofizika **17**, 907—908 (1972).

Silman, I., Karlin, A.: Acetylcholine receptor: covalent attachment of depolarizing groups at the active site. Science **164**, 1420—1421 (1969).

Smoluchowski, M. von: Versuch einer mathematischen Theorie der Koagulationskinetik kolloider Lösungen. Z. physik. Chem. **92**, 129—168 (1917).

Sturtevant, J. M.: The fluorescence of α-chymotrypsin in the presence of substrates and inhibitors. Biochem. Biophys. Res. Commun. **8**, 321—325 (1962).

Theorell, H., McKinley, J. S.: Liver alcohol dehydrogenase. Acta chem. scand. **15**, 1797—1810 (1961).

Theorell, H., Nygaard, A. P.: Kinetics and equilibria in flavoprotein systems II. Acta chem. scand. **8**, 1649—1658 (1954).

Thron, C. D.: On the analysis of pharmacological experiments in terms of an allosteric receptor model. Molec. Pharmacol. **9**, 1—9 (1973).

Thron, C. D., Waud, D. R.: The rate of action of atropine. J. Pharmacol. exp. Ther. **160**, 91—105 (1968).

Waltz, F. G.: Kinetic and equilibrium studies on the interaction of ribonuclease A and 2'deoxyuridine 3'phosphate. Biochemistry **10**, 2156—2162 (1971).

Waud, D. R.: Pharmacological receptors. Pharmacol. Rev. **20**, 49—88 (1968).

Waud, D. R.: On the measurement of the affinity of partial agonists for receptors. J. Pharmacol. exp. Ther. **170**, 117—122 (1969).

Webb, G. D., Johnson, R. L.: Apparent dissociation constants for several inhibitors of acetylcholinesterase in the intact electroplax of the electric eel. Biochem. Pharmacol. **18**, 2153—2161 (1969).

Weber, G.: The binding of small molecules to proteins. In: Pullman, B., Weissbluth, M. (Eds.): Molecular Biophysics, pp. 369—396. New York: Academic Press 1965.

Werman, R.: An electrophysiological approach to drug-receptor mechanisms. Comp. Biochem. Physiol. **30**, 997—1017 (1969).

Young, J. M., Hiley, R., Burgen, A. S. V.: Homologues of benzilylcholine mustard. J. Pharm. Pharmacol. **24**, 950—954 (1972).

Conclusion

J. M. VAN ROSSUM

A drug administered to man or animals elicits a number of effects which vary in intensity, depending on the dose. These various effects depend on its pharmacokinetics and pharmacodynamics. With regard to the kinetic aspects of drug action, the following features may be considered:

1. *Pharmacokinetics*, processes governing transport through the body from the locus of application to tissue(s) in which the receptors are situated.
2. *Membrane transport*, drug transport through membranes of cells both in the process of absorption and elimination, and with regard to distribution towards the immediate environment of the receptors.
3. *Receptor interaction*, the interaction of drug molecules with the receptors leading to the ultimate effect.
4. *Consequences*, the reactions of the individual or the animal to the effects, his past experience, setting of regulation systems, health state, disease condition etc., which all may greatly influence the final outcome of drug action.

The intensity of a particular pharmacologic effect of a drug changes as a function of time, depending on the drug concentration in the receptor compartment, the time-dependent process governing regulation mechanisms, and the interaction between the possible other effects induced by the drug. Depending on the time constants of the various processes involved, certain processes may be rate limiting, whereas others are in a steady state. For instance, drug receptor interaction may be a very fast process with regard to the processes governing distribution of the drug throughout the body.

In this volume, primary attention has been focussed on time-dependent processes in membrane transport, distribution throughout the tissues, and the drug-receptor interaction.

1. Transport through membranes constitutes the basis of the access of drug molecules to the receptors and of the macrotransport in body fluids. The treatise by SCHELER and BLANCK discusses the physicochemical problems of membrane transport of drugs, based on the morphology and architecture of membranes and an irreversible thermodynamic approach to transport of matter and solutes. This basic treatment is applied to various forms of membrane transport as encountered in biology. The critical treatise by SCHELER and BLANCK not only discusses drug transport through membranes that are fixed equilibrium structures themselves, but also through membranes that are dynamic organizations.
2. Pharmacokinetics provide a formal treatment of drug transport, which in many ways has important practical consequences not only in pharmacotherapy but

also for the rational design of experiments with drugs in both animals and man. A critical discussion of the kinetics of absorption, elimination and distribution of drugs has therefore been included in this volume by KRÜGER-THIEMER and by VAN ROSSUM et al. Both linear pharmacokinetics and nonlinear kinetics

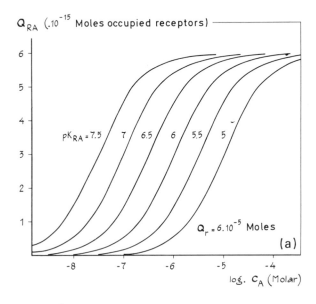

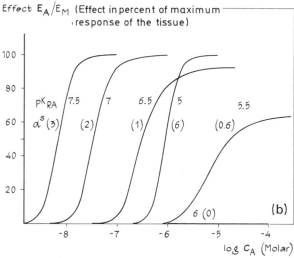

Fig. 1. (a) The occupation of receptors by drug molecules as a function of the logarithm of the concentration based on the Langmuir adsorption isotherm for drugs with different affinity constants. 50% Receptor occupation is reached when the concentration equals the dissociation constant (pK_{RA} is neg. log of the dissociation constant). (b) Theoretical dose-response curves based on the receptor occupation of Figure 1a and a nonlinear stimulus-effect relationship. The curves are steeper while the position no longer corresponds to the dissociation constant

has been dealt with. The experimental data at present available do not need us to include nonlinear thermodynamics at the level of the membranes. The time constants encountered are usually longer than several minutes, and often involve even hours or days. This may imply that these macrokinetic processes largely determine the kinetic behaviour of the pharmacologic action of a drug in vivo.

3. Drug-receptor interaction is in general based on the reversible binding of drug molecules with receptors, according to the LANGMUIR isotherm (see Chapter VAN DEN BRINK and Fig. 1a). This implies that drug-receptor interaction is studied under conditions of equilibrium, or at least it is assumed that this is the case. Since drug transport over the entire organism (pharmacokinetics) and transport through membranes in the target tissue is a slow process with respect to the rate of drug-receptor association and drug-receptor dissociation, it is reasonable to assume that equilibrium conditions are met for the drug-receptor interaction (see Chapters 1, 2, 3 and VAN GINNEKEN, Chapter 7).

Various drug-receptor theories such as the occupation theory and the rate theory lead to exactly the same dose-response curve in equilibrium conditions (see MACKAY, Chapter 5). It is, however, not certain that in all cases conditions of equilibrium are met. For instance, a transient maximum may resemble an equilibrium leading to incorrect conclusions (see GOSSELIN, Chapter 6).

It must be emphasized that drug-receptor interactions can only be measured indirectly via a response of the tissue. This is the case even for isolated organs. The relation between receptor interaction and the final effect that is the so-called stimulus-effect relation.

It is hardly possible that the relationship between receptor occupation and effect is a linear one. It is even unlikely that a linear stimulus-effect relation holds for drug effects in simple isolated organs.

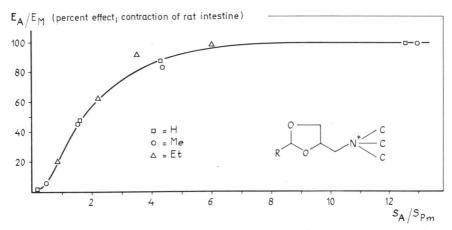

Fig. 2. Stimulus-effect relationship for cholinergic drugs studied in a piece of rat intestine. The three different drugs, which have different affinity and intrinsic activity, appear to manifest their effects via the same stimulus-effect relationship. This is a rather strong argument that such a stimulus-effect relationship is valid. This stimulus-effect relation is in agreement with a log-normal distribution

Experimental evidence for a nonlinear relationship is abundant, as the dose-response curves under the precondition that equilibrium conditions are met differ from the receptor occupation curves. Compare Figure 1a and b. The curves in Figure 1b have been derived from the occupation curves by assuming a

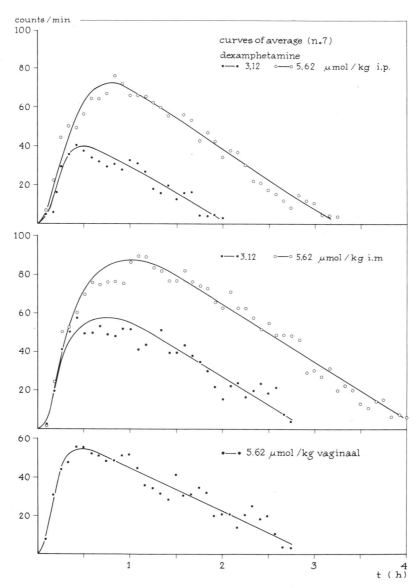

Fig. 3. Locomotor activity scores following injection of dexamphetamine in different doses and via different routes. After the peak, activity decreases linearly with time. It is therefore likely that in the given concentration range the effect is linearly proportional to the log concentration, while the latter falls off linearly in time. (Reproduced after van Rossum and van Koppen, 1968)

nonlinear stimulus-effect relation. The shape of the curves as well as their position differ from the corresponding receptor occupation curves. Since it is possible to calculate the affinity constant from the dose-response curve by using irreversible antagonists in combination with an agonist, it is also possible to calculate the relative intrinsic activity (see VAN DEN BRINK, Chapter 4 and MACKAY, Chapter 5).

It should then be possible to access the stimulus-effect relation. This has been done for three cholinergic drugs using the same piece of rat intestine (see Fig. 2). In fact, the three different agonists, which differ both with regard to affinity and intrinsic activity, agree with the same stimulus-effect relationship. This stimulus-effect relationship corresponds to a log normal distribution. It should be realized that the shape of the dose-response curve for certain drugs (those which have a high intrinsic activity, so that maximum effect already occurs when only a small fraction of the receptors is occupied) is determined by the stimulus-effect relationship rather than by the LANGMUIR isotherm.

The dose-response curves of drugs in isolated organs are in general S-shaped, so that there is a linear relationship between log of the drug concentration and the effect over a limited concentration range. Often over the traject from 20—80% of the effect the linear relation holds. The limited concentration range may occur over a change in concentration of a factor of 10. In this linear concentration range, therefore, the effect decreases linearly with a fall of the log of the drug concentration.

The log of the drug concentration decreases linearly with the time after administration (see KRÜGER-THIEMER, Chapter 2 and VAN ROSSUM et al., Chapter 3). This would imply that the effect in vivo may linearly decrease in time, at least over a limited concentration range (e.g., a factor of 10).

It is known from the pharmacokinetics of amphetamine in man that for this drug the log concentration decreases linearly with time over more than a factor of 10. The effect of amphetamine can easily be quantified in rats by measuring the increased locomotor activity (see Fig. 3).

Indeed, it appears that the amphetamine action is a linear relation of the time after administration. Furthermore, the same relation is encountered by using a different dose and a different route of administration.

It must be stressed that, since the effect is proportional to the log concentration, and the log concentration is proportional to the time, it is not possible to calculate the biological half-life from a time-effect curve. It is, however, possible to calculate the half-life if two time-effect curves are used (VAN ROSSUM and VAN KOPPEN, 1968; LEVY, 1967).

It is perfectly clear that conclusions from time-response curves in vivo contain a large number of uncertainties. Considering the various time constants involved, it seems, however, justifiable to consider the drug-receptor interaction to occur in equilibrium conditions.

A more serious challenge is the fact that in the intact animal or in the patient, a large number of regulation mechanisms are involved, so that a drug-induced change may be compensated by a number of processes.

In order to study drug effects successfully, it is advantageous to keep the drug concentration constant over sufficiently long periods of time, for instance by constant infusion or repetitive administration.

The use of dynamic systems analysis (as e.g. applied in economics, weather predictions and blood pressure regulation) may be extremely helpful. It is anticipated that such an approach will successfully be applied in the study of the action of drugs in man and animals.

References

Levy, G.: Kinetics of pharmacologic activity of succinylcholine in man. J. Pharm. Sci. **56,** 1687—1688 (1967).

Rossum, J. M. van., van Koppen, A. T. J.: Kinetics of psycho-motor stimulant drug action. Eur. J. Pharmacol. **2,** 405—408 (1968).

Author Index

Page numbers in *italics* refer to bibliography. Numbers shown in square brackets are the numbers of the references in the bibliography.

Subject Index

Handbuch der experimentellen Pharmakologie
Handbook of Experimental Pharmacology

Heffter-Heubner, New Series

Springer-Verlag Berlin Heidelberg New York

Reviews of Physiology, Biochemistry and Pharmacology

Ergebnisse der Physiologie, biologischen Chemie und experimentellen Pharmakologie

Editors: R.H.Adrian, E.Helmreich, H.Holzer, R.Jung, K.Kramer, O.Krayer, F.Lynen, P.A.Miescher, H.Rasmussen, A.E.Renold, U.Trendelenberg, K.Ulrich, W.Vogt, A.Weber

Springer-Verlag Berlin Heidelberg New York